# A SPY In The House of Medicine

by GEORGE A. SILVER, M.D.

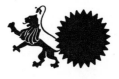

Aspen Systems Corporation
Germantown, Maryland
1976

"This publication is designed to provide accurate and authoritative information in regard to the Subject Matter covered. It is sold with the understanding that the publisher is not engaged in rendering legal, accounting, or other professional service. If legal advice or other expert assistance is required, the services of a competent professional person should be sought." From a Declaration of Principles jointly adopted by a Committee of the American Bar Association and a Committee of Publishers and Associations.

*For Rachel, Sara and Daniel*
*That their medical care won't need such explanation*

# TABLE OF CONTENTS

# Preface

Most Americans are convinced we need to fashion a more serviceable medical care system. We are tired of being victimized, tired of being unable to exercise any control over costs, over availability, over access, over quality. None of us wants to regiment medicine, but none of us wants to continue this kind of enslavement either, forced to pay whatever is demanded and forced to accept whatever is given. The doctors and administrators are behaving too much like the royal governors before the American Revolution.

Yet we have been so frightened by the complexity of the medical care system and the solemn pessimism of the experts that we have become immobilized. Economists, busy with economic formulas warn of inflation; medical professionals warn of system overload and quality deterioration; medical teachers threaten production of second class doctors; and medical researchers predict a dwindling of inventions and discoveries.

We have been deluged with books and articles in recent years documenting the deficiencies and defects of the medical care system. These defects and deficiencies are real, and they are serious. Along with these we have been barraged with the antidotes—usually single-barreled solutions promoted by enthusiastic partisans—and simultaneously with gloomy prognostications of the evil effects of the application of such antidotes.

Scholars often know so much about their subject that they can sense threats from any kind of change, and such threats tend to immobilize them and their readers, too, when they write of their doubts and the consequences. I am told that engineers have a mathematical formula relating weight to wing-span that proves conclusively that a bumblebee cannot fly.

Scholars and experts are, after all, technicians, and they can dazzle you with their technical expertise. But Americans from the earliest times have behaved in accordance with a much more practical philosophy—a "can do" philosophy that has consistently confounded the experts and resulted in the superb technical achievements for which we are admired all over the world. The motive force of American progress has always been a challenge: we wanted something and we found a way to get it.

Too many people are deprived, mistreated, or untreated in the present medical care system. A democratic people, with a deep-rooted respect for one another and for our democratic traditions cannot tolerate the iniquities and inequities of the present medical care system much longer.

Reluctance to change is born of fear and that fear is born of ignorance of the workings of the system. This book attempts to put every reader on the same footing with the experts in the knowledge of how the medical care system works. You can see for yourself what parts of the system are not working; which ones deserve to be retained, which discarded; what can be changed, which elements substituted. Once we understand the machinery, no matter how complicated the design, we are on the road to setting things right.

Fair shares, easy and equal access to decent quality medical care is what we are after. This is not too difficult an achievement. This book is about our medical care system, its elements, and how it works. If equity in medical care is what you want, knowing these things should help you get it.

George A. Silver, M.D.

# ACKNOWLEDGEMENTS

*My gratitude to my wife Mitzi, who outlined what ought to be said; to Anella Short, Myra Brunswick and Barbara Hall, who patiently deciphered the hieroglyphics.*

# Chapter 1
# Some History

---

To understand something about any institution in a society, it is well to know something about its history. History as related to medical science and care must be seen from a number of different perspectives because medical science has roots in a number of different disciplines. To understand its history one has to look at many things, such as the scientific revolution of the 17th and 18th centuries and the industrial revolution of the 19th century. Furthermore, the origins of the various sciences many years before the industrial and scientific revolutions have to be reviewed in order to recognize their association with, and their place in, the development of current medicine and medical practice.

## UNIVERSALITY VS. NATIONALISM

Medical care grew from several roots, some of which touch upon aspects of science in general and on the specific sciences related directly to medicine. Some relate to national and social developments unique to particular countries. There isn't such a thing as a German chemistry, a Russian chemistry or an American chemistry. Chemistry is a universal science. The laboratory sciences are generally denuded of any nationalist content with the exception of emphasis. When we come to medicine, the body of knowledge included in the diagnosis, care and treatment of patients, we do find some differences, though relatively small ones. We cannot honestly discuss English medicine, Austrian medicine or Italian medicine as being substantially different from American medicine or Russian medicine in theory. However, in the training of the physician, the kind of efforts put forth to establish a diagnosis, the decision making as to what shall be done, or between diagnosis and treatment, there may be a considerable national coloration. Americans offer more bedside teaching in training centers. Europeans put less emphasis on laboratory tests in office practice. French doctors prefer to ensure compliance by giving medicine by injection. However, the textbooks of medicine, translated from one language into another, have such approximate similarities that for all practical purposes one can talk about world medicine and see each national coating as being somewhat superficial.

When we come to medical practice, however, this is not the case at all. There are very great national differences with regard to both expectation and models of practice; one can truly speak about a Russian medical system, Chinese medical system, American medical system, etc. The differences here are truly derived from characteristic, historic, national, social, economic and political aspects; and as such are idiosyncratic and unique to the individual country. This is one of the reasons why it is almost impossible to transfer medical care systems from one country to another. For a long time in the United States there was a terrible fear, encouraged by professional medical organizations, that we were going to become the victims of "Bolshevization" of American medicine. It was threatened that if we would adopt a system of national health insurance, for example, we would become exactly what Russians have become; and our doctors and patients would interact as Russians do in their medical care system. The vision portrayed in the press to Americans of a Bolshevik medical care system was naturally in tune with the image of the Soviet Union at the time: grim. The likelihood of such a transfer or "transplant," which is a more popular and understandable modern term, was very remote indeed. Like many transplants in the human body, countries tend to reject foreign institutions.

For a significant historic evidence of this, we need only look at what has happened to the countries in eastern Europe that came under Russian influence after World War II. Most of them had had some system of social insurance in which was imbedded some modified form of the Bismarckian national health insurance. When they came under the dominant influence of the Soviets, who had an established medical care system whose form had been frozen in the 1920's, all of the eastern European countries adopted a form of socialized medicine very similar to the Russian model. It was even reported that the Czechs, through the good offices of the government in exile in London, had very carefully translated Henry Sigerist's book *Socialized Medicine in the Soviet Union* into Czech to be used as a model for the organization of their medical care system to be developed once the war was over. Andrija Stampar, the famous Yugoslav public health statesman who had spent many years in exile in the United States because of his revolutionary, antiroyalist and socialist principles, once returned to Yugoslavia as the director of their health services after the war, moved to put into operation a Yugoslav modification of the basic Russian organizational plan for health services delivery.

It is unlikely that the various governments tried to copy the Russian system with every letter and punctuation mark in place. And it is interesting that in the twenty-five years since then, each of the eastern European countries has taken on a socialized medicine scheme different from the Russian, intimately related to the system of medical practice that was in operation in the country before the Second World War, and adjusted to the postwar cultural, social and political aspects of the individual country. Poland, for example, has a government-operated medical care system with a hierarchic arrangement not too different from the Russians. But since agriculture continues to be essentially a private enterprise in Poland, Polish farmers have to pay fee-for-service for their medical care or buy voluntarily into an insurance scheme. Doctors, therefore, are permitted to continue some private practice. That is, of course, each doctor provides required time in government service, for which the government pays a basic salary.

The "polycentric planning" of Yugoslavia (which was the cause of the bitter feud between Stalin and Tito), an essential difference between the Russian and Yugoslav brands of communism, has resulted in the idiosyncratic, localized form of medical service delivery control in that country. It is quite different from the overall hierarchic planning of the Soviet Union.

I expatiate on nationalistic tendencies in medical care primarily to show how important it is to note the origins of *American* medicine. When we understand the influences and bases of our current system, we will also have a platform from which we can guage the future — how much we can do to the system or what kind of change we can hope for in the system. The light of historical experience in the development of our present medical care delivery system will illuminate future possibilities.

## ORIGINS OF AMERICAN MEDICINE:
## EUROPE'S POOR RELATION

American medicine was an offshoot of European medicine, particularly the English. In the early days, because most of the people who emigrated to the new, strange world tended to be those who were less well-rooted in the old country or who were having difficulty adjusting there, physicians were very few. The country was rich in virgin land and natural resources but there was very little cash flow. As a consequence it was extremely rare for people in America to get to school in England or Holland (the preferred centers for medical education); most medical education, therefore, was acquired on an apprenticeship basis. It is true that some of the apprentices then went off to get themselves "finished" in Scotland or in Leiden, but for several hundred years the basic training of doctors was in this country, from other doctors. After a couple of generations it meant that being trained in medicine as an apprentice was to be trained among doctors who themselves were trained as apprentices. Respect for academic training, which was the hallmark of European medical education, became less important in the American colonies. For example, in Boston, perhaps the largest American city in the early 18th century, only six trained physicians were available for a population of about 100,000 people. There were others who called themselves "doctors." Whereas in Europe only an earned university degree allowed one to be called "doctor," anyone who had any medical training in America (and some without!) called himself "doctor." Since there were no licensing boards and no university in which medical education was a characteristic element out of which a doctor's degree could be given, it was a perfectly simple and understandable process. This rudimentary beginning automatically affected medical education and consequently medical practice. This ruled the way in which physicians were looked upon by themselves, by their patients and by the populace at large in this country.

In Europe, the 17th and 18th centuries were also a time of great change and shifts. Medicine was just coming out of the Middle Ages, during which time those who practiced the different arts and crafts related to medicine were in different guilds. For example, the physician was a part of the Artists' Guild; and the apothecary, the dispenser of medicine, a part of the Grocers' Guild. The 17th century saw the beginning of science, the pursuit as we today view it, and the beginning of medicine as a scientific profession. Specifically, the 17th century saw the discovery of the circulation of blood; the publication of the first modern anatomy book; the invention of the microscope; the publication of Sydenham's *Great Systematic Text Book of Medicine.* There were "doctors" trained as apprentices also, and certainly the apothecaries and surgeons were so trained, but there were also learned physicians who obtained their degrees by studying in the universities.

The 18th century saw the struggle among these various skills beginning to be straightened out in Europe. The apothecaries, who had fulfilled the role of "general practitioner," were more and more constrained to their shops and the role of the general practitioner was taken over by the educated physician. The surgeon began to get more of his training in the same curriculum as the physician, with part of his education in the teaching hospitals; soon the surgeon was an educated professional.

## AMERICAN MEDICAL EDUCATION

In 18th century America, the first medical schools were established in 1765 in New York and Philadelphia and the first public hospital in 1752 in Philadelphia. Even with these accomplishments, graduates of medical schools couldn't supply the physician needs of the country, growing rapidly through immigration and growth in size (doubled in 1803 by the Louisiana Purchase). Therefore, apprenticeship continued to be the most important mode of producing doctors. The Americans then accomplished the unique invention of a new kind of medical education, the proprietary medical school. This was nothing more than a combination of physicians to train apprentices. They could in this fashion greatly increase the number of apprentices each could take under supervision and, of course, increase their income appreciably. The first of these schools was established in Baltimore in the early 19th century but similar institutions multiplied across the country rapidly as the United States grew toward the Pacific. There was no need to make distinctions among apprentice-trained, proprietary medical school-trained or university-trained physicians ("Democratic Vistas"); there was no way to establish quality or suitability standards. Anyone who had a few years of experience with one of the proprietary schools, or the fixed four years of the university education, called himself "doctor" and practiced in a fairly similar way and had equal claim on community support.

Between 1800 and 1900, the United States saw the development of about 176 medical schools. Some were nothing more than diploma mills in which there were no laboratory facilities or even running water available; no effort to provide experience in any of the scientific disciplines basic to medical practice; and only very limited opportunities for learning about the clinical experiences of the doctors with whom they were associated. In some of the schools there was a blatant chicanery, allowing students to register and so long as they paid their tuition, not overseeing that they appear in class. These "diploma mills" existed right up until the 20th century.

The result was that there were many doctors. We entered the 20th century with about one physician for every five hundred people, a better ratio than we have today, and proportionately even more because there were fewer specialists among them; they were predominantly family doctors and general practitioners. They were of enormously uneven quality, since some were graduates of diploma mills, and others were the graduates of apprenticeships of varying quality, and a few were the graduates of medical schools and universities where they had to have some reasonable experience and the best training of the time. To be accurate, however, according to Abraham Flexner in his examination of some of the medical schools which are today quite famous and prestigious, in 1910 they weren't much better than the diploma mills in their education, training facilities and faculty. ("Medical Education in the United States and Canada," Bulletin No. 4, Carnegie Foundation for the Advancement of Teaching, 1910.)

The varying quality of the physicians gave rise to a considerable amount of justified complaints and satires at their expense. Since one couldn't tell from the name plate whether the doctor was from one of the better or one of the worse educational situations, this did provide for a fairly equitable distribution. Neither rich nor poor had a better chance for good treatment.

The presence of many doctors in the cities limited individual practices; there was too much competition for patient confidence. Doctors of whatever training were motivated to drift out of the cities to rural and frontier areas. The doctors followed the pioneers westward and became part of the adventures of the American frontier. You may recall in some of the Bret Harte stories of the mining camps in the frontier west, there was always a character named "Doc." He may have been drunk and incompetent, but he was there. In 1910 when the Flexner Report came out, it reported that rural areas, with populations of 80 to 100, had three or four physicians.

The fact that science and scientific training in medicine hadn't quite reached American shores in the middle of the 19th century meant that most of the doctors were practicing second rate European medicine and were perhaps fifty years behind the average European practitioner. European physicians and teachers looked upon the American scene with some of the same contempt and irritation with which some U. S. physicians now look upon foreign medical school graduates.

There were efforts to change this. Daniel Drake, an apprentice himself at the age of sixteen at the beginning of the 19th century, eventually was "finished" in Edinburgh, and came back to agitate for improved medical education in this country. In his own lifetime he established seven medical schools and wrote a definitive textbook on the diseases and treatment of the time. His book, *The Diseases of the Interior Valley of North America,* is as much a classic for its observations and for its intuitions and analyses as that of any of the great European writers of his time. A number of the medical schools he established are still prominent. One of them, St. Louis University in Missouri, is the largest Catholic medical school in the world.

Oliver Wendell Holmes, the physician father of the more famous justice with the same name, a renowned author and essayist, was also professor of anatomy at Harvard and diligently strove to upgrade and improve the teaching of medicine there. He fought valiantly to establish the principle of contagion and transmission of infection. He was the leader of the American physicians who strove to change the horrible infant death rate and his essay, "On Puerperal Fever," is as much a classic as the essay of Semmelweis. Holmes was able to make changes in his own immediate vicinity at Harvard, so that the doctors did not come from the autopsy room with their dirty and infectious hands to the delivery room. But he was not able to effect much change in overall practice in the United States. America's medical leadership was in the years ahead. Antiseptics and aseptic surgical practice were twenty-five years ahead. But in the 1850's, Harvard and Michigan represented *European* islands of excellence in medical education in the United States.

## AMERICAN HOSPITALS

Much as with doctors, the hospital situation was also somewhat different in the United States. The early hospitals were associated with poor houses or were set up by communities for the care of the sick poor. This is similar to what had happened in Europe and some of the same tradition carried over in the beginning. The physicians who tended the poor people were paid by the community as they were in Europe. However, in the late 18th century, as a result of cyclical economic depression and tremendous financial reverses, the citizens of Philadelphia were no longer able or willing to pay the physicians who attended the sick poor at Pennsylvania Hospital, and prepared to close the hospital. The physicians, unwilling to see this one institution where the sick poor could be tended closed, volunteered to serve without pay. Thus began the tradition of voluntary service by physicians in American hospitals with associated admitting privileges, whereby they could take care of their private patients in the same institution if they so chose.

This was totally different from Europe, where particular physicians were paid to serve in public hospitals. They might, if they chose, take care of their patients there, but only the paid physicians could take care of the patients admitted. Doctors had to build their own private institutions to provide care to their private patients. In the United States from the start, therefore, hospitals were public hospitals in which unpaid doctors worked. Later in the 19th century, when hospitals began to be built in response to growing needs for more facilities, the religious, fraternal or other community groups who constructed them arranged for the institutions to be non-proprietary (not owned by the providers, not in business for profit). Doctors worked there, on patients who couldn't pay, to earn the privilege to care also for their paying patients there.

At the beginning of the 20th century, therefore, American medicine was already different from European medicine in important ways:

(1) The quality of medical education and resultant patient care was not as good. American physicians who were stirred by the scientific revolution and the burgeoning revolution in the medical sciences, and who wanted to be part of this — to learn and to be able to do more and different things — had to go abroad to study.

(2) There were twice as many physicians relatively in the United States as in Europe, and because they were all "doctors" without regard to whether their training was from apprenticeship, a proprietary medical school, diploma mill, or university, and competition ensued, it was easier to develop specialty training in this country. This is, in a sense, a paradox because American medicine was basically inferior to European medicine in the training and the education of the practitioner. But it was easier to specialize and practice the more modern categorical kind of medicine in the U. S. because of the larger pool of doctors and the competition. If there were lots of doctors, it would be no hardship on the community for one to leave to train as a specialist. And if the competition was keen among general practitioners, getting a specialist rating guaranteed a different, more expensive clientele.

(3) The hospitals in this country were almost entirely nonprofit institutions run by community groups either on a public or voluntary basis. From the standpoint of future developments, it was easy to see that American medicine could very easily jump into the lead in terms of quality and training, but that it would also be more difficult to control medical practice because of the intimate association of the hospitals with practitioners, and the relative ease with which physicians could become specialists.

## DEVELOPMENT OF MODERN AMERICAN MEDICINE

The rest of the history is probably better known and needs no long elaboration. America was becoming wealthier. The technical genius of America adopted and adapted to the scientific revolution in a national industrial advance. Medical science was not far behind. In the 1890's, the great prototype of modern medical education was established in Baltimore at the Johns Hopkins University. The flow of black gold and the conscience of John D. Rockefeller had established a General Education Board (a philanthropic foundation) which aimed to raise the level of American medical education at every medical school to that of Hopkins. The beginnings of consumerism were evident in the Pure Food and Drug Act, state licensing laws and energetic action by the American Medical Association to eliminate quacks and inadequate practitioners. By the 1920's, the hundreds of medical schools had been reduced to only fifty and the number of annual graduates from 7500 to 2500. All the medical schools strove to establish themselves as centers of clinical excellence and to attract foundation money and high quality students.

All sorts of other things were happening in our society as well, which also had an impact on the idiosyncratic development of American medical practice. For example, group practice began in the United States. Its beginnings can be traced to the 1860's with the building of the Southern Pacific Railroad, because it was necessary to supply medical services for the mobile groups of workers and the attendant camp followers. As they drove their way across the country with the iron rails, through forest and farm land, there were few settled communities from which medical care could be obtained. The railroad owners hired physicians at fixed salaries to move to communities where the railroad workers were located. These groups of physicians would then move ahead after a time, but they moved and worked as a group.

As the Northern Pacific struck out across the prairies they followed this example, and other railroads did the same. Thus group practice was born. Shortly thereafter, the Mayo brothers set up their clinic for group practice as a diagnostic center; a number of other experimental groups of practitioners set themselves up for easier access by patients and more satisfactory scientific practice by the professionals.

In summary, the 19th century saw American medical practice grow away from the European parent for geographic and historic reasons. The resulting forms were basically influenced by Europe, but they were different: the doctor's education and background were different; the medical schools were different; the hospitals were differently organized, sponsored and funded. And America invented group practice.

By the 1930's, many of the problems related to getting and giving medical care were well established in this country. The decline in the number of practitioners trained shifted the scale of competition. Rapid urbanization after 1900 reduced the number of doctors willing to move out into rural communities or practice in impoverished areas. The increasing numbers of specialists changed the ratio of patients to family doctors drastically. And the cost of medical care was rising.

The discontent was abetted by the democratic ideology of the American political system. There was an increasing move toward trade unionism and more agitation for improvement in labor legislation. We saw the beginning of increased federal domination and responsibility in the Income Tax Law of 1913. We saw the establishment of a Department of Labor, with a separate Women's Bureau and a Children's Bureau. These were efforts to restrict the exploitation of women laborers and the shocking abuse of child laborers prevalent at the turn of the century. An organization called the Association for American Labor Legislation agitated for these improvements and tried to obtain legislation for Social Security and compulsory health insurance to protect workers against the cost of medical care particularly when they were ill and couldn't work. There had been advances like this in Germany as far back as the 1880's. The English passed a National Health Insurance act in 1911. As a matter of fact, national health insurance was an item in the political platform of Teddy Roosevelt and the Bull Moose Party of 1912. The American Medical Association, which prior to 1920 was one of the more active participants in the movement to improve the health conditions of American workers, actually had a committee report approving compulsory health insurance in 1916, just before the United States entered World War I. The emphasis was on *compulsory* health insurance because the committee felt voluntary health insurance would be unAmerican since only those people who could pay for it would be able to buy it. (A rather ironic comment on the position that professional organizations of physicians have taken since that time.) The union movement, growing as it was, strongly supported this health insurance approach. The Epidemiologic Laboratory Service of the United States Public Health Service, investigating health and disease problems, provided a supporting document in 1916 on how health insurance could be organized in this country on a national basis.

The entry of the United States into the First World War put an abrupt stop to these activities since everything had to be concentrated on the war effort. The unpopularity of World War I and President Wilson's illness combined to drive America into an isolationist posture. Industrialists and financiers, who saw the rise of a proletarian revolution in Russia as the forerunner of a worldwide revolution, began beating the drums against Bolshevism. The Democratic Party was in disarray, defeated at the polls in 1920, and the Republican Administration which took office after that was solidly and almost hysterically anti-Bolshevist. The idea of making any change in the delivery system of medical care that would in any way resemble what was being done in Bolshevik Russia, was an anathema. In 1932, when the Committee on the Costs of Medical Care urged rather mild changes such as increased group practice and voluntary health insurance, the uproar raised by the professionals and professional spokesmen drowned out the recommendations.

Despite the fact that the chairman of the Committee on the Costs of Medical Care was Ray Lyman Wilbur, president of Stanford University, a practicing physician who had been president of the American Medical Association, the organization and its program were vituperatively attacked. When John Kingsbury, an official of the Milbank Memorial Fund, returned from the Soviet Union in 1934 to write a laudatory book about medical practice there called *Red Medicine,* he was denounced. A campaign was mounted by physicians to stop ordering Borden's milk. (The Milbank Memorial Fund was headed by Albert Milbank, who with his sister, Elizabeth Milbank Anderson, had established it. Albert Milbank was also president of Borden.) The boycott had an effect.

The taint of Bolshevism associated with any recommendation for improved organization of medical practice and/or government financing of the cost of medical care has remained to this day.

In a more subtle way, somewhat greater evils were perpetrated in the loftier name of science and research. Rigid application of developing scientific theory, and approval and almost worship of medical science as an ideal, resulted in the emergence of more laboratory-oriented, fewer patient-oriented and practice-minded physician graduates from the medical education establishment. When, after World War II, it became possible for the United States government to provide substantial support in the medical field, the black mark against support to medical education for fear that it might lead to government control and therefore Bolshevization of medical practice, resulted in the pouring of federal funds into biomedical research. This had the effect of distorting the direction of medical education, so as to keep it only minimally concerned with the development of physicians for the care of the American patient at an affordable price.

The great watershed is always dated 1910, when the Flexner Report, *Medical Education in the U. S. and Canada* appeared. It created a sensation at the time, with its harshly critical descriptions of the poor quality of medical education generally and the shockingly poor quality of teachers and practitioners.

The Flexner Report gets a lot of the credit (and blame!) for the events that resulted after its publication. The report had been ordered by the Carnegie Foundation, an *educational* rather than medical foundation, for the purpose of improving education. Abraham Flexner, author of the report, was not a physician; he was an educator. His approach and emphasis derived from what he thought modern times, scientific development and the needs of the medical field required in the way of medical educational opportunities. No one can fault him for his notions. However, the emphasis was such as to disestablish whatever values there were in the traditional schools and shift the pendulum totally in the other direction. Again, this is not to say that the Flexner Report was the actual trigger that resulted in the changes, or the only factor that brought about change in medical education. The soil was already prepared in that the changing nature of American society at the time, with urbanization, industrialization and mechanization as the seeds. The worship of science and its application; technology; the new developments in engineering and instrumentation; and the rising expectations of the American people for modern and improved services of all kinds had laid the groundwork. It was inevitable that there would be some kind of emphasis on laboratory and scientific *practice* of medicine as on scientific *education* for medicine. The enormous production of doctors in 19th century America also laid the groundwork for a labor pool that could be readily blanketed into the specialist fold. Science, particularly the scientific method, almost compelled specialism in the developing fields associated with it. How could a generalist embrace all the new knowledge? Or contribute to the new, narrowing, deepening channels of knowledge? Everything about the climate was right. The Flexner Report was essentially a declaration of principle of what was already on the way rather than a fuse touching off an explosion.

There are legal maxims in this vein, such as "law follows custom," indicating that only after society has tested and put certain behavior into established use does a law appear and validate it. And so it can be said of the Flexner Report. It didn't initiate the scientific change in medical education with all the consequent changes in medical practice; it announced it, described it and predicted it.

In summary, the kind of doctor we have today; the way in which he is paid; his status in society; the way he is educated; what he expects of patients, of hospitals, of insurance companies is the fruit of past developments. So too, with patients: what he expects in care; how he expects to be treated in the doctor's office and in the hospital; what and how he expects to pay for medical services — all of these have roots in the past.

# Chapter 2
# Staying Alive and Well
# in Our Medical Care System

---

## ISSUES IN HEALTH CARE: COSTS

### MEDICAL CARE

In the United States today, medical bills are paid mostly by the person getting the medical care. True, we talk about "third party payments," meaning that someone pays on our behalf, such as an insurance company or a welfare fund of a trade union. But it is *our* money, out of our pockets, through premium payments to the insurance companies; or by way of wage deductions (even the employers' contribution in an employer-employee welfare fund, is the employees' money — "our money" — since it would have been negotiated for as a wage increase if it weren't sequestered into the health insurance benefit). These out-of-pocket expenses, "direct" (from our wallets or bank accounts) or "indirect" (insurance or welfare funds), have to be distinguished from government-paid medical services in public hospital clinics or by way of government insurance programs like Medicare, Medicaid or the military dependence program. True, the tax funds come from our pockets ultimately as well, but Congress appropriates and assigns the funds and negotiates the arrangements.

Our "direct" medical bill payments come to more than $35 billion and "indirect" to about $25 billion for a total of over $60 billion, while the *government* (federal, state and local) puts up more than $40 billion. In other words, 60 percent of medical bills are paid by the person receiving the medical care.

We will see that this is unevenly divided among the elements of medical care costs: 80 percent of hospital costs are paid by insurance on the private expenditure side; but only half of the visits to doctors in their offices are covered by any insurance — and not all the costs even of those visits.

There are other differentials as well. For those over 65, because of the Medicare program, 30 percent of medical costs are "direct" and 6 percent

13

covered by private insurance; while for those under 65, "direct" costs are 37 percent of expenditures and private insurance covers another 33 percent for a total of 70 percent of all medical care costs.

Put another way, 20 percent of the population, those over 65, pay 40 percent of the cost of medical care directly or through private insurance; while the other 80 percent of the population pays 70 percent of the costs themselves! If we look at it in dollar costs, however, because of the greater amount of illness and greater demand among the elderly, it comes out shockingly different.

Those over 65 average more than $1,000 in costs per person per year, of which almost $400 comes out of their own pockets — not from government or private insurance. For those under 65, average expenditures per year per person is only $300, of which a little over $100 is out of pocket, and another $100 from private insurance.

It is true that the government is paying an unequal percentage of the cost for the elderly in relation to other citizens. But the difference is minimized in terms of the greater needs of the elderly so that despite this, older people on an average are paying 4 times as much out of their own pockets for medical care than other segments of the population, and older people generally are poorer than the rest of the population — 30 percent as against 20 percent below the designated poverty level.

So that is where the money comes from. And it is paid out, very largely, in piecemeal chunks — hospital services as provided, prescription drugs and fee-for-service to physicians. For most people, the big area of concern in regard to medical care, is money. Of course there are other problems — access, quality, impersonality of treatment — which impress different groups in society as being of greater or lesser priority. But of this variety of issues about the medical care system, the one that touches the most people, is irritating and frightening and has certainly stimulated the greatest effort to reform or change the medical care delivery system, is *cost*.

The economists use the term "costs" in a production sense — that is, what it costs to produce a service. By "prices" we mean what the producer charges for that which he has produced. These are not unfamiliar concepts. If we think of medical care as a product, in the same way that we consider other products that we purchase, "expenditures" for medical care would therefore be the total cost of what we buy. The "price" of a physician's visit, for example, may be $10; our "expenditures" for physicians' services may come to $1,000 — if we use 100 visits. It is not so much "costs" or even "prices" that may upset us as it is the "expenditures," the total, that can have such a staggering effect.

When it comes to medicines, a company in the drug business may have to provide information about its costs and it will be relatively easy to see the difference between "cost" and "price" and recognize how our expenditures

FIGURE 2-1:  Per Capita Expenditures for Personal Health Care Met by
Third Parties and Paid Directly, by Age Group, Fiscal
Years 1966 and 1974

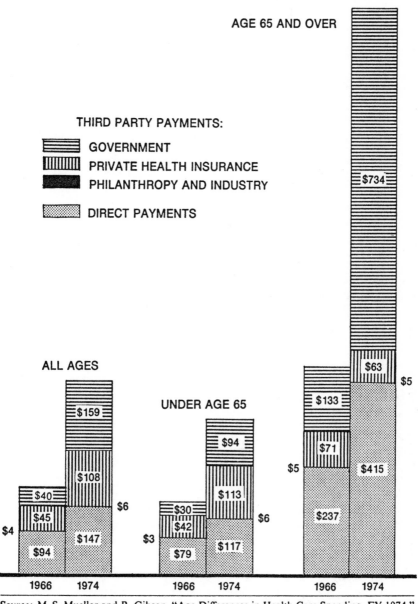

*Source:* M. S. Mueller and R. Gibson, "Age Differences in Health Care Spending, FY 1974,"
*Social Security Bulletin,* June 1975, p. 15.

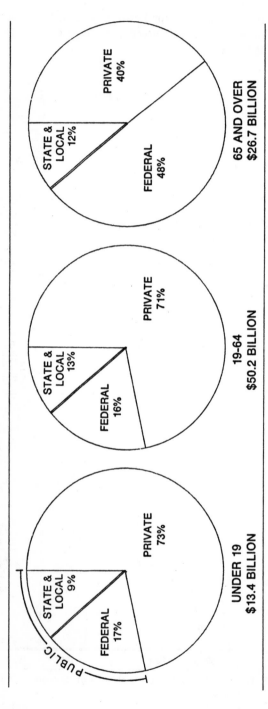

FIGURE 2-2: Percentage Distribution of Expenditures for Personal Health Care, by Source of Funds and Age Group, Fiscal Year 1974

*Source:* M. S. Mueller and R. Gibson, "Age Differences in Health Care Spending, FY 1974," *Social Security Bulletin,* June 1975, p. 6.

are related to this. We can see the "profit" and the discrepancy between "cost" and "price." In the nonprofit system, the cost of production of a hospital bed day, for example, is presumably the same as the price, so that our expenditures can be reckoned simply by adding up our days of care. The same holds true for physicians' services. In the profit-making area, we may take issue with the producer's prices on the assumption that these are inflated by unreasonable profits; and by utilizing public and private pressures, try to bring costs and prices more realistically in line. In the nonprofit area where costs and prices are the same, efforts to control expenditures have to be directed at reduction of costs (assuming utilization as fixed): more efficiency, better productivity, economies of operation and management. The producers (managers, administrators, doctors) will indignantly assure you that the efficiencies and economies are of the highest order in *their* system. It is *utilization* that needs to be reduced. Stop asking for so much service!

Clearly, in addition to holding costs down to reduce expenditures in the nonprofit area, one might well think of squeezing overall use or reducing total use of services, since prices multiplied by usage equals total expenditure. In order to reduce total expenditures we can either reduce costs where possible or reduce utilization where possible.

### PRESCRIPTION DRUGS

Within the medical care industry, a look at the drug industry, in which the product is a substance, not a service, makes it easier to recognize the overall problem and the possibilities of solution. The extreme profitability of the pharmaceutical industry, which returns almost twice as much to its shareholders than the average for the rest of the American manufacturing industry (15.1 percent as compared with 9.1 percent returned in 1971) is an easily visible case (Sciences and Society Series, "Issues of Health Care," No. 1, November 1973.)

We can see that, over time, drugs and drug sundries have gone down from 13.9 percent to 9.3 percent of total individual medical expenditures. We may be confused enough to believe that drug companies are providing drugs more economically, that prices are lower or profits less, whereas the very opposite is the case. 13.9 percent of $25.8 billion, the total medical expenditure for 1960, is $3.58 billion; this is considerably less than the 9.3 percent of $94 billion ($8.74 billion) of 1974. As a matter of fact, the expenditure is almost three times more. Inflation would account for only half of that increase.

There are many good source books for information on prescription drug manufacture, promotion and sale. Aside from reports of hearings before various Congressional committees, with a special fascination for those who

TABLE 2-1: National Health Expenditures, by Type of Expenditure and Source of Funds, Fiscal Years 1972-74

(In millions)

| Type of expenditure | Total | Source of funds | | | | | |
|---|---|---|---|---|---|---|---|
| | | Private | | | Public | | |
| | | Total | Consumers | Other [1] | Total | Federal | State and local |
| | | | | 1974 [1] | | | |
| Total | $104,239 | $62,929 | $58,043 | $4,886 | $41,311 | $28,343 | $12,968 |
| Health services and supplies | 97,183 | 59,815 | 58,043 | 1,772 | 37,369 | 25,335 | 12,034 |
| Hospital care | 40,900 | 19,272 | 18,759 | 513 | 21,628 | 14,845 | 6,783 |
| Physicians' services | 19,000 | 14,476 | 14,462 | 14 | 4,524 | 3,277 | 1,248 |
| Dentists' services | 6,200 | 5,858 | 5,858 | — | 342 | 210 | 132 |
| Other professional services | 1,990 | 1,629 | 1,591 | 38 | 361 | 226 | 136 |
| Drugs and drug sundries [2] | 9,695 | 8,900 | 8,900 | — | 795 | 404 | 391 |
| Eyeglasses and appliances | 2,153 | 2,065 | 2,065 | — | 88 | 50 | 38 |
| Nursing-home care | 7,450 | 3,504 | 3,474 | 30 | 3,946 | 2,208 | 1,738 |
| Expenses for prepayment and administration | 4,224 | 2,934 | 2,934 | — | 1,290 | 1,042 | 247 |
| Government public health activities | 2,126 | — | — | — | 2,126 | 1,234 | 892 |
| Other health services | 3,445 | 1,177 | — | 1,177 | 2,268 | 1,840 | 428 |
| Research and medical-facilities construction | 7,056 | 3,114 | — | 3,114 | 3,942 | 3,008 | 934 |
| Research [2] | 2,684 | 205 | — | 205 | 2,479 | 2,395 | 84 |
| Construction | 4,372 | 2,909 | — | 2,909 | 1,463 | 613 | 850 |
| Publicly owned facilities | 1,112 | — | — | — | 1,112 | 277 | 835 |
| Privately owned facilities | 3,260 | 2,909 | — | 2,909 | 351 | 336 | 15 |

[1] Preliminary estimates.

[2] Research expenditures of drug companies included in "drugs and drug sundries" excluded from "research expenditures."

Source: N. L. Worthington, "National Health Expenditures 1929-1974," Social Security Bulletin, February 1975, p. 9.

TABLE 2-2:  Aggregate and Per Capita National Health Expenditures, by Type of Expenditure, Selected Fiscal Years, 1929-74

(In millions)

| Type of expenditure | 1929 | 1935 | 1950 | 1960 | 1966 | 1970 | 1974 |
|---|---|---|---|---|---|---|---|
| Total | $3,589 | $2,816 | $12,027 | $25,856 | $42,109 | $69,202 | $104,239 |
| | | | Aggregate amount (in millions) | | | | |
| Health services and supplies | 3,382 | 2,788 | 11,181 | 24,162 | 38,661 | 64,065 | 97,183 |
| Hospital care | 651 | 731 | 3,698 | 8,499 | 14,245 | 25,879 | 40,900 |
| Physicians' services | 994 | 744 | 2,689 | 5,580 | 8,865 | 13,443 | 19,000 |
| Dentists' services | 476 | 298 | 940 | 1,914 | 2,866 | 4,473 | 6,200 |
| Other professional services | 248 | 150 | 384 | 848 | 1,140 | 1,385 | 1,990 |
| Drugs and drug sundries | 601 | 471 | 1,642 | 3,591 | 5,032 | 7,114 | 9,695 |
| Eyeglasses & appliances | 131 | 128 | 475 | 750 | 1,309 | 1,776 | 2,153 |
| Nursing home care | — | — | 178 | 480 | 1,407 | 3,818 | 7,450 |
| Expenses for prepayment and administration | 101 | 91 | 290 | 807 | 1,446 | 2,115 | 4,224 |
| Government public health activities | 89 | 112 | 351 | 401 | 731 | 1,437 | 2,126 |
| Other health services | 90 | 63 | 534 | 1,262 | 1,620 | 2,625 | 3,445 |
| Research and medical facilities construction | 207 | 58 | 847 | 1,694 | 3,448 | 5,137 | 7,056 |
| Research | — | — | 110 | 592 | 1,545 | 1,846 | 2,684 |
| Construction | 207 | 58 | 737 | 1,102 | 1,903 | 3,291 | 4,372 |

TABLE 2-2 Continued:    Aggregate and Per Capita National Health Expenditures, by Type of Expenditure, Selected Fiscal Years, 1929-74

(In millions)

| Type of expenditure | 1929 | 1935 | 1950 | 1960 | 1966 | 1970 | 1974 |
|---|---|---|---|---|---|---|---|
| | | | Per capita amount [1] | | | | |
| Total...... | $29.16 | $22.04 | $78.35 | $141.63 | $211.56 | $333.57 | $485.36 |
| Health services and supplies...... | 27.48 | 21.59 | 72.83 | 132.35 | 194.21 | 308.81 | 452.51 |
| Hospital care...... | 5.29 | 5.66 | 24.09 | 46.56 | 71.57 | 124.74 | 190.44 |
| Physicians' services...... | 8.08 | 5.76 | 17.52 | 30.57 | 44.54 | 64.80 | 88.47 |
| Dentists' services...... | 3.87 | 2.31 | 6.12 | 10.65 | 14.40 | 21.56 | 28.87 |
| Other professional services...... | 2.01 | 1.16 | 2.50 | 4.65 | 5.73 | 6.68 | 9.27 |
| Drugs and drug sundries...... | 4.88 | 3.65 | 10.70 | 19.67 | 25.28 | 34.29 | 45.14 |
| Eyeglasses & appliances...... | 1.06 | .99 | 3.09 | 4.11 | 6.58 | 8.56 | 10.02 |
| Nursing home care...... | | — | 1.16 | 2.63 | 7.07 | 18.40 | 34.69 |
| Expenses for prepayment and administration.. | .82 | .70 | 1.89 | 4.42 | 7.26 | 10.19 | 19.67 |
| Government public health activities...... | .72 | .87 | 2.29 | 2.19 | 3.67 | 6.93 | 9.90 |
| Other health services...... | .73 | .49 | 3.48 | 6.91 | 8.14 | 12.65 | 16.04 |
| Research and medical-facilities construction...... | 1.68 | .45 | 5.52 | 9.28 | 17.32 | 21.76 | 32.85 |
| Research...... | — | — | .72 | 3.21 | 7.76 | 8.90 | 12.50 |
| Construction...... | 1.68 | .45 | 4.80 | 6.04 | 9.56 | 15.86 | 20.36 |

[1] Based on January 1 data from the Bureau of the Census for total U. S. population (including Armed Forces and federal civilian employees overseas and the civilian population of outlying areas).

Source: N. L. Worthington, "National Health Expenditures 1929-1974," Social Security Bulletin, February 1975, p. 13.

are interested in full details, there are two interesting, well-written books on the subject: Richard Harris's *The Real Voice,* about investigations carried out by Senator Estes Kefauver in the 1950's; and Silverman and Lee's *Pills, Profits and Politics,* a very up-to-date review of the entire topic.

We can be content with a brief summary of costs, prices and expenditures.   Naturally the manufacture and sale of prescription drugs is a competitive business.  Business in the United States allows itself any action to maximize profits.  It sees its responsibility primarily to the shareholder or owner, not to the consumer.  In the customary picture of the "adversary relationship" as seen in U.S. business life, the slogan is "caveat emptor" — let the buyer beware.  If the consumer wants protection, he must get it from a specially designated consumer representative — not from the owners and manufacturers.  Short of breaking the law, the business owner's role is to use all the strategies he can to sell his product, to win out over a competitor's product, and make as much profit as possible.

In the clothing or furniture business, while hardly pardonable, this point of view with regard to business ethics may do little damage.  In housing or bridge building this attitude may be criminal and even murderous.  Similarly, in the matter of prescription drugs, which involves life and death, destructive side effects, and the sometimes lethal effects of useless drugs only to mention a few possibilities, a "caveat emptor" philosophy becomes dangerously unethical.  Drugs must be safe, properly compounded, and effective.

There are laws to protect us, and the federal Food and Drug Administration to oversee the industry and regulate manufacture and distribution with safety and effectiveness in mind.  These factors don't work as well as they ought to because regulating agencies and the laws they enforce tend to become captives of the regulated.  The manufacturers have the money and knowledge and usually employ or train most of the experts.  So when a regulating agency is set up it is natural that former employees or consultants of industry are the most promising and qualified candidates.

But to return to the cost/price/expenditure area, the manufacturers would all like to have a special product of which they are the sole supplier, one that every doctor would have to prescribe for every patient every day.  If they can't realize such utopia, they would like to get as close as possible.  So they do research on finding new drugs, not all for treatments for dangerous and widely prevalant diseases.  Mostly they have their researchers working on a competitive alternative to an already popular drug marketed by another firm.  Then they inflate the value of their "discovery" compared to the drug already in use and spend much advertising overhead persuading the doctors (who write prescriptions) and pharmacists (who stock the medicine) that this particular medicine and no other should be prescribed and sold.

The doctors play a part in this, too; some innocently and some not so innocently. The clinical trial of drugs often determines how widely a drug can be or may be used, and industry uses the results in pushing the merchandise. So medical journals are full of such articles and drug companies like to advertise in them. Doctors can receive publicity (and money) and trips to conferences to report on experiments utilizing new drugs, or prestigious lectureships in medical schools, and some doctors will court drug companies for research funds, travel grants, subsidies for reprinting and redistributing their articles. And the companies innundate doctors with samples of drugs, multicolored advertisements, toys, gifts,

TABLE 2-3: The American Drug Industry: Sales, Research, Promotion and Profits, 1950-1972 [1]

| Year | Sales Worldwide (millions) | Sales U. S. (millions) | Worldwide Research and Development (millions) | % of Sales | Promotion (U. S. only) (millions) | Net Profits (millions) | % of Sales |
|---|---|---|---|---|---|---|---|
| 1950 | $1,430 | $1,013 | $ 39 | 2.7 | $203 | $ — | — |
| 1951 | 1,485 | 1,148 | 50 | 3.4 | 230 | — | — |
| 1952 | 1,540 | 1,175 | 63 | 4.1 | 235 | 129 | 8.4 |
| 1953 | 1,595 | 1,213 | 67 | 4.2 | 243 | 129 | 8.1 |
| 1954 | 1,650 | 1,252 | 78 | 4.7 | 250 | 152 | 9.2 |
| 1955 | 1,815 | 1,457 | 91 | 5.0 | 291 | 191 | 10.5 |
| 1956 | 2,090 | 1,676 | 105 | 5.0 | 335 | 250 | 11.9 |
| 1957 | 2,420 | 1,742 | 127 | 5.2 | 348 | 283 | 11.7 |
| 1958 | 2,640 | 1,802 | 170 | 6.4 | 360 | 301 | 11.4 |
| 1959 | 2,750 | 1,805 | 197 | 7.2 | 361 | 319 | 11.6 |
| 1960 | 2,860 | 1,905 | 212 | 7.4 | 381 | 306 | 10.7 |
| 1961 | 2,992 | 1,954 | 238 | 7.8 | 391 | 314 | 10.5 |
| 1962 | 3,236 | 2,199 | 251 | 7.8 | 440 | 317 | 9.8 |
| 1963 | 3,469 | 2,317 | 282 | 8.1 | 464 | 354 | 10.2 |
| 1964 | 3,717 | 2,479 | 298 | 8.0 | 496 | 401 | 10.8 |
| 1965 | 4,219 | 2,779 | 351 | 8.3 | 556 | 464 | 11.0 |
| 1966 | 4,660 | 3,011 | 402 | 8.6 | 602 | 503 | 10.8 |
| 1967 | 5,102 | 3,226 | 448 | 8.8 | 645 | 515 | 10.1 |
| 1968 | 5,665 | 3,655 | 485 | 8.6 | 731 | 545 | 9.6 |
| 1969 | 6,208 | 4,008 | 549 | 8.8 | 811 | 596 | 9.6 |
| 1970 | 6,853 | 4,322 | 619 | 8.8 | 864 | 664 | 9.4 |
| 1971 | 7,383 | 4,667 | 684 | 9.0 | 933 | 721 | 9.5 |
| 1972 (est.) | 8,070 | 5,031 | 728 | 9.0 | 1,006 | 734 | 9.1 |

[1] *Worldwide Sales:* Data shown for human and veterinary products, dosage and bulk forms. Figures for years 1961-1972 taken from Pharmaceutical Manufacturers Association, *Annual Survey Reports,* Washington, D. C. Figures for years 1950-1960 derived from PMA data on dosage forms only plus 10 percent to represent estimated bulk forms.

*Source:* M. Silverman and P. R. Lee, *Pills, Profits and Politics.* Copyright © 1974 by The Regents of the University of California; reprinted by permission of the University of California Press.

FIGURE 2-3:   Distribution of Manufacturer's Sales Dollar [1]

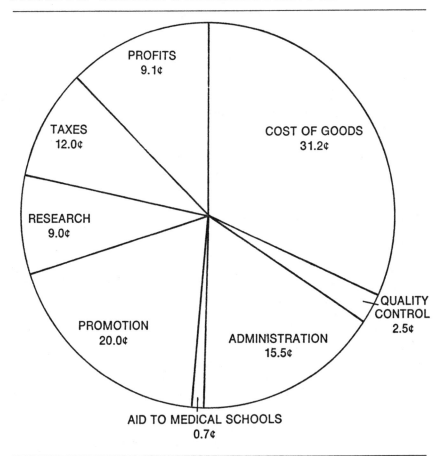

PROFITS
9.1¢

TAXES
12.0¢

COST OF GOODS
31.2¢

RESEARCH
9.0¢

QUALITY
CONTROL
2.5¢

PROMOTION
20.0¢

ADMINISTRATION
15.5¢

AID TO MEDICAL SCHOOLS
0.7¢

[1] Derived from extrapolation of data in U. S. Department of Health, Education, and Welfare, Task Force on Prescription Drugs, *The Drug Makers and the Drug Distributors* (Washington, D. C.: U. S. Government Printing Office, 1968), p. 13.

*Source:* M. Silverman and P. R. Lee, *Pills, Profits and Politics.* Copyright © 1974 by The Regents of the University of California; reprinted by permission of the University of California Press.

models of parts of the body, desk ornaments, calendars, and free magazines on medical topics. In addition "detail men," carefully trained salesmen, visit doctors repeatedly to persuade them to buy, use and dispense the company's products.

The effect of all this on *cost* is plain. It will cost more to do the product development research and if that is really not entirely necessary, it adds unnecessary costs. Selling and advertising are expensive. It is estimated that drug companies spend about $6,000 per year per doctor! All of this jacks up the *prices*. And this is before the very generous profit the companies allow themselves. Also, the encouragement to prescribe may increase the number of prescriptions and the amount of drugs prescribed and sold. All this adds to *expenditures.*

One hears a great deal about "generic prescribing." This has to do with the chemical nature of a drug and its chemical name, as opposed to its brand or patented name. The drug company wants the drug to be known best by its brand name rather than the chemical (generic) name. That way whenever it is prescribed, their product will be ordered. If you ask for "acetyl-salicylic acid" you may get a chemical substance which is aspirin for a few pennies. If you ask for "aspirin" it may not cost much more. But if you ask for a particular *brand,* such as Bayer, you will pay a much higher price.

Manufacturers resist cost controls that will reduce their profits, their opportunities to promote their own products, their "research, product development and medical education" efforts that are so costly.

Yet, $5 billion could be saved from the prescription costs and drug sales in the United States by reducing production and distribution costs, eliminating the competitive advertising and substituting generic prescribing. The arguments against this, as offered by the industry and their professional supporters, are not without merit:
- not all companies are equally reliable
- not all mixtures are equally effective, even with the same essential ingredients
- product development sometimes leads to significant new medications and not just competitive alternatives or novelty products
- without profit stimulation, the industry would wither and die

*Expenditures* are high in prescription drugs because of high *prices* solely reflective of high production *costs* and high *profits.* It is not utilization by the consumer that can be regulated to reduce expenditures. After all, the consumer only buys what the doctor orders. And he orders what the industry provides. Expenditure control is clearly a matter of *cost* control.

RISING HEALTH CARE EXPENDITURES

Figure 2-4 shows that health expenditures have gradually crept up from 3.6 percent of the gross national product in 1929 to 7.7 percent of the gross national product in 1974. This doubling of the percentage is a vast increase in total expenditures considering the vast increase in the Gross National Product (GNP). It also has to be seen in the light of the other things we've discussed: greater numbers of specialists working in the health field; new machines that have been invented for better diagnosis and treatment; increased numbers of beds for hospitals and nursing homes and long term care of all kinds; "miracle drugs" and "miracle surgery." Prices have gone

FIGURE 2-4: Annual Expenditures for Medical Care, Selected Years

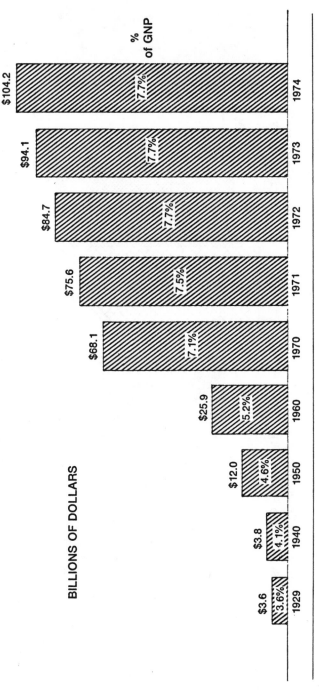

BILLINGS OF DOLLARS

% of GNP

| 1929 | $3.6 | 3.6% |
| 1940 | $3.8 | 4.1% |
| 1950 | $12.0 | 4.6% |
| 1960 | $25.9 | 5.2% |
| 1970 | $68.1 | 7.1% |
| 1971 | $75.6 | 7.5% |
| 1972 | $84.7 | 7.7% |
| 1973 | $94.1 | 7.7% |
| 1974 | $104.2 | 7.7% |

*Source:* Cooper, Barbara S., Worthington, Nancy L., and Piro, Paula A. "National Health Expenditures, 1929-73" *Social Security Bulletin,* February 1974, U. S. Department of Health, Education, and Welfare.

*Research and Statistics.* Note No. 32-1974, Department of Health, Education, and Welfare, *Social Security Administration,* Office of Research and Statistics, November 29, 1974.

*Source: Basic Charts on Health Care,* Subcommittee on Health, Committee on Ways and Means, U. S. House of Representatives, July 8, 1975, p. 5.

FIGURE 2-5:   Hospital Cost Comparisons

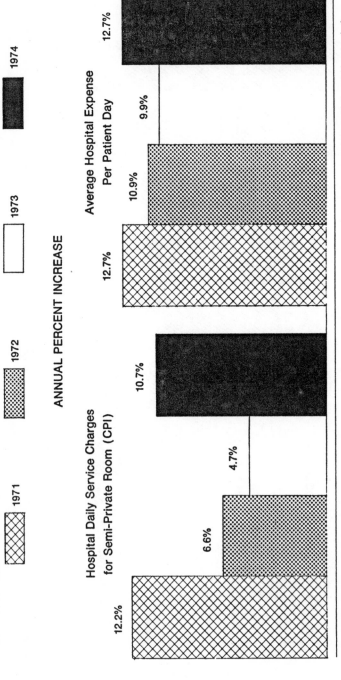

*Source:* Consumer Price Index. Bureau of Labor Statistics, U. S. Department of Labor. Journal of the American Hospital Association, American Hospital Association, April 16, 1975.

*Source: Basic Charts on Health Care,* Subcommittee on Health, Committee on Ways and Means, U. S. House of Representatives, July 8, 1975, p. 13.

up generally, too. So the total bill, including higher cost, labor, technology and price overheads results in the huge expenditure of over $104 billion in 1974 for all health services.

Hospital care represented a little under 40 percent of the total expenditures, physician services just under 20 percent. This is quite a change from 15 years ago when hospital expenditures were only 30 percent higher than expenditures for physician care; now hospital expenditures are double the expenditures for physician services. As was stated previously, this is a product in part of the increasing cost of the new and improved kinds of equipment, the increased numbers of personnel, and the large number of facilities in use. There is much more utilization of hospitals today as compared with 15 years ago. This is not to say, however, that hospital expenditures are completely justified in terms of cost or that economies could not be introduced, but only to make the point that it is not simply the total costs in a hospital that have gone up from an average of $30 a day to $100 a day.

Of course, all expenditure eventually comes out of our pockets, some indirectly from federal, state or local tax funds. In 1974 the federal government was responsible for about 25 percent (over $25 billion); state and local authorities 12 percent ($12 billion) of the $37 billion which was the total public expenditure. (These expenditures are up since the 1960's, when the United States government first undertook considerably more in the way of paying for medical care. Prior to that, federal expenditures approximately equaled state and local expenditures and the total public expenditure was closer to 24 percent of all expenditures for health services.)

Of *personal* health care expenditures, private health insurance pays $23 billion worth, roughly 23 percent of all expenditures. Putting all this together, it appears that our out-of-pocket expenditures (other than public or private insurance) for personal health care comes to $32 billion. Of this $32 billion, $4 billion is for hospital care, or a little bit less than 10 percent of all the monies paid out for hospital care come out of the patient's pocket directly. However, about 40 percent of the money paid for physician services comes out of the patient's pocket directly and 86 percent of the expenditures for dental services and an equivalent amount for drugs and drug sundries. In other words, while almost 90 percent of the hospital bills are paid by the federal government or through health insurance, only 60 percent of doctor bills are paid this way, and only about 14 percent of dental bills and drugs.

See how this pattern of payment has changed over time: In 1929 there were practically no insurance benefits. Of the $3 billion spent for personal health care, less than 10 percent came out of the public sector. In 1940, this had increased to 15 percent, and by 1965 when the first federal programs of any magnitude came into being, the public share had gone up to 20 percent. Since then this has risen to almost 40 percent.

Looking at the sums spent from an individual standpoint, personal health care expenditure has increased from an average of $29 in 1929 to $485 per person in 1974. However, the private pocket part of this has gone down from 86 percent to 60 percent of the bill, while the public sector part has gone up proportionately to 40 percent. Nevertheless, 85 percent of $29 is considerably less than 60 percent of $485!

While one can see that drug prices seem to have declined in the Consumer Price Index, this is not a true reflection of changing drug prices on the patient's purse. It is well known that the Consumer Price Index is constructed without regard to the rapid change in the use of drugs or the introduction of new ones. And these are usually the very expensive ones. The decline in price reflects only that an *established* drug (such as aspirin) has declined, so it tells you nothing about the prescribing habits of physicians in using new drugs that are not included in the Consumer Price Index.

Viewing costs from the perspective of the past half century, it is clear that science and technology have imposed a heavy burden of cost and consequent expenditures upon the American people. To a considerable degree the burden has been minimized by the gradual increase of public expenditures (that is, by the use of tax dollars), which lessens the impact on the individual at the time of required service. In addition, gradual introduction of insurance against some of the heavier burdens of health costs, as in hospital costs, since the 1930's, has also tended to mitigate the impact of increasing costs. This does not take into account, however, the effect of inflation, of course, or the unequal distribution of public funds, which are largely directed toward the payment of health insurance costs for the aged (Medicare) and the payment of health services for the poor (Medicaid). These two items together comprise 22½ percent of the $37 billion dollars spent under public programs, or 60 percent of all public money and even more than that of the federal contribution toward the payment of these costs. So the vast majority of Americans do not benefit directly, therefore; only something like 15 percent have all or part of their medical care bills paid with public money.

The great mass of middle income Americans see no personal benefit in the many billions of dollars that public agencies spend for medical care. Furthermore, private insurance is sufficiently comprehensive neither in scope nor in percentage of payment to alleviate the burden of increased costs and inflation for the majority of Americans.

Somewhere between 76 percent and 87 percent of the population are covered for some part of hospital costs. (There is some variation in the quoted percentage, depending on whether the federal government through

TABLE 2-4:  Percent Population Covered by Insurance for Indicated Costs

| Type of plan | Hospital care | Surgical services |
|---|---|---|
| Total, all ages..................................................... | 100.0 | 100.0 |
| Blue Cross-Blue Shield................................. | 36.0 | 35.7 |
| Insurance companies.................................... | 60.1 | 58.9 |
| Group policies............................................ | 39.4 | 43.4 |
| Individual policies ..................................... | 20.7 | 15.5 |
| Independent plans....................................... | 3.9 | 5.4 |

*Source: Medical Care Costs and Prices,* Department of Health, Education and Welfare (SSA) 72-11908, January 1972, p. 93.

its Office of Research and Statistics of the Division of Health Insurance Studies of the Social Security Administration makes the estimate or whether the Health Insurance Association of America makes the estimate!) Overall 75 percent of all consumer expenditures for hospital care are covered. While about 73 percent of the population are covered for medical or surgical care given in hospitals and about 38 percent have coverage for office and home visits to or by a physician, only about 48 percent of the costs of these services are met by insurance. So basic health insurance plans do not reach all the people and do not cover all the costs incurred during illness and hospitalization.

Further, meeting even 25 percent of hospital costs is frightening. When hospital costs were $40 per day, meeting 25 percent of the cost for a ten-day stay would come to $100. Now that hospital costs are over $100 a day, a ten-day stay will mean an average out-of-pocket cost of more than $250.

There are refinements hidden in these figures which come to much more out-of-pocket expenditure than appears on the surface. For example, 15 and 20 years ago the surgeon's fee would be $100 for an appendectomy and anesthesia was charged as part of the hospital cost. Today the same surgery would cost $250 to $350, and an anesthesiologist would be paid as well. The more complex kind of medical and surgical care for which people are now hospitalized also involves many more consultations with subspecialists and this means added fees. It is not unusual, therefore, for hospital bills to run to thousands of dollars for special kinds of care — coronary or intensive unit care, for example — and added consultant services.

To cap this, hospital insurance has a terminal date so that hospitalization after 30 or 60 days will add to formal costs, which mount steadily and heavily. All in all, while most of the scare stories about family bankruptcy and the headlines relating to the outrageous costs to which patients are subjected affect only a minority of people (about 1 percent), the majority are affected enough so as to resent and become angered by the mounting cost of insurance associated with mounting out-of-pocket costs.

## ISSUES IN HEALTH CARE: CONTROLLING COSTS

How can we control costs? When we looked at prescribed drugs, a visible, three-dimensional product, cost control was to be resolved through one of two processes: cut away the carelessly competitive aspects which add so much to the cost; and/or reduce or eliminate the profits.

What can we do about medical care costs? Are they competitive? Do competitive aspects add to the costs? Are they necessary to proper performance of service? How can we judge? Since services are "non-profit" there's no need to add a point on the elimination of these nonexistent elements.

In brief, will we get good service (prompt, efficient, effective) if we make changes? And the corollary: are there changes that could bring this about?

These questions summarize 50 years of criticism, study and recommendations for our medical care system. That's what all the books on the market deal with, in attacking or defending our medical care system. That's not really what *this* book is about because I'm hoping to offer you information from which you can design your own solutions.

The following breakdown lists the major defects that inhibit control or reduction of medical costs and expenditures.

1. *The hospitals:*

   • Too many beds
   • Patients kept longer than necessary
   • People who could be cared for in other, less expensive ways
   • Too many people working in hospitals; inefficient management
   • Overuse of equipment (too many x rays, laboratory examinations, etc.)
   • Too much consultant and subspecialty use for teaching and research purposes
   • (the opposite accusation) Not enough consultant use and too many diagnostic tests, because of inadequate training and ignorance of doctors
   • Superfluous surgery
   • Insufficient coordination of related services (such as pediatrics and obstetrics)
   • Lack of inter-hospital sharing of expensive, rarely used capabilities (neurosurgery, cardiac surgery, or complex radio therapy), that are never used to capacity in any one place
   • Cost-plus reimbursement system giving no incentive to change
   • A system in which the doctor orders (admits and discharges) while the patient pays, so that doctors don't feel the spur

• A system in which 40 percent of the costs are paid by government or through an intermediary (Blue Cross or other insurance companies) and the evidence or stimulus for change is obscured

The criticism summarized is: (a) competition (hospitals don't coordinate); (b) lack of community services as alternatives to hospital care; (c) lack of interest on doctors' part; and (d) lack of supervision by paying agent (insurance company). From that vantage point, it shouldn't be any more difficult to control costs in hospitals than in the prescription drug business.

2. *The doctors:*

• Contribution to hospital inefficiency and lack of economy (mentioned above)
• Failure to accomplish services in the office or create community structures to avoid patient hospitalization
• (the opposite) Unnecessary visits, tests, consultations, surgery

3. *The insurance companies:*

• Insuring in-hospital costs fairly completely, but out-of-hospital care minimally, driving most care unnecessarily into the hospital
• Failing to set standards for reimbursement that would encourage efficiency or economy
• Failing to mandate uniform medical quality standards, thereby automatically inflating costs of care by incompetent doctors and inadequate institutions.

4. *The community and Congress:*

• Unwilling or too intimidated to challenge the professionals to arrange a compromise system
• Continuing to tolerate poor practices even when the inefficiencies and diseconomies are revealed

Given this laundry list of villains and villainous practices, it is no wonder so many different recommendations for change have been made. Many of the villainous aspects of these charges have been examined earlier but Congress and most of the public tend to see both the problem and solution in terms of the insurance area and programs.

## ISSUES IN HEALTH CARE:
## FINANCING AND REIMBURSEMENT

### PUBLIC AND PRIVATE HEALTH INSURANCE

Some of the pressures for changing the medical care delivery system, or at least changing the financing mechanisms in order to control the inexorable rise in costs, emphasize the inequities of *private* insurance as currently operating. The increasing role of *public* financing of medical care is an effort to use both approaches to some limited degree: there is expansion of public sector funding for medical care through Medicare and Medicaid; civilian health and medical care programs for dependents of the uniformed services (CHAMPUS); the Veterans' Administration program; and payments made for services under state disability insurance programs or Workmen's Compensation. So we continue to try to get 100 percent population coverage by either public or private health insurance.

It is almost impossible to estimate how many people today are without insurance altogether. We know that there are 41 million Americans under age 65 who have no economic protection against the cost of hospital care through private insurance. Roughly half of this number, about 20 million people, have Medicaid payments made on their behalf. But some significant percentage of this number are over 65 and covered by Medicare in part, so that the Medicaid payments are supplementary. Therefore, perhaps 30 million people are not covered by Medicaid or Medicare and have no private insurance either. The plight of those poor who are not eligible for Medicaid and cannot afford private insurance is a terrible one and will need to be met in some fashion by the government.

It is the plight of the 75 percent, those who do have private insurance but for whom that insurance is inadequate in scope or coverage, that is the cause of the largest public concern, since it involves the largest number of people. Also, Medicare pays less than 40 percent of personal health expenditures for the aged, which creates very real and difficult problems that will have to be improved through Medicare legislation. And finally, it is the majority of Americans, those under 65 with a sizable proportion of their hospital, physician and drug bills unpaid by insurance or the government, who are urgently demanding attention and relief.

We will discuss the government's payment programs and the opportunities for improvement or modification of payment programs a little later. At this point let's spend a little time on insurance generally — the principles involved and the possibilities.

In the early 19th century when the arithmetic of life tables and the theory of probability were first being widely considered, prototypal principles of insurance against the cost of medical care were also being developed.

There are basically two areas of insurance: protection against the risk of something that may or may not happen (illness), as opposed to protection against an eventuality that is certain to happen although one may not be able to say quite when (death). In the case of an event that may or may not happen, the insurer (the agency that does the insuring) makes the best possible guess as to how many such events will occur and what the average price of each event will be. This is the role of the actuary. In this way the presumed losses will be divided up among those seeking protection. In the case of the certainty, (death) the costs are divided as to expectancy of the duration of payments.

The difference between *insurance* and *prepayment,* although the definitions have been blurred, lies in this theoretical difference between possibility and certainty. In both instances the purpose of the policy is to take the weight of cost off the individual at the time an event actually occurs. There is a difference in cost, also, between the two. The *insurance* policy may not equal the actual cost of medical services, which are so variable in amount or price; whereas under a *prepayment* system, the insured individual benefits to the full extent of the services provided. Blue Cross coverage, guaranteeing a semiprivate room, would be *prepayment.* A policy for $25/day while in the hospital would be *insurance.*

Insurance and prepayment programs have a substantial history. We have records of hospital insurance dating back to the 17th century in Quebec where the community taxed itself to pay for the use of the local hospital, basing taxes on the overall costs. In the late 18th century the United States government went into the health insurance business, charging the members of the Merchant Marine a flat monthly sum to cover the cost of their medical care. This was particularly necessary then, to insure their being treated decently if they became sick in foreign ports and required hospitalization. This was at a time when the United States was still sailing to "foreign ports" in Florida and Louisiana as well as to the Carribean. And if the American sailors could not pay foreign medical bills, when recovered they would find themselves "pressed" into a foreign navy.

The health insurance principle on the largest scale as applied to the working population was undertaken in Britain and on the continent at the end of the 19th century. As the impact of the Industrial Revolution broadened and deepened, unionization created the opportunity for union members and the "Friendly Societies" (cooperative working or neighborhood groups) to insure themselves against the cost of illness for a modest weekly or monthly contribution. These insurance and welfare plans eventually resulted in more comprehensive state health benefit programs under Social Security; first in Germany, then in other parts of the continent, and eventually as a National Health Insurance system in England in 1911.

Insurance against the cost of hospital or physician medical care was not an important part of the American scene until long after it had become established as an integral part of the European scene. Undoubtedly this was related to the important differences between American and European social attitudes and welfare commitment; America's strong individualistic, entrepreneurial, frontier type of philosophy as opposed to the closed, more group-related philosophy on the European Continent. It wasn't until the Great Depression in the early 1930's that private insurance against the cost of hospital care began to gain interest nationally.  Prior to that there were small "Friendly Societies" and cooperatives in the United States, but with little consequence and very little subsequent growth.

Prepaid group practice has a longer, more durable history in the United States than private health insurance for either hospital or physician services. I do not mean the federally prescribed marine hospital service in 1798, but the prepaid group practices like the Northern Pacific group practice plan which developed out of the building of the transcontinental railroad; the group health cooperative in Elk City, Oklahoma; and even the paternalistic Endicott-Johnson factory program in Binghamton, New York.

With the onset of the Depression, nonpayment of bills caused several hospitals to go into bankruptcy, and an imaginative hospital administrator, Dr. Justin Ford Kimball in Dallas, Texas, undertook to write insurance policies against the cost of hospital care for a group of teachers.  Teachers, of course, faced with widespread unemployment, were desperately anxious to avoid the possibility of becoming public charges.  That was the beginning of Blue Cross, the nonprofit pacesetter for the *private* health insurance industry.  As Blue Cross grew, private insurance companies recognized an opportunity to get into the field and began to sell similar health insurance policies.

In the late 1930's and early 1940's as the United States built up defense manufacturing activities prior to entrance into the Second World War, booming employment and the fixing of wages and prices resulted in "fringe benefits" being discussed in labor negotiations.  Employees bargained only for benefits outside the wage package.  The net effect of this was to increase real wages substantially, while not disturbing the wage pattern that was being set by the government and maintained in the actual salary levels. The most common element bargained for at that time was "health" insurance (really only hospital insurance).

The resulting competition worked out to the benefit of the commercial insurance carriers; by the 1950's they had outrun Blue Cross and covered better than 60 percent of all subscribers covered for hospital costs.  Over the next fifteen years a reverse began and with the big leap provided by Medicare legislation in 1965, Blue Cross forged ahead.  Currently, Blue Cross and commercial insurance carriers share equally in the number of subscribers covered.

"Number of subscribers" does not, however, present a fair picture.  The commercial carriers tend to sell packages of insurance to employer-employee welfare funds, the biggest purchasers of group insurance.  The packages usually include pensions, Workmen's Compensation, life insurance and other types of benefits in addition to the health and hospital coverage.  In order to get business the insurance companies tend to price their hospital insurance below that of Blue Cross in the same way that department stores advertise "loss leaders." They advertise some items below cost, since they are willing to give up some of the profit on that particular item, expecting to make so much more on the other things they sell. Since those covered in the employer-employee welfare funds tend to be younger, the likelihood of their using medical services is less; they are the best risks. This kind of "experience rating" results in the worst risks gradually accumulating under Blue Cross coverage. Blue Cross, originally a community rated plan (one in which everyone paid the same rate regardless of his own experience or preexisting illness) was at a disadvantage, and forced to raise rates constantly. So Blue Cross began experience rating in order to compete; both Blue Cross and commercial carriers continue to practice experience rating.

TABLE 2-5:   Health Insurance: Income and Expenditure

| Type of plan | Subscription or premium income | Claims expense | Operating expense |
|---|---|---|---|
| | Amount (in millions) | | |
| Total | $17,184.8 | $15,743.5 | $2,402.5 |
| Blue Cross-Blue Shield | 7,370.9 | 7,060.2 | 534.3 |
| Blue Cross | 5,147.1 | 5,009.3 | 290.0 |
| Blue Shield | 2,223.8 | 2,050.9 | 244.3 |
| Insurance companies | 8,746.0 | 7,656.0 | 1,786.1 |
| Group policies | 6,774.0 | 6,510.0 | 867.1 |
| Individual policies | 1,972.0 | 1,146.0 | 919.0 |
| Independent plans | 1,067.9 | 1,027.3 | 82.1 |
| Community | 445.1 | 425.0 | 32.0 |
| Employer-employee-union | 544.5 | 536.0 | 42.0 |
| Private group clinic | 15.0 | 12.3 | 2.1 |
| Dental service corporation | 63.3 | 54.0 | 6.0 |
| | Percent of premium income | | |
| Total | 100.0 | 91.6 | 14.0 |
| Blue Cross-Blue Shield | 100.0 | 95.8 | 7.2 |
| Blue Cross | 100.0 | 97.3 | 5.6 |
| Blue Shield | 100.0 | 92.2 | 11.0 |
| Insurance companies | 100.0 | 87.5 | 20.4 |
| Group policies | 100.0 | 96.1 | 12.8 |
| Individual policies | 100.0 | 58.1 | 46.6 |
| Independent plans | 100.0 | 96.2 | 7.7 |
| Community | 100.0 | 95.5 | 7.2 |
| Employer-employee-union | 100.0 | 98.4 | 7.7 |
| Private group clinic | 100.0 | 82.0 | 14.0 |
| Dental service corporation | 100.0 | 85.3 | 9.5 |

*Source: Medical Care Costs and Prices,* Department of Health, Education and Welfare (SSA) 72-11908, January 1972, p. 99.

The effect of experience rating is to make for uneven premiums and also total expenditures in different covered groups. Blue Cross, dealing with different, often worse risk population groups, may handle a larger amount of money, given the same number of subscribers. Because the experience of their subscribers would be worse, the estimated costs would be greater; the premiums would therefore be higher and actual expenditures greater.

Blue Cross, as a nonprofit plan, is expected to have a "retention rate" (the amount retained from the premiums as overhead and operating expense) considerably lower than that of the commercial companies who expect to make a profit on health insurance. Blue Cross also has lower operating expenses (a 5 percent operating rate). So do some commercial insurance carriers, but on the average, in 1973 profit making companies selling individual health insurance policies paid out only 53¢ on every dollar taken in, while Blue Cross paid out an average of 95¢.

Insurance, therefore, is not an altogether inexpensive way of protecting against sudden overwhelming costs of hospital and medical care. The "net cost" (the difference between subscription income and claims expense) of private health insurance in 1973 was $2.9 billion. Net cost includes overhead and profit. In the same year, private health insurance was meeting 25 percent of the total cost of personal health care in the United States.

TABLE 2-6:    Health Insurance: Premium Income, Benefit Payments and Retention (1972)*

|  | Commercial | BC/BS | All |
|---|---|---|---|
|  | | (Billions of Dollars) | |
| Premium Income | 15.2 | 11.5 | 26.7 |
| Benefit Payments | 10.6 | 10.4 | 21 |
| Retention | 3.7 | 1.0 | 4.7 |
| (Rate) | 26% | 8% | 18% |

* 1972 premiums are earned premiums.

Source: *Source Book of Health Insurance Data 1974-75,* Health Insurance Institute, pp. 41, 47.

TYPES OF POLICIES

There are many different kinds of private insurance policies dealing with the types of medical care costs that may arise. Earlier I illustrated the fact that private insurance varied widely in scope and coverage. The premiums therefore vary in the same way. For example, one can buy an *indemnity* type policy against the cost of medical care, which reimburses the individual a fixed amount of $20 a day or $100 a week for an illness requiring medical or hospital care. Another type of insurance is the *service* policy (like Blue Cross) in which the individual who requires medical or hospital care is guaranteed a certain kind and amount of service at full and actual cost. Under Blue Cross the client is promised a semiprivate room and certain other privileges associated with hospital services for a fixed period of time — 21 days, 30 days, 90 days, etc. Under the service plan the individual is less likely to have an out-of-pocket expense than under the indemnity plan. Also, indemnity plans tend to foster inflation more than the service plans, because in service plans those providing the care have to make arrangements to budget for a fixed amount of money for the service covered. In indemnity plans where the individual makes his arrangements with the provider (e.g. the hospital) and receives cash with which to pay the bill, there is theoretically no limit on what the provider may charge. It is quite possible, of course, that the individual arrangements with the doctor or hospital will result in substantially lower charges or expenditures. However, history dictates otherwise. What happens as a rule is that the charges are considerably more than the indemnification. As a consequence, most people with indemnity policies are more dissatisfied with their insurance than those with service policies.

A modification of the indemnity type of plan that has found greater favor is one in which cost sharing is an element. This is something of a compromise between service and indemnity plans. The insured is guaranteed service, but pays something at the time of use. Medicare has such a feature. But there are also full indemnity insurance policies of this kind. An outstanding example of such cost sharing is "major medical insurance." An individual who incurs a medical expense agrees to pay a fixed sum — the first part of those costs — in a "deductible" of $50, $100, $250, or whatever. Thereafter, he is guaranteed that he will only have to pay a fraction of the remainder, 10, 20 or 25 percent, with the insurance company paying the rest. This is, of course, equally as inflationary as the other indemnity type programs, but is less likely to be an irritant. Of course, the following year his premium will probably go up and he will be irritated at that!

WEAKNESSES OF INSURANCE PROGRAMS

The disadvantage for national programs of medical care in using insurance companies is that insurance companies were never intended to be more than bill paying mechanisms, whether it was to pay cash to the customer or to pay the provider for bills rendered, on estimated budgets or negotiated costs. The insurance companies have traditionally seen themselves in this light. As a consequence, those aspects of the medical care provision that required supervision lest they be abused or deliberately manipulated for profit, were specifically eliminated from the concern of the insuring company, whether it was Blue Cross or a commercial carrier. This role definition fostered abuse, encouraged inflation and created a pattern that obstructed any rational control, or even a semblance of responsibility for cost control.

Health insurance is a big business. In 1974 it was a $25 billion business. In 25 years it has grown from 9 percent of the share of financing of personal health care to 25 percent. Private health insurance now pays over 35 percent of all costs of hospital care and 37 percent of all costs of physician services, particularly in hospital physician care (but only 8 percent of dental costs and 5.7 percent of drug costs). And the insurance companies, clinging to almost $3 billion of this, are still unready or unwilling to assume responsibility for controlling the circumstances under which the costs were incurred — to set and supervise standards of acceptable medical practice as a prerequisite for coverage and payment.

Insurance companies also display a surprising lack of enterprise for a capitalist endeavor. While the manufacturing industry prides itself on continuing investment in "risk" capital (taking chances in order to enlarge their market and broaden profit), insurance companies take no such risks. Their policies tend to be restricted to the safest, most actuarially sound forms of coverage — the events most easily predictable and the risks most easily covered. Hospital care is the easiest medical care product to predict and protect against. Out of the early experiences with service benefits, it was in-hospital insurance that got the greatest emphasis, and ambulatory services were slighted. The natural effect of this, as could have been easily predicted, was that if a medical service was needed that would be paid for *in* hospital but not *outside* the hospital, the insured would prefer — in many instances demand — that the service be performed *in* hospital. This tended to drive services into hospitals. As the hospital grew technically, employing more people to service the new complex and expensive machines, operating costs naturally rose and insurance costs rose with them to meet consequent rising medical care costs. And since the insurance benefit package depended on cost and the companies did nothing to supervise the management or operation of the institutions where benefit packages were being arranged, the result was a typical cost plus situation. The hospital hired people, bought equipment and made whatever improvements or modernizations thought necessary or desirable; Blue Cross and the commercial insurance carriers met the charges competitively; premiums continued to rise. As more hospital services were used, more hospital services were demanded. We had arrived at a state of development where Medicare could do a lot and people wanted it done; the hospital was the place to do it. The insurance companies saw no reason to change the situation.

### EFFORTS FOR IMPROVEMENT

Over the years the disparity between what could be done by health insurance and what was being done was pointed out continuously, in private consultants' studies, community investigations, Congressional hearings, etc. But it was not until Congress, heavily involved in multi-million dollar expenditures by way of Medicare and Medicaid, imposed legislative controls, that insurance companies reluctantly began to pay attention. Even so, they have not shown traditional American venturesomeness and the field has suffered heavily as a consequence. Probably, had the insurance companies been more socially responsive, cooperating in an effort to keep costs and prices down, the entire situation today would be different; but they have been and continue to be overcautious.

### NATIONAL HEALTH INSURANCE

The private health insurance companies should not be concerned that passage of a national health insurance bill will undermine or destroy their business. The experience in both Britain and Canada, after the passage of national health programs, shows that public policy usually leaves a broad area of expenses, up to 25 percent of health service costs, which can be covered by insurance; this represents a profitable field for the companies to till. The difficulty, of course, is the present size of the health insurance market and the question as to whether equal profits can be met under lesser circumstances. It is very likely, because of the pressures imposed by the vast wealth and power of the $25 billion insurance business, that in some fashion the private companies will be afforded a continuing large business regardless of the degree to which the government gets into national health insurance. If so, it would be good to recommend national circulation of something on the order of "A Shopper's Guide to Health Insurance," which was published a few years ago by the unintimidated insurance commissioner of Pennsylvania, Herbert Denenberg. His guide fully describes the different types of policies and explains how you can tell from the insurance company's financial report whether or not you're getting your money's worth. He shows how the language of various policies can limit your access to reimbursement. As an example, if the illness is covered when it is first *manifested* after the effective date of the policy, then it makes little difference when you contracted it as long as the symptoms for which you are to be treated don't show themselves until *after* the policy goes into effect; but if the language says the disease has to be *contracted* after the policy goes into effect, then you could find that your very expensive illness (or pregnancy) isn't covered by the insurance.

Denenberg wanted all insurance policies written in *English* rather than *"legalese."* This is an important point; as Denenberg emphasized, knowledge on the part of the consumer is the key to the improvement of health insurance policies. (This theory could well be applied to other aspects of the medical care system as well.) If the professional jargon were reduced so that laymen could understand exactly what was involved (how much it would cost to do this rather than that, and why it would be more to their advantage to have this instead of that) there would be less confusion and more quality control and fair competition. If people could understand the practical aspects of what is involved in getting and giving service; getting and giving payment; what the insurance policy, the provider, and the system offer; it would be a lot easier to make mutually satisfactory arrangements and adjustments in the medical care system.

In this section, we have discussed financing of medical care costs by way of the American health insurance system, and some of the historical reasons why insurance has failed to meet needs. It would appear on one hand that insurance is essentially a benefit, affording protection against unexpectedly large and frightening health expenses. On the other hand, it would appear that our health insurance programs are unbalanced so that insurance is not as effective a protection as it should be. The private carriers have not always demonstrated social responsibility; set standards of control; or exercised any kind of restraint on expenditures, duplication of resources or useless and costly devices. In these areas of weakness, they are responsible to a considerable degree for the inflationary costs which have brought us to our present unhappy situation. Therefore, insurance is essentially a neutral economic mechanism that can be protective or destructive, depending on how it is used. If some of the more arrant exploitation could be controlled, perhaps the current health insurance program would be more useful.

### REIMBURSEMENT MECHANISMS

From the standpoint of costs, it would seem that the reimbursement mechanism by which hospitals or providers are paid has an important influence on whether or not hospitals will manage their "business" with efficiency and economy. If they are paid simply on the basis of expenditures as billed, there is no incentive for either economy or efficiency. In the hospital the use of "prospective budgeting" (budgeting for personnel and equipment costs in advance) might help to improve management efficiency. As for the other providers, such as independent physicians, advance budgeting is difficult. It would require some kind of reimbursement arrangement in which either the total amount of money to be paid or total amount of services to be rendered could be agreed upon in advance. But doctors resent and reject such arrangements.

Experience here and abroad shows us that there are at least four separate ways in which physicians can be reimbursed (as well as combinations not listed):

1. *Fee-for-service:* payment upon rendering of each medical service.
2. *Capitation:* payment of a fixed sum per month or year per patient, who then receives all services needed without any charge; the British general practitioner is reimbursed this way.
3. *Salary:* full-time payment for agreed upon hours, working conditions, etc.; this is common for specialists' reimbursement in socialist countries and many other parts of the world.
4. *Session payments:* a salary reimbursement, for a fixed piece of time; this is common in England for specialists.

Budgeting in advance for physician costs is possible under any of these methods except fee-for-service. And even fee-for-service, if there is a fixed fee schedule, can be handled through prospective reimbursement also.

Brian Abel-Smith, an internationally famous health economist, once observed that most nations find that their national medical organization insists upon reimbursement mechanisms that maximize their income. If there are many doctors, as in Israel, the Israeli Medical Society is on record for *salaried* service, guaranteeing income. If there are too few patients per doctor, or a large unmonied population with not enough money to support the doctors, a government service capitation, which allows the physician some degree of freedom in negotiation, is preferred, as in England. If, on the other hand, there is a very wealthy community with not too many physicians, fee-for-service is most rewarding. The doctor can then dictate how many visits the patient makes and what his price per visit should be. On the surface, then, fee-for-service tends to increase utilization, thus maximizing the physician's income. Capitation may be less satisfying to the doctor even though it guarantees his income, since frequency of patient service will not increase his income; a preordained ceiling has been imposed. From the doctor's standpoint, utilization may be maximized, but income remains unchanged.

Under the salary system, physicians are also guaranteed their income; here there is danger that they may not elect to give the patient as many services as the patient would like to have. And again, the doctor may feel that the lack of a financial barrier may "maximize utilization."

On the session basis, in which a doctor is employed to work a fixed number of hours for a fixed fee, and see whatever patient comes to him, the number of patients seen can be manipulated either by the employer (who pays the doctor's session fee), or by the doctor himself, by seeing patients for longer or shorter periods of time.

Of these reimbursement mechanisms, there does not seem to be one in which both doctors and patients can be uniformly satisfied. Most countries use some combination of these methods. In the Scandinavian countries a fixed capitation is combined with a small charge to the patient to create a satisfactory cost sharing mechanism. The amount of the charge at the time of service is sufficiently small so as not to inconvenience or frighten off a patient from making appropriate use of the service; at the same time fixed capitation satisfies the doctor that he is receiving an adequate income, and the added charge controls overutilization.

Reimbursement mechanisms can have a profound influence on whether insurance is cost and quality protective, is fair to patients and provides doctors or hospitals with an adequate source of income.

## SOLUTIONS FOR HOSPITAL COST CONTAINMENT AND LOWER PATIENT EXPENDITURE

It is a very common complaint made against the hospital system that it tends to be more a competitive rather than a cooperative system. The services provided should relate to the needs of the community and the patient rather than solely to those of the provider. In many ways the hospital is still the doctor's workshop, as we discuss, and as a consequence there are things that hospitals do in order to satisfy physicians that have nothing whatever to do with community needs or patient needs. Expensive equipment proliferates when it could be localized; expensive hospital units proliferate when they could be centralized.

Actually, the common criticism of too many neurosurgical or cardiac surgery units, the multiplication of cobalt bombs for the treatment of cancer, or pediatric beds in more than one hospital, is hardly the major cause of difficulty. Basically, hospitals cannot be utilized as community resources because of the private practice of medicine. Physicians have to maintain hospital visiting and admitting privileges in a particular hospital to earn their livelihood. If a patient wants to be cared for by *his* doctor then he has to be hospitalized in the particular hospital in which *his* doctor works. His doctor then wants all the equipment and specialized personnel and complex materials available in the institution where he takes care of his patients. This is the basic cause of the multiplication. A hospital's board tends to reflect the hospital doctors' interest; the hospital's management in response tends to reflect the doctors' interests and so the patient is forced to pay twice — taxes and increased costs of hospital insurance or through out-of-pocket payments — for the rapidly rising cost of hospitalization resulting from this duplication.

This duplication is not only expensive; just as important, it discourages centralized cooperative specialist groups. I have reference here to cardiac surgery and neurosurgery particularly.  It is well known that in order for cardiac surgeons (and teams) to be competent in their activities they need to carry on a certain number of procedures per week or per month to maintain their requisite skills.  Where cardiac surgery is not that prevalent, more than one or two hospitals, even in a borough the size of the Bronx in New York, may "stock" very expensive personnel and equipment sitting on the sidelines, performing one or two services a year at which they cannot be terribly proficient.  But as long as private practice by physicians is encouraged, they will compete in these specialties, and as long as specialists are turned out by the medical schools without limit this kind of competition is inevitable.

Another complication in this cost problem is that the hospital and its ambulatory services, separated as they are from the physicians' offices and other aspects of medical care, tend to be skewed in their use.  What could be looked after in the office is seen in the hospital.  Hospital clinics tend to be more expensive than necessary because, when physically located on the hospital premises, managed by the hospital, they tend to reflect the overhead cost of the institution as a whole rather than the appropriate overhead that would be their cost if they were free standing.  Hospital clinics' overhead may be five or ten times the overhead of a doctor's office.  The skewed insurance coverage, driving people into hospitals for care, has an added inflationary effect there.

There is evidence of provider cost containment through strict controls in the prepaid group practice systems where the volume of hospitalization is tied to the income of physicians (the patients' premium includes both hospitalization and physician services).  The more the doctor hospitalizes the patient, the greater the hospital costs, the less money there is available for physician salaries.  In situations like the Kaiser Plan (prepaid group practice), hospitalization tends to be at 25 percent to 30 percent, or at most 50 percent, of that in communities in which there is no relationship between hospitalization and the physician's income.

A second lesson is found in Europe where there is a clearer relationship between budgeting and hospital personnel.  There are only two persons per bed working in Swedish hospitals and over three persons per bed working in American hospitals.  The difference, of course, with about a million American hospital beds, is an added one million American hospital workers.  Since personnel costs represent 66 percent of hospital costs, a million added workers represents 20 percent of the total cost of hospital care.  In 1974, this came to $41 billion and 20 percent of that is over $8 billion.

I am reminded of an old Persian tale in which a prince of great wealth had two sons who were constantly quarreling.  Being afraid that after he died they would quarrel over the estate and incite civil war, he left a will in which everything was to be divided equally between them.  One son was to do the dividing and the other to have first choice.  It would seem that something of this sort arranged among the providers might have a significant inhibiting effect on the rate of inflation.  Perhaps the insurance money should be given to the hospitals with instructions to pay the doctors according to a system they would work out cooperatively on a budgeted basis.  Or else the money should be given to the doctors as a group, with instructions to work out a system for reimbursing the hospital.

# Chapter 3
# Access and Availability

---

## THE RISE IN MEDICAL CARE DEMAND

The increasing difficulty of many Americans to obtain medical care when they want or need it is related to many factors, some of which are only partly the result of inefficiencies and inadequacies in the medical care system. For example, in proportion to the population, there are not fewer hospital beds, doctors, nurses or other kinds of health workers. But there has been a very great increase in the *demand* for medical services.

Until the beginning of this century, most people did not have very much confidence in doctors and relied far more heavily on home remedies that were considered very helpful; pharmacists were able to dispense just about anything across the counter legally. At least half the surgery and more than three-quarters of the deliveries were done at home. The hospital was looked upon as a place where only the gravely ill were sent and certainly not a place where the middle class or wealthy people would want to go. They were seen as public or charitable institutions for the poor. Even more recently, the Queen of England has had her babies in Buckingham Palace rather than in a hospital. The Washington Hospital Center has built a deluxe floor for the special care of the wealthy, emphasizing that there has to be something special in a hospital that is supposed to be for the rich as against one that is supposed to be for the poor.

Lawrence Henderson, a physician and Harvard professor, is supposed to have said, that 1915 was probably the first year in human history that the average patient consulting the average physician had a 50-50 chance of benefiting from the encounter; this was the great watershed at which point patients began to think it desirable and necessary to consult a physician when they were ill.

People were becoming more aware of a scientific, rational approach to health and disease. Medicine was becoming more specialized. There were now people who knew a great deal about specific kinds of illness and could probably do something helpful about some of them.  By the 1930's new kinds of drugs and more daring and sophisticated types of surgery were known and available.  After World War II, the new drugs being introduced not only became desirable and necessary, but there was a feeling of frantic compulsion for care by the physician; that now it was a matter of life or death.  And, as a result of the technological developments and advertising of "miracle cures," pressures for care in the hospital were evident as well.  There was, in other words, a complete reversal of attitude: people *wanted* physicians and hospital services; and demanded more resources to be made available.  No more home deliveries; no more kitchen surgery.

Futhermore, many of the things that had been conducive to maintaining the patient at home had disappeared.  The large family homes had become apartments.  The extended family setting with aunts or cousins who could act as nurses was disappearing.  It was now necessary to provide institutional care for people who had been looked after at home.  There was no more looking after feeble old relatives — they had to be in nursing homes.  More people were living into the age groups where they were most susceptible to chronic illnesses, so there was more need for doctors, hospitals and nursing homes.

## LACK OF ACCESS AND AVAILABILITY

### PHYSICIAN SPECIALIZATION AND SUBURBAN MIGRATION

There continues to be an increasing demand for the services of physicians and the added different kinds of health workers, and for the services of institutions; more belief in all kinds of medical care.  This might be called "patient pressures."

On the other hand, there have been factors in medicine itself moving in the same direction.  Medicine was becoming increasingly specialized; it was necessary for doctors to have more specialized equipment and the institutions in which to work.  The same drive toward specialism was drawing doctors out of neighborhood practice where they had been general practitioners and making them into in-hospital specialists: surgeons, neurosurgeons, dermatologists, cardiologists, etc.  There was no longer the kind of quality physician available in terms of family care that had been available at the time the scientific revolution began, at the turn of the century.  Then there were 150,000 American physicians for 75,000,000 people, or roughly one for every 500, of whom 90 percent were family physicians; this made it possible for there to be a doctor readily available for most people no matter where they lived.  Fifty years later it was altogether different.  The doctors were specializing and becoming concentrated into hospital medical facilities.

In the 1970's, we are about 210 million people with almost 350,000 doctors in private practice, or roughly one to every 600, not too different from the distribution in 1900. But now almost 100,000 of them are interns, residents, fellows, teachers and out of the mainstream of private practice, which reduces the ratio to about 1:800! And 70 percent of them are specialists, which leaves only 30 percent as family physicians or general practitioners, so that there are really only 60,000 doctors in primary care for 200 million people; approximately one for every 3,000 people, only one-fifth the number of family physicians that there were at the turn of the century.

Furthermore, 80 percent of the population is now urban; there is a disproportionate distribution of physicians in urban and suburban areas as opposed to rural areas. We find that while 20 percent of the population is in rural areas only about 17 percent of the doctors are. While 25 percent of the population is in suburban areas, some 40 percent of the doctors are. If we look at this from the standpoint of family practitioners, the situation is

FIGURE 3-1:    Percent Distribution of Non-Federal Physicians in United States and Possessions by Activity. December 31, 1973

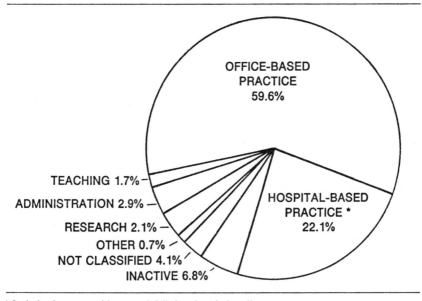

\* Includes interns, residents, and full-time hospital staff.

NOTE: Percentages may not add due to rounding.

*Source: Profile of Medical Practice,* American Medical Association, 1974, p. 107.

somewhat different.   There are more general practitioners in rural areas proportionately than in urban/suburban areas.   Nonmetropolitan counties with 50 million people have 8 percent of the physicians but 23 percent of the general practitioners.   Many of the general practioners, however, who still remain in the rural areas, are ten years older on the average than their colleagues in the city, and there is a concomitant deficit of specialists in the rural areas.   In the suburbs there is a plethora of specialists and large numbers of young interns and pediatricians carrying the brunt of what used to be the general practitioner's family doctor role.   In the inner cities, however, there is a lack of both specialists *and* family doctors in office practice.

Access to medical care is limited by the changes in medical practice — the flocking of young practitioners into the suburban areas and the medical centers, with an associated drain of physicians from the rural areas and the inner cities.   Ironically, at the turn of the century there was apparently a better representation of physicians in the rural areas than in urban areas; so was the greater percentage of patient population.

TABLE 3-1:   Non-Federal Physicians, Hospitals, Hospital Beds, Population, and Income by Metropolitan and Non-Metropolitan Areas

| | Total | METROPOLITAN | | Non-METROPOLITAN | |
|---|---|---|---|---|---|
| | (100.0%) | Number | Per-cent | Number | Per-cent |
| Total Physicians (12-31-73) | 333,966 | 288,424 | 86.4 | 45,542 | 13.6 |
| Total Patient Care | 272,850 | 234,640 | 86.0 | 38,210 | 14.0 |
| Office Based Practice | | | | | |
| General Practice | 47,195 | 32,384 | 68.6 | 14,811 | 31.4 |
| Medical Specialties | 48,185 | 42,964 | 89.2 | 5,221 | 10.8 |
| Surgical Specialties | 63,234 | 54,170 | 85.7 | 9,064 | 14.3 |
| Other Specialties | 40,520 | 36,099 | 89.1 | 4,421 | 10.9 |
| Hospital Based Practice | 73,716 | 69,023 | 93.6 | 4,693 | 6.4 |
| Other Professional Activity | 24,748 | 23,018 | 93.0 | 1,730 | 7.0 |
| Inactive | 22,624 | 18,402 | 81.3 | 4,222 | 18.7 |
| Not Classified | 13,744 | 12,364 | 90.0 | 1,380 | 10.0 |
| Hospitals (12-1-73) | 5,937 | 3,052 | 51.4 | 2,885 | 48.6 |
| Hospital Beds (12-1-73) | 914,839 | 684,589 | 74.8 | 230,250 | 25.2 |
| Resident Population (12-31-72) | 209,448,200 | 156,922,400 | 74.9 | 52,525,800 | 25.1 |
| Income (1972) | | | | | |
| Per Capita | $ 3,779 | $ 4,073 | | $ 3,001 | |
| Per Household | 11,617 | 12,418 | | 9,220 | |

* Includes Medical Teaching, Administration, Research, and Other.

*Source:* G. N. Roback, *Distribution of Physicians in the U. S., 1973,* American Medical Association, 1974, p.15.

As changes in living habits and specialism of physicians were taking place those people who didn't have access to the office-based doctor began to use the hospitals more. Today community hospitals, with almost a million beds, represent 6,000 of the 7,000 hospitals in the United States. They almost doubled their out-patient visits from 94,000,000 in 1966 to 171,000,000 in 1974. Over the same time period, their in-patient admissions increased only 20 percent, from 27,000,000 to 33,000,000. Emergency room visits show an equally astounding leap in numbers of people cared for and number of visits made. The conclusion is clear. Access and availability have been transformed at the same time that perceived need and demand were augmented. The "new" medical care was wanted. If family physicians weren't locally available to provide it, hospitals were expected to take up the slack. The change in medical education and medical practice increasingly benefited the monied, able-to-pay, suburban dwellers; the doctors gravitated to them. Entrepreneurial values overcame professional values. This is not to say, of course, that this happened everywhere simultaneously or to the same degree, but the statistical evidence makes it clear that access to medical care for certain segments of the population was gradually restricted.

### GEOGRAPHIC DEPRIVATION

For some members of the population groups and specific populations, restrictions were even greater. There had been limited services before but the belt was tightened. Geographically isolated places have been even less likely to retain the services of a physician and people living there have increasing difficulty in finding their way to a hospital. In the 1940's, recognition of the trend resulted in the passage of the Hill-Burton Act which provided for federal participation in the cost of construction of hospital facilities in rural and isolated areas. Over the next 25 years thousands of hospital beds were provided. Many small hospitals were built in rural areas according to plan, with the participation of state governments, although it was very largely a federal program with an enormous investment of federal money.

The rural areas benefited to the extent that the hospitals were built. But the purpose behind the law didn't quite develop as it was intended. At the time the program was being discussed in the Congress, the point was made that one of the reasons for building the hospitals was to attract physicians. Physicians presumably didn't want to practice in rural areas because they couldn't get enough professional stimulation or opportunities to do modern medical work in the rural areas, without modern hospitals. While that may

FIGURE 3-2:   Doctors Per 100,000 Population in Appalachian States by Wealth of County (1967)

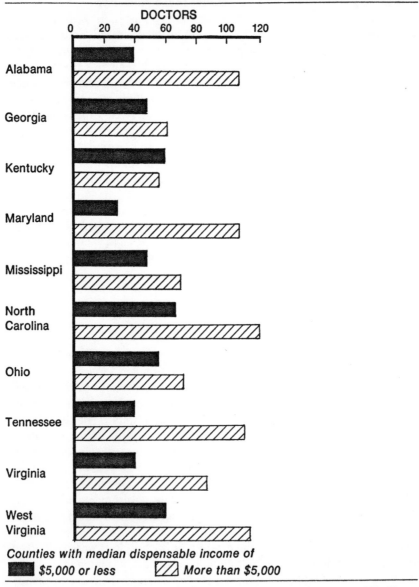

Counties with median dispensable income of
████ $5,000 or less      ▨ More than $5,000

*Source: Towards a Comprehensive Health Policy for the 1970s.* Department of Health, Education and Welfare, May 1971.

*Source:* R. Maxwell, *Health Care: The Growing Dilemma,* McKinsey & Company, 1974, p. 21.

have been true the hospital construction did not attract the numbers or quality of physicians that were needed.

As we point out in the discussion on medical education, the purpose and direction in the training of physicians after World War II militated against the possibility of their wanting to place themselves in socially necessary practice situations. The emphasis in medical education was to stimulate the physician to display his vast skills and to give him the personal satisfaction of being able to deal with complex cases requiring specialized services. For these reasons he preferred to remain in contact with people who could afford to buy those skills and understand them; to remain in constant touch with the situation in teaching hospitals. There he could offer his skills and carry out his activities under the best possible circumstances. So the new specialists did not flock to the rural areas. They flocked to the nearby suburbs or remained in teaching hospitals. General practitioners were not being trained at all and the few who did take it up or did return to rural areas or the inner city were inadequate to make up the deficit of the outward migration.

## MINORITY DEPRIVATION AND DISCRIMINATION

There are other types of deprivation from access to medical care. Access to effective medical care by the minority, 20,000 blacks living in the ghettos and the rural South; 10,000,000 Spanish-speaking Americans in the rural and poverty ridden Southwest or the ghettos of California cities; and newly immigrating Puerto Ricans in the ghettos of New York City and other eastern cities had been sharply limited by their minority status from the beginning. The increasing migration of specialists and family doctors to suburban areas and teaching centers meant that the already limited availability was being dissipated further. Poorer than most and with more illness, because poverty and illness go together, their situation became intolerable.

From the data it can be seen that geographic location, minority status, and poverty are the prime attributes of lack of access and availability. The grim irony is that these three factors of limited access are usually found together. Further, epidemiological studies have shown us that these factors are conducive to greater medical needs. Add to this the evidence from the previous chapter, and we see that despite the fact that they're poorer, they will have much larger expenses for hospital and physician care. These are the very people who will hesitate to go for early care out of fear of anticipated expense; when they do go, the medical care given may be too late, more difficult and painful, leave more disability, and, of course, be even more expensive.

And there is evidence of a pattern of discrimination as well, even when patients do have insurance coverage (as in Medicaid or Medicare) in that there is a significantly different utilization by the nonwhite as opposed to the white patient. Even without financial obstacles, the discriminatory character of access to services is evident. Medicare pays larger sums for outpatient services for minority groups than for physician services in the office. Medicaid shows a substantial differential in payments for the aged, paying for twice as many white as nonwhite patients. Different sections of the country list a sharp distinction between white and nonwhite reimbursement under Medicaid.

### MINORITIES AS MEDICAL PROFESSIONALS; DISCRIMINATION AND UNBALANCE

Some other evidence of a discriminatory pattern can be seen in the fact that only 75 percent of hospitals indicate minority patients on their census; about the same number show appointment of minority group interns or residents. Only about half the hospitals in the United States give staff privileges to minority physicians. This is certainly also a reflection of the fact that only 2 percent of the physicians in the United States are of a minority group; they might not be distributed well enough to admit patients in all hospitals, or to request admitting privileges to 100 percent of the hospitals. While this is being remedied to a degree, the number of minority students enrolled in health professional schools has not increased so markedly as to forecast that that proportion will be modified significantly in the near future. Data for 1972-1973 show that only 8 percent of medical students were of minority origin. This shows itself also in the distribution among other health care professions; while 17 percent of those students enrolled in associate degree (2-year) nursing schools are minority students, only 13 percent enrolled in baccalaureate (4-year) nursing programs are.

The disproportionate distribution of physicians is related to their selection of where to practice and specialize. Physicians make these selections based on professional interests rather than our society's needs. The storm of demand for additional physicians makes it appear that the shortages are real, actual shortages rather than artificial ones imposed by the lack of distribution. W. I. Thomas, the celebrated American sociologist, pointed out many years ago that if a proposition were considered to be true, the consequences were real. In other words we would behave as if the proposition *were* real and so it would have real effects. Merton's "self-fulfilling prophecy" is similar in that he adds that by believing something to be true, we act so as to make it come about! The United States is attracting large numbers of foreign medical graduates in an effort to meet the needs resulting from lack of physician distribution. We want to assure an adequate supply of professionals within the hospital system. We try in this way to meet demands of communities for additional doctors. However, the foreign medical graduates tend to practice very much in the same areas and in the same specialities as their American counterparts; the situation is not modified, but intensified and exaggerated.

Attracting foreign medical graduates into the United States has an additional element of injustice. There are 9,500 native Philippine trained physicians licensed and practicing in the United States. There are only 5,200 native American black physicians.

## SOLUTIONS TO MEDICAL DEPRIVATION

The problem of restoring the balance in medical resources is obviously not one of more physicians or more hospital beds. It would appear that in order to restore some balance, there has to be a redistribution of physicians; and better transportation and more efficient and economic use of the existing facilities and resources. And there has to be some change in the current economics of medical practice, so that patients may take advantage of available resources without being inhibited by financial barriers.

Concerned people have come up with many different solutions to these problems, and Congress has passed laws and appropriated money to try to solve the problem in accord with some of these suggestions.

### INCENTIVES AND DISINCENTIVES TO MEDICAL GRADUATES

One effort is focused on the deprived areas. The National Health Service Corps offers salaries and jobs in such places. Young doctors who have borrowed money to complete their educations and want a guaranteed salary for a while to pay off heavy obligations can enlist. At one time, when there was a doctor draft, a limited number of doctors could volunteer for such duty instead of military service. Now specific scholarships are offered, whereby the graduate will pay back year for year each year of education paid for by the government. A new law is pending to make this compulsory for most students that their education be paid for entirely, after which they must accept assignments for service in medically deprived areas. Another offered solution provides for monetary bonuses to practitioners in underserved areas.

Legislation makes it possible for some underserved areas to obtain federal funds to set up experimental programs, and so attract physicians.

There is also a general kind of appeal to the idealism and democratic aspirations of young people through magazine articles and television programs describing the kinds of needs. Efforts are also made to modify medical education in order to produce the desired effect:

- selection of more candidates from deprived areas in the belief that they are more likely to return there to practice
- incentive payments to medical schools to offer courses in family medicine
- bonuses to medical schools for students interested in family practice or work in deprived areas
- withdrawal of support for specialty training

Similar pressures are suggested to be put on specialty boards and hospitals to reduce specialist production and employment of foreign medical graduates.

In addition to the federal government, states are employing financial incentives and disincentives to try to change the direction and momentum of distribution of physicians and other medical care resources.

It may not be possible to accomplish redistribution of physicians and resources without altering significantly the traditional entrepreneurial character of medical practice. There will have to be a *social* decision as to whether physicians can be ordered to certain areas to practice for a specified amount of time (considered by some people indentured servitude) after they have been educated at public expense; or, whether certain medical specialties can be restricted in numbers so that some physicians will not be able to move into more lucrative, more desirable or more comfortable practice, specialties and locations.

The problems raised by lack of medical access and availability are the problems of our society generally, as well as the specific problems of medical practice. While cost is an important item and cannot be overlooked in a reshaping of medical services in the United States, the deficiencies of access and availability are far more than economic problems; they stem from many sources, some cruelly created by social barriers, and, to be solved, will require much thoughtful concentration and social responsibility.

Even with laws dictating that medical school graduates were to spend time in under-doctored areas, the likelihood that they would remain there would be remote unless some of the social and cultural deficiencies were relieved, as well as transportation, educational facilities, and housing. The fact is that the impoverished areas lack educational, cultural, and social facilities and activities that would attract a doctor's wife and family, would also be an impediment to his deciding to practice there, in addition to the lack of professional stimulation and opportunity.

### HELP TO MINORITY GROUP PHYSICIANS

We might wonder whether the effort to obtain more minority candidates for medicine derives from our sense of fairness alone: an effort to equalize

the proportion of minorities in the profession to their demographic proportion in the population, perhaps; or simply to end the discrimination in
admission policies by a kind of retributive justice, admitting more
proportionately, qualified or not.  There is also a belief that by admitting
more minority candidates and providing more minority physicians, the poor
distribution of physicians will be rectified.  Black doctors will go to ghetto
areas in the cities, or to the rural south where the black population tends to
be concentrated; chicano physicians will practice in East Los Angeles and
the rural southwest.  To accept the premise that this is what ought to
happen is inherently undemocratic.  Doctors, of whatever race, color or
religion, should serve all patients, not tribal groups, in a democratic society.
And if there are problem areas, a more democratic distribution system
ought to be devised.

Additionally, the intensive medical school training and education, exposure to classmates and faculty with a profoundly professional ethos and
motivation, is bound to have an effect on the minority candidate admitted.
He will have an effect on his classmates; some of the appeal for equity will
be transmitted as the minority student expresses the social needs of his race
or geographic life experience.  But the classmates will have an effect on the
minority student as well.  After four years of medical education and four
more years of hospital and specialty training, the minority student will
undoubtedly have absorbed a conception of role that will make the underserved areas as unappealing to him as to the majority students.  I suspect he
will be more "doctor" than "minority."  Lack of professional contacts, or
teaching hospital relationships; inadequate schooling for his children; and
decreased cultural advantages and social opportunities will find him equally
reluctant to undertake that life as a long-term career.

## SUMMARY

The poor distribution of doctors has many causes — professional, economic, social, situational.  It is doubtful that a single solution is feasible.
Until all of America is more nearly equal in housing, job availability,
educational opportunities, cultural resources and transportation, the solution to full medical care resource equalization will be unattainable.  It may
be that roads, helicopters and closed circuit television may be more likely
answers in the short haul and require closer attention than complex schemes
for getting doctors into underserved areas — schemes often based more on
faith than fact.

In short, the rise of specialism and the strengthening of the ties between
the graduate and the institution; diminution of numbers of family practitioners; the association of physicians with more well-to-do areas; the
gradual deemphasis on rural living as a way of life; the lack of cultural

amenities, educational facilities, housing and transport to attract professional people and their families in underserved areas, all resulted in reinforcement of selective deprivation of parts of the country and groups of people.

The poor native Americans, chicanos, blacks in urban ghettos and the people of isolated rural areas suffer most keenly from the deprivation of access and availability of medical care. The middle income people are principally harassed by costs. Resources have gradually increased; there are no fewer doctors today than there were 100 years ago, proportional to the population, but they are mostly specialists; we lack family doctors. They are unevenly distributed, and they are expensive.

# Chapter 4
# Medical Care — General and Specialized

---

## AMERICAN PLURALISM: DEMOCRATIC?

Americans are generally proud of the pluralism that freedom of expression and entrepreneurial drive encourages and sustains. This pluralism is supposed to facilitate competition because it gives people choice, another aspect of American life that, in theory, sets it off from many other countries not so rich in resources and not so inclined to allow individuals the opportunity to express themselves. It is true that in many instances the apparent pluralism is quite superficial and the choices meaningless. But when pluralism allows relatively ineffective methods, procedures or institutions to continue to survive and compete, it is actually a social deficit rather than a gain; a democratic ideal that manifests undemocratically. Similarly, if a needed article or service is expensive or located only in specific places, as is medical care, it really exists only for those who can attain it. It cannot be *freely* chosen because it is not *freely* available.

Luxury items such as caviar, Cadillacs and mink coats may simply be the expression of choice. After all, you can buy foods that are as tasty and as nutritious as caviar but much cheaper and more easily available. You can get transportation at considerably less cost than a Cadillac; and you can keep warm with something that costs far less than a mink coat. Society acts to aid people at poverty level who are prevented from getting food, transport or warmth. We aim at full employment, for one thing, so that everyone ideally has an opportunity to get a job and earn the money to buy what is needed; or we try to provide public services from tax money to support those who are unable to hold a job. Our society expects the able to get what they need for themselves, to the degree they work for it. And it says it will supply for the helpless what they cannot provide for themselves.

## MEDICAL PLURALISM: LACK OF FREE CHOICE

In medical services, however, the matter is more complex. There are sophisticated reasons why the pluralism for which we aim is not only ineffective but essentially undemocratic and dangerously inadequate for dealing with situations of medical need. The model of medical care is a physician, hospital and prescribed medicines. There are a few million people outside this system who are attended by other "medical" services. There are those who attend chiropractors, naturopaths, herb doctors, etc.; there are those who do not seek traditional medical care because of religious belief. The probability is that about 10 percent of the American people will regularly get their medical care outside the system of accepted medical practice. There may be slightly more who do not use the existing services because of financial reasons, lack of access, etc. This is not *choice* on their part; the vast majority of Americans who would want medical care would choose the traditional doctor-hospital-druggist system.

### THE FINANCIAL AND GEOGRAPHIC VARIABLES

For all practical purposes, therefore, medicine is a monopoly. The choice one has is essentially limited to location and price. And since we have whittled down the numbers of medical school graduates in proportion to the population over time (although this is building up again), and since the bulk of those educated in our medical schools choose to be specialists, the choices that most people have in getting medical care are fairly limited.

If you happen to be rather wealthy, and a member of the majority community, and if you live in a well-to-do suburb, you will have access to a large number of physicians and a large number of different kinds of specialists; you may truly have choice. You cannot know much about their quality, because there is not any "gourmet's guide" to physicians or hospitals as yet. It is true that in the wake of consumerism a few guides have been prepared, but these are rather rough indicators and not very specific in general descriptions. You cannot get the four star-, three star- or two star-type ratings applied to restaurants. The guide that has been developed in Prince George's County, Maryland, for example, tells you only limited things about the doctors: where they were trained; what their office hours are; and how much they charge. These may be tentative indications of quality, but they can hardly be described as definitive. In most instances and in most places we do not even have that amount of information about doctors. As far as hospitals are concerned, the only thing that we can know is that they have been accredited by a private organization called the Joint Committee on Accreditation of Hospitals, run by the American Hospital Association, the American Medical Association, the American College of Physicians and the American College of Surgeons. These are "friendly" critics, with a stake in the hospitals and their own professional interests, so the question as to whether it is a suitable hospital for your individual needs is not really what concerns the accrediting body. What further hampers hospital choice is that you will be admitted to the hospital where your physician has privileges, if you want him to take care of you; it may not necessarily be the one that you wish to attend nor may it necessarily be the best.   However, the fee-for-service nature of medical practice makes it necessary for your doctor to insist on your going to that hospital in order that he may attend you and collect his fee.  The system also makes it necessary for hospitals to limit their attending staff so as to be able to keep bed space available for the members of their staff.

Circumstances like this make a mockery of "free choice," of course.  But for the less wealthy minority persons living in other places the lack of choice is even more glaring.  In isolated geographic areas or in the inner city where minorities and the poor live, the representation of doctors is far less and the probability that patients have any choice is remote, even if they could afford it.  The same holds true of hospitals.  So that on close inspection, we are faced with the fact that the traditional concept of pluralism and free choice for most Americans is a myth when related to health care.

### THE ACCEPTED VS. THE UNORTHODOX

For some Americans the choice is not among traditional types of physicians, but between the traditional and the unorthodox — chiropractors, spiritualists, naturopaths, etc.  While only a fraction of the American people are attended by such practitioners, they do have a choice.  It is surprising that more people do not select such practitioners or go to them in frustration or urgent need.  But they do not.

It was not always so.  In the middle of the 19th century many American patients were dissatisfied with their doctors who, as they became more scientific and rational, refrained from making quick diagnoses and prescribing wild mixtures and experimental drugs; with increased scientific knowledge, they would only prescribe a drug when they *knew* it suited a disease for which they had made an appropriate diagnosis.  As a consequence the best physicians did very little diagnosing or prescribing.  The patient in despair consequently turned to cultists, and the unorthodox practitioners multiplied in this country.  There was, for example, the growth of an herbal healing group called Thomsonian botanism, a sort of prepaid group practice in which subscribers paid $5 a year for a book in which symptoms were diagnosed and curative herbs prescribed.   Lincoln subscribed to the Thomsonian book, in addition to having a personal physician in the White House.

## THE IDEAL VS. THE REALITY

The "standard" pattern in the United States for the delivery of medical services has been, from the beginning, a solo practice relationship of an individual traditional type of physician with an individual patient.  It not only seems to be the most preferable today, but has been the most prevalent over the years.  Up until recently it would have been hard to figure out why it *should* have been otherwise.  There wasn't enough specialist knowledge that would require more than one skilled person to attend to all medical concerns of the patient.  The doctor carried in his head all the medical knowledge that there was.  He had in his bag all that was required in the way of instruments for diagnosis, as well as pills, powders, liquids, plasters and other medicines in the way of treatment.

It was discussed in Chapter 1 that American medical practice reflected differences in medical education and social attitudes between Europe and the United States.  The pioneer tradition, lack of educational institutions and the extraordinary mobility of both the physicians and the patients contributed to a situation in which the classical pattern of hospital, physician, pharmacist and the subpractitioners: (uroscopist, midwife, bone setter and other "paraprofessionals") commonly evident in Europe were not so evident in America.  The American physician, without university education or experience, was called upon to do everything: to pull teeth, to perform surgery, to dispense pills, to deliver babies, to diagnose and treat ordinary illnesses of people of every age and occupation.  He really was a *general* practitioner.  It also imbedded in the American consciousness an established method of practice, a polyvalent person as the doctor.

This essential American tradition, based on large numbers of physicians and the less frequent availability of other kinds of practitioners, engraved the pattern of role expectation on the part of patients before science, industrialization, urbanization and technical development undermined the possibility of maintaining or even achieving such a goal.  But the ideal remained fixed in the minds of both patients and physicians, so as eventually to create a discordance between the ideal and the reality, which was (and is) very frustrating.  Furthermore, when the situation did change, so that even the *ideal* of the physician was transformed, the patients' expectations remained fixed in the past; this created an additional conflict among disparate elements: patients' expectations, the realities of practice, and physicians' expectations.

# THE ORIGINS OF MEDICAL PLURALISM

### THE "SLIDING SCALE"

For the most part, poor people received care from the same physicians who took care of the well-to-do in the cities and rural areas of 19th century America. The mix of income groups among the population in small towns and even in the cities was such that rich and poor could be living next door to one another; neighborhoods were not as clearly segregated as they are today, even though there might have been "good" and "bad" parts of town. As the doctor tended to serve the people in a given neighborhood of varying income, the technique of physician payment called "the sliding scale" was created. Those who could pay the full fee did so; others paid less according to how much they could afford; and some paid nothing at all. Depending on what collections were like, the physician's "full fee" might have been quite high, and in some instances he might even have had a sliding scale of what constituted his "full fee," charging wealthy people considerably more than he would charge the average person. In time this grew to be known as the "Robin Hood" system of fee scales — robbing the rich to look after the poor.

### CLINICS, DISPENSARIES AND GROUP PRACTICE

The growth of clinics in the United States paralleled development of "sliding scales." Free clinics and dispensaries in association with the work house or other welfare establishments were set up so that those who could pay nothing to the physician would be segregated from the physician's private office and concentrated elsewhere. The purpose of this was probably dual. First, it may have stemmed from characteristic Calvinist attitudes which in many ways formed so much of American social institutions; the insistence on the fact that being poor was at least a sin, certainly the impoverished one's own fault, and perhaps even a crime. Under these circumstances the poor ought to be segregated and punished to show that he was inferior and also to give him a goal. Second, the doctor might have wanted to segregate those patients who were not paying, so that they would not clutter up his office, taking up the time that he could be devoting to paying patients. He was willing to set aside a separate piece of his time during which he could take care of the poor; in another setting altogether, and with someone else paying the "overhead" on *that* office practice.

Later in the 19th century, as the burgeoning science of medicine encouraged physicians to look more deeply into various aspects of their craft, and specialism began to be something more than simply a word in medical practice, those physicians who wanted to see a particular kind of patient used the clinics as an opportunity for setting up such segregated sessions.  It was easier and more scientific and efficient to group those patients with a singular affliction, so as to keep their records together, make comparisons and draw conclusions.

Of course the clinic was an ideal site for medical care of the poor for other reasons.  Poor people were not considered to have the same rights over their bodies as the well-to-do, who paid for services.  If you were getting free care, the doctors in the clinic had the right to ask you to do things they might not ask their paying patients; they could even order you to do them or lose the privilege of the care you were receiving as a benefit from the doctor and the community.  Clinic patients thus became "teaching material."  As the scientific aspect of medical service became more important to the doctor and more interesting and exciting to the profession as a whole, and specialism grew and flourished, the clinics became the important seedbed of knowledge and "practice" not only in the delivery of services but in the trial of new procedures and drugs.

As medicine became more and more expensive, more and more people found it necessary to use the clinics because they could not afford to pay a doctor.  The doctors wanted more people to go to the clinics, in part to foster specialism and improve their training opportunities, and in part not to have to take care of nonpaying patients in their offices.  They did not expect patients who could pay to want to go to the clinic; that only became a problem only after the Great Depression.  They did not feel that they were losing trade by sending patients to the clinic since these were patients who could not pay anyway.  The clinic assumed the burden of easing the doctor's conscience by maintaining the tradition of "free" service that had been the hallmark of the profession.  Doctors boasted that they took care of people without regard to income.  That they might take care of the poor differently or in different places or give them a different amount of time or concern was not so obvious and was denied absolutely if such a charge were made.  One would commonly hear that "poor people and rich people get the best medical care."  The implication of this was that in a clinic setting or in the wards of a public hospital (which corresponded on an inpatient basis to the outpatient clinic), the solicitious care and attention by doctors who gave their time without compensation, along with the growing numbers of house staff associated with increasing hospital services, provided such a rich mixture of modern medical care for poor patients that they were just as well off as the wealthy, who had to pay large sums of money for the same kind of attention and care.

Like so many other myths, there are some actual roots of fact in historic reality.  However, while this may have been true for a time, and in some places, it certainly was not true everywhere nor did it continue to be true. As medical practice became increasingly complex, larger numbers of physicians in training — interns, fellows, residents — had to be employed in order to look after the larger numbers of people who required care in clinics or hospital wards. After World War II, when medicine became increasingly laboratory-oriented, the practice of medicine turned increasingly inward. The major focus was then on the technical mechanism of medical practice: "learning" and "teaching" supplanted patient-oriented aspects and attitudes. As a consequence, clinic patients became more and more objects of study "cases," bags of organs and tissues in which the disease was inspected and treated; "future reference" seemed of a higher priority than the immediate individual patient. Among the many ironies engendered by the situation was the one of medical "charity." The profession gradually lost its tradition of free care as a means of social philanthropy; the clinic ceased to be a service function by the doctor for the poor and became a teaching function for the students.

As medical care became more and more expensive and America became more and more affluent, doctors wanted to share in that affluence. The casual character of payment for medical care was lost. It was replaced by a great concern for payment.

Then, the large numbers of people affected by the Depression had to get their care free from clinics; this threw an added financial burden on the clinic and dispensary system. Private philanthropy, which had been the mainstay of these rather small hospital and clinic operations up until the 1930's, was unwilling to cope with the increasing burden of simultaneous income tax and continued philanthropic contributions. The 1930's saw a reduction of the lavish character of philanthropic support of hospital operations that had been the earlier mode. Furthermore, the Depression had made inroads among the wealthy themselves. The state had to take over some part of the burden of hospital deficits.

The state, in turn, began to be rather sticky about who received medical benefits; "means tests" were established, of a fairly rigid character, to be sure that those who received free care actually deserved it. Clinic patients who were not under the defined category, "entitled" to free care, had to pay something. As medical costs increased, the "something" increased along with it. In a pattern thus set, no care was actually free. Those patients who were "entitled" were paid for by the state. Those patients not so entitled had to pay.

But the sliding scale for the physician's office continued. The physician, however, did not have to bear the burden of the low-paying or nonpaying patient; the hospital, and eventually the state, did. The high-paying patient continued to pay the doctor. Among the doctors the validity of the sliding scale remained, even though the low end was no longer his obligation or responsibility. He continued to charge high fees to the well-to-do to offset the "free" care that he still presumably gave. However, he no longer gave free care. In public hospitals the services were paid for by the public, and if the physicians were not paid (employed) to provide the services, the house staff provided them. No one provided care without charge.

In the private voluntary and community hospitals, attending physicians gradually reduced their time and services in the clinic, leaving them to be served by the house staff. They continued to pay attention as required to the specialized clinics, seeing the particular patients in which they were interested. They would select cases generally that increased their capabilities as specialists, giving them the prestige, cachet and experience they needed. Clinic service therefore increased their professionalism and earning capacity; it was not really a donation.

Further, when the states were no longer capable of meeting the increasing cost of medical care in the clinics, the federal government began to take over costs, first in the way of vendor payments and then later through Medicaid, making possible the large scale reimbursements to institutions.

Clinic costs were inflated additionally because the clinics were part of hospitals and hospital costs themselves were inflated. The clinic was saddled with hospital overhead, hospital costs and the expensive requirement of maintaining a "readiness to serve" the sickest possible patients. This caused outpatient visits to jump to three and four times the cost of a visit to the physician's office. However, the tradition had been set and so poor people, although permitted to do so under Medicaid, did not flock into the physicians' offices. This may have been partially because the physicians discouraged their attendance or actually refused to accept Medicaid patients, but also it was partially because they were accustomed to getting their care in the clinic. For the limited care they were providing to poor people, hospital clinics thus were paid more than physicians were paid for similar care in their private offices.

The two methods of practice described, solo fee-for-service in the doctor's office and hospital clinic practice, have been the major sources of delivery of medical care for individual patients over the past 200 years. Even in the usual group practice, one or the other of these was the customary pattern for providing care. In some instances the individual physician would carry his own patients within the group as if it were a private office, so that only administrative matters were handled on a group basis systematically. All other arrangements with the patient were made by the individual doctor. In other instances the groups operated as if they were clinics and the patient had no specific doctor; the group at large was his physician. The difference in the group practice was that *all* the patients were paying patients and *all* the patients were treated alike in either case. Some of the problems of group practice may have been derived from the fact that patients expecting the solo-type of relationship who were subjected to the clinic-type relationship resented and rejected it. The administrative operation of registration, appointment making, record keeping, cost accounting, supplies purchasing, etc., could be highly efficient in a group, but if the doctors operated as if it were a hospital clinic in which patients were not to receive the personal care and solicitude that they expected from the solo practitioner, the group foundered.

### HIGHER MEDICAL FEES THROUGH GUARANTEED PAYMENT

Past tradition has now been turned around. There are to be no more nonpaying patients in our society. Either the individual or the state will pay medical bills. This expectation has a corallary. If everything will be paid for, the rates established for payment will have to be the same for those going to the physician or to the hospital providers. If not, the same familiar disparity in access will appear. Furthermore, the idea that poor people pay less and wealthy people pay more for their services so as to make possible a compensatory average for the provider (the physician), is gone. The sliding scale has now been replaced. The government is expected to pay "reasonable and customary charges" in all instances in which there are federally supported payment programs for medical care.

The net effect is to create an inflationary spiral with the floor always being what had been last year's ceiling. In normal times as costs go up for food, clothing and housing, medical care costs usually go up, too; wages follow. The difference is that in earlier times medical care costs were built around a floating average in which there was an expectation that some people paid nothing. In these days with the government paying for those who otherwise *could* not pay, and insurance paying for those who otherwise *might* not pay, the physician has a guaranteed income and the customary and prevailing charges will be at a much higher level proportionately than they would have been earlier. In other words, physicians' fees as well as medical care costs generally have jumped ahead of the general cost of living in the inflationary upward spiral. It is true that hospital costs have increased at an even greater rate than physicians' fees, but as we shall see when we discuss hospitals, that in part may also be ascribed to the practices and charges of physicians.

## THE TWO-CLASS SYSTEM OF MEDICAL PLURALISM

American society has settled into a two-class system of medical care: the doctor's office for those who pay their own bills; the clinic for those who do not. In many parts of the country this cannot hold true because there are no hospital clinics. Specialism never made a foothold or local physicians are afraid that if hospitals go into clinical practice, this would drain off not only the poor but some of the paying customers. In those places doctors actively oppose establishment of clinic services. It is also true that in some parts of the country the local physicians have continued to look after the poor in their offices. And, sad to say, in some parts of the country, particularly those where the minorities are heavily represented, there is neither clinic service nor a private physician's office for most of the poor.

### THE GHETTO CITIZEN

As we have come to learn from the rebellions that have taken place in the past ten years in our cities, there is no such thing as *a* city dweller, but congeries of *people* living in the city; occupying different qualities of housing; living in neighborhoods that represent different cultural traditions, opportunities for employment, transportation, education and health. We are accustomed today to hearing about the "ghetto," a word never used until the 1960's except to describe the enclaves in which Jewish people were segregated at various times in history. Now we think of the ghetto as that area of the city to which the poor, and more generally the minorities, are relegated. The ghetto was formerly known as "slum" and sometimes euphemistically as "the inner city." In earlier days people spoke of "across the tracks," meaning the poorer parts of the town, but it did not have the same implication, nor perhaps the reality, of confinement, frustration, filth and decay, extensive oppression or explosive hostility. In such a setting, one can easily believe that if there had been medical care resources — hospitals, physicians and pharmacies — they would have fled, and so they have.

In Boston at one time a physician-population ratio of 1:600 would have meant a fairly even distribution of physicians throughout the community. A quick look at census checks within the city, however, shows it to be quite otherwise. Within the "inner city" the ratio is 1:2,000 and in the suburbs, 1:500. The great hospitals of Boston remain as they were, large flourishing enterprises with huge clinics, but the population served has shifted. The ward population is from the "inner city," even as the population in the suburbs fills its own recently built community and proprietary hospitals.

The same story is repeated in every large urban center — Philadelphia, Baltimore, New York, Chicago, Detroit. We are familiar with the shift that has taken place in the population of the urban public schools, where the majority are minority group children; the well-to-do white majority attend private and suburban schools. The same holds true for medical care services. The resources have fled to the suburbs along with their middle and upper income white clientele and the inner cities are left with inferior and inadequate resources. City hospitals, when not overcrowded, are still underfinanced. The physicians who used to serve in them have gone to the suburbs; few are left to carry out community medical care obligations. Internships and residencies in the inner city areas are no longer as desirable as they once were and the teaching hospital units in the inner city hospitals acquire an inadequate supply of American medical school graduates. It is worse if the hospitals are not strongly affiliated with universities. The places of American trained doctors are taken by foreign medical graduates, many of whom have some difficulty with the English language. The inner city inhabitants, (often immigrants,) might be having some difficulty with standard American English themselves; they will have much greater difficulty with the English of the foreign medical graduates. Furthermore, cultural differences create added gulfs in understanding between patient and doctor.

### THE URBAN AND SUBURBAN RICH

The well-to-do who do remain in the city in comfortable neighborhoods and high-rise apartments, or those in more luxurious suburban homes, do have access to their own physician, a solo or group practitioner associated with hospitals that continue to serve this clientele of interest. Within limits they receive the best of modern medical care, but at fairly high prices for which they are covered by insurance. Of course in some ways the rich suffer some of the consequences of the systematic disorganization and inequities of medical care that the poor do. After all, many of the people who live in the suburbs work in the cities. If they get sick downtown while they are at work they have to take the kind of medical care that the poor get — emergency rooms, clinics, foreign medical graduates, older and old-fashioned general practitioners. It is one of the risks of two classes of medical care.

## DISSOLVING THE TWO-CLASS SYSTEM OF MEDICAL PLURALISM

### AID TO THE GHETTO

In a discussion once on the need for encouraging more minority group members to enter the medical profession, Chester Pierce, a professor of psychiatry at the Harvard Graduate School of Education, pointed out that as the gulf between the rich and the poor widened in terms of medical care services, it was increasingly important that minority group members be trained for medical service with the hope that they would practice in the inner city to serve the minorities there. This is perhaps a not too likely hope, but more likely than the hope that middle-class white youths entering medicine might do that. He said he thought the white majority should understand the need for turning out more black (and other minority) physicians; if for no other reason, than when their children or grandchildren were taken ill or involved in an accident in the city, and needed to be treated in one of these inner city hospitals, they would find a well-trained doctor.

The numbers of physicians working in the inner cities has declined not only because the doctors have followed their clientele or seek that upper middle class clientele; the physical situation in the ghetto is unattractive and frightening. Perhaps if medical students were selected differently or if education for medical practice would have continued to foster its traditional commitment to social responsibility, a number of young graduates would want to remain with inner-city medical care services. The likelihood, however, has diminished as the recruiting process for medical education has emphasized scientific responsibilities, along with changing expectations and conceptions of role by physicians. At the moment it is unlikely that medical schools would select even from among minorities a cadre of recruits who would not be devoted to the current role model of doctor, or who would not become dedicated to this role model after exposure to the intensive socialization process of medical education.

Objectively, it is hard to understand why the poor and the black should have reserved to them the responsibility for serving the poor and the black. In any case, the numbers of doctors continue to dwindle and the other types of health workers associated with physicians' services working in those areas dwindle concomitantly. Hospitals, unless they are strongly affiliated with teaching institutions and need the "teaching material" in the ghettos, decay. Visiting nurse services are reduced to a few hours a day, as rapes, robberies and muggings discourage the visiting nurse from making calls. Julian Tudor Hart, an English physician, has designated this ghetto situation as the "Inverse Care Law:" the more services that are needed the less likely it is the services will be given.

AID TO THE RURAL AREA

Rural areas have suffered to an extent the same consequences as the inner city effect of centripetal force on the physicians who concentrate around the teaching hospitals and in the suburbs. Rural patients are restricted to the care of fewer general practitioners, somewhat older than their colleagues in the city, with fewer specialists.

There are perhaps 1,000 communities in the United States (20 percent of the population) that have no physician at all; although they may be on "trade routes" so that by traveling 40 or 50 miles they can reach a physician, they remain deprived locally. In many parts of these isolated communities, roads are bad or nonexistent. A good many minority group people live in such isolated areas; their deprivation is thus compounded. But even for relatively well-to-do Americans who live in isolated rural areas, the situation is perilous when it involves accidents or medical emergencies such as heart attacks, strokes or hemorrhages.

While Children's Bureau activities and national funding have caused many states to undertake special programs to assist in the care of "high risk" patients, only a few hundred thousand people benefit. Special services have been set up for transport of high risk mothers to hospital centers and premature babies to urban intensive care and premature units. But these are limited programs; not all mothers or infants needing such services receive them.

As for emergency medical care in general, the whole country is at a disadvantage as far as access to good quality facilities is concerned, particularly involving road accidents, and rural people more so. A national emergency service requires a nationally controlled network of transportation, communication and 24-hour medical care services. That is a long way off, despite federal and foundation support to local communities. National centers for head injuries, burns and orthopedic reconstruction are also in the distance.

There is no dearth of models as to what could be done for the medically deprived if an effective *national* health program were in existence. Organization of doctors into groups has been shown to be effective in rural areas through the use of both added transport and what are known as "satellite" clinics. The Rip Van Winkle Clinic, established in Hudson, New York, served all of Columbia County. The physicians who were located in the satellite offices were part of the Group. They came in once each week to make rounds in the county hospital, attended meetings with their colleagues, and would also come for some time during the year to spend a week or so in residence. Their colleagues and the specialists who worked in the group center in Hudson would go out to visit and consult regularly, so that hardly a day would pass but that the "isolated" physician in the satellite clinics could communicate with his colleagues either personally or by telephone.

While it may be true that the kind of physician who would have joined the Rip Van Winkle Clinic may not be the prototype of the kind of physician who graduates from medical school, sufficient numbers of these might be found to populate clinics and satellites of this kind set up in relation to rural areas in various parts of the country. Dr. Michael Shadid established a farm cooperative for medical care along these lines early in the century in Elk City, Oklahoma. Caldwell Esselstyn, from a long established New York patron family, built and developed the Rip Van Winkle Clinic in Columbia County, New York. With support and help from the government, medical educators and the medical profession, this probably could have been done in the hundreds of places requiring it in other parts of the country. However, both the incentive and the stimulus were missing; government financial support was not forthcoming; the Elk City Cooperative and Rip Van Winkle Clinic are no more, victims of rural poverty and professional insensitivity. Some private clinics that attempt the same services, but with a narrower focus, continue to exist. The Marshfield Clinic in Wisconsin still serves a large rural community.

In other countries the emphasis has been more on transport of the patient to the medical center rather than putting a doctor into the isolated area. The Highland and Island Service in Scotland, for example, provides motor and air transport for patients from the isolated mountain areas and Scottish Isles. The Flying Doctor service in Australia brings the physician by plane to the isolated branches. The Australians also use a short wave radio system for instant communication with isolated areas. In Swedish Lapland physicians and specially trained nurses travel over long distance by car or bicycle in summer weather and by sled in the winter to make periodic visits, and with added transport, bring patients to hospital centers when necessary. Norwegian physicians visit the isolated island areas off the coast by boat on a regular schedule.

Except for some experimentation with closed circuit television for both information and diagnostic and therapeutic advice, the United States has done very little in the way of national health services for isolated areas.

To summarize, the average rural resident, if he is within reasonable distance of a medical center, can get *some* of the best of modern medicine provided he can afford it, just as the city dweller of modest or reasonable income can. True, the rural resident is less likely to have the kind of insurance the city dweller has, who, through his employment, is covered by group insurance. Group insurance is far cheaper than individual insurance, so rural people are 50 percent less likely to have insurance coverage, which also makes it less likely that they will use the services or be able to pay for them if they do.

Isolated people have great difficulty in obtaining medical services, or paying for them, and very little is being done to create a system for providing them with medical services.

## MEDICAL SERVICES TO PEOPLE OF SPECIAL NEEDS

### THE ELDERLY

Old people in the United States, because they have special needs and are so strongly dependent on their community and on society generally for help and support, are at a particular disadvantage in the face of the entrepreneurial, individualistic philosophy so powerfully paramount in the medical care system. They are at a special disadvantage because of social changes that have failed to influence our social philosophy.

A century ago, the "family" tended to be much larger than what sociologists refer to today as the "nuclear family" — mother, father and a child or two. The family was a living arrangement including sometimes brothers and sisters, aunts and uncles, grandfathers and grandmothers, even distant cousins — the "extended family." Carving farms and ranches out of the vast land required large numbers of people. Large families were not only useful but necessary. In such a setting sick people could be looked after by other family members. Handicapped people, mildly mentally retarded, even the psychotic, and especially the old, were looked after at home. There was always someone available — older children not yet at work, unmarried aunts and uncles, grandfathers and grandmothers — to care for them; they did not have to be institutionalized if they were not totally capable of looking after themselves. Institutional care was really not an option; it existed only sparsely. Gradual urbanization; the reduction of the rural population; the rise of apartments and small houses; increasing numbers of working mothers and increasing prevalence of small families of one or two children destroyed this family care capability. At the same time, the scientific developments aiding public health, such as chlorination of water, immunizations that eliminated infectious disease, development of drugs and chemicals for many common diseases, resulted in increased life expectancy.*

Because the increase in life expectancy means that more people will live to a normal life span, there will be more older people proportionately in the

---

* "Increased life expectancy" is usually erroneously taken to mean that people are going to live to be 80, 90 or 100. It means instead that more of the people born in a particular year can expect to live an allotted life span of *70*. While the *average* life expectancy has increased since 1900 from 47 to 70 years, those people who were born in 1900 maintain the 47-year life expectancy. Fewer of them will live to be 70 than the children born in 1970. The life expectancy — *to* age 70 — was increased for succeeding generations by reducing deaths in adulthood. Nothing we have invented or discovered will allow more people to live beyond age 70. For example, despite all the new drugs, operations and immunizations, after age 45 one has little more chance of living any longer than if one had been born 100 years ago.

population. In 1900, for example, when the population was 76 million, only 4 percent were over 65. Today with 220 million, 10 percent are over 65. You can readily understand the magnitude of this change. Three percent of 75 million is 2¼ million people. Ten percent of 220 million is 22 million. The total population has only tripled but the population of old people has multiplied by ten.

TABLE 4-1:    Population by Age, Selected Years

| Year | (Millions) Total Population | Under 19 | % | Over 65 | % |
|------|------|------|------|------|------|
| 1900 | 76 | 34 | (45) | 3 | (4) |
| 1910 | 92 | 39 | (42) | 4 | (4) |
| 1920 | 106 | 43 | (41) | 5 | (5) |
| 1930 | 123 | 48 | (39) | 7 | (6) |
| 1940 | 132 | 46 | (35) | 9 | (7) |
| 1950 | 151 | 51 | (34) | 12 | (8) |
| 1960 | 179 | 69 | (39) | 17 | (9) |
| 1970 | 203 | 77 | (38) | 20 | (10) |

*Source:* United States Census, U. S. Dept. of Commerce, U. S. Population Vol. I, Part 1, June 1973.

More people are living into those age groups where they are more likely to be exposed to the hazards of chronic disease. At the same time, the kind of family structure and situation needed for their care if they are handicapped or ill has disappeared. American medical care has a dual problem: first, there is an enormous difference in the amount of medical care services and resources needed because old people require more medical services; second, there is greater need for adding institutional services or some kind of social care for the elderly who cannot now be looked after in their own homes by their own families. Similar needs are evident for the care of handicapped children.

Old people do need more medical services, as is illustrated in Figure 4-1. Only one third of all those over 65 have no chronic illnesses and are able to look after themselves. Another third are periodically in need of care or attention because they suffer from a chronic illness. The other third, however, have fairly severe illnesses, require fairly constant attention and are in and out of hospitals; a portion of them are constantly institutionalized because there is no other way of caring for them. They cannot look after themselves and their families are unable or unwilling to look after them. They represent less than 10 percent of the elderly population. A million of them will be in nursing homes or equivalent institutions, a half million or more in mental hospitals or general hospitals from which they cannot be

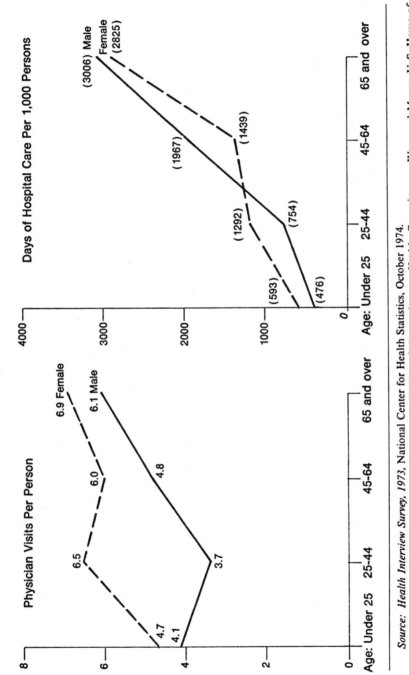

FIGURE 4-1.   Utilization of Medical Services, by Age, in 1973

**Physician Visits Per Person**

**Days of Hospital Care Per 1,000 Persons**

*Source:* *Health Interview Survey, 1973*, National Center for Health Statistics, October 1974.
*Source:* Congressional Source Book, *Basic Charts on Health Care,* Subcommittee on Health, Committee on Ways and Means, U. S. House of Representatives, July 8, 1975, p. 65.

discharged because there is no place to send them. And unknown thousands who remain somewhere in the community are inadequately cared for and more or less neglected.

The basic problem for the old people in that latter situation is that again there is no national program for assuring that they get the service, supervision and solicitous attention that they need. We are familiar with the periodic nursing home scandals. To a large extent these represent not just the greed of entrepreneurs, but the sad state of the conscience of the American people that permits this neglect and poor treatment. The nursing homes, or whatever other euphemism is used — old people's home, extended care facility, chronic disease hospital, convalescent home — offer varying professional attention. They vary from very fine institutions with highly professional care and attention, excellent food and accommodations, recreational and occupational activities under the auspices of nonprofit agencies or profit-making institutional managers, to the most viciously neglected, unsafe, firetraps where the innocent victims are abused. At present the annual institutional cost for nursing home care runs to approximately $7.5 billion — $4 billion of this from public sources — and these costs are rising.

Historically, nursing homes developed as proprietary institutions. Cities also built hospitals as adjuncts to their poorhouses, and the destitute elderly needing care were admitted. As hospitals gradually became places where people other than the sick poor received care, they grew either directly under public auspices or as a magnanimous effort of voluntary groups: fraternal organizations, religious groups, and community philanthropists. The institutions that were established for the care of the incapacitated elderly, however, were developed as substitutes for family care, and it was families who sought them out and offered to pay in order to have these surrogate services provided. The earliest nursing homes were actually boarding homes that older nurses or even neighborhood women or "nurses" without nursing degrees would operate out of their own homes or somewhat larger home-like buildings, servicing six or so inmates. They were proprietary from the start.

Today, although 10 percent of hospitals are proprietary institutions, 80 percent of nursing homes are. Nursing homes grew slowly through the 1920's and 1930's, but even by 1960 there were only 400,000 nursing home beds in the United States. However, under the impetus of the Medicare program, which allowed for the payment of several months of posthospital care in "extended care facilities," nursing homes multiplied quickly all over the country. "Extended Care Facilities" (ECF) were defined by law and regulations in such a fashion as to allow payment for the better professional types of nursing homes only. The proprietary homes which did comply with regulations and looked after these government-paid cases flourished.

In addition, the simultaneously implemented Medicaid program, undertook to pay for the state share of the care of the sick poor. Those who needed nursing home care, but who were not eligible for the "ECF," wound up in the less desirable nursing homes that did not qualify for Medicare reimbursement. Patients who were incapacitated, did not need hospitalization, had no homes or could not be looked after at home, became Medicaid charges. Changes in welfare philosophy eliminated "relative responsibility," a rule that had governed welfare eligibility for centuries, providing that the *family* had the primary responsibility for care; the state would only pay if it could be shown that the family was unable to pay. Once this rule was abrogated, *all* old people were found to be poor. A study in the 1960's showed that 50% of the people over 65 had incomes below $3,000 a year. It was inevitable that there would be some degree of "dumping;" that families would put their old people away in institutions and let the state pay the bill.

The increase in construction of nursing homes after 1965 was paralleled by an increase in the expenses of Medicaid. Most Medicaid money nationally goes for the payment of services in hospitals, nursing homes and extended care facilities (augmenting the payments of Medicare). Old people are 20 percent of the population; but 30 percent of all Medicaid payments are on their behalf. Half of all Medicaid money is paid out for nursing home care.

The nursing homes have become an albatross around the neck of the American people. We are unwilling to practice the "Eskimo Decision;" to put the old people out on an ice floe to wander off and die. We feel we have *some* social responsibility, but society as a whole is unwilling to meet the real costs, or would like to forget that inadequate payments to greedy owners must result in inadequate facilities, inadequate feeding, neglect and ill-treatment. Last year I spoke to a hospital group and criticized nursing home care and management rather strongly. A man in the audience took issue with me and we had a somewhat acrimonious debate. He identified himself as the owner and manager of a nursing home in New York City. Last week's New York *Times* carried two stories concerning that nursing home. In the latter one, a patient was found dead on the roof. He had been there about three days. His absence was unnoticed in the home during that time.

Medical and institutional care of old people pleads for orderly social management and control. There would be greater efficiency and effectiveness, and probably less expense, with greater satisfaction to both the old people and their families, who often suffer unnecessary guilt because of the neglect and mistreatment. It requires only organized community action. That handicapped people or older people who cannot look after themselves require attention does not necessarily mean that they require large nursing care institutions with 100 or 200 beds, with their impersonality, bureaucracy and emphasis on profit. In many instances old people could be looked after relatively easily in their own homes or in the home of a neighboring family, if additional services were available to them in the home so as to take some of the burden of responsibility from the family. If the medical services were guaranteed; if needed periodic nursing care and supervision could be provided; if some sort of home-help activities could be made available on a regular basis, such as assistance in shopping, cooking, and cleaning; many families could continue to look after an old person at home. This would provide the necessary structured team service; all the varieties of needed care provided in a routine formal way with full understanding on the part of the family as to what would be required and how help could be obtained in an emergency.

Such a home care program has been in operation out of the Montefiore Hospital in the Bronx, New York, since 1946. It is very successful, and much cheaper than either hospital or nursing home; part of the cost is borne by the family itself in contributing shelter and food. More flexibility in the Medicaid system or in the community's welfare system would even allow for family support funds for families who could not afford to provide continued shelter and food. It is true that supervision would be needed to make sure that the patient was not neglected at home. But this would be relatively simple, involving routine telephone calls and visits.

The Montefiore Home Care Program in its heyday provided a bridge between hospital and community with a strong emphasis on the patient's needs rather than the institution's needs. For example, hardly any diagnosis was excluded, if the family was willing. Patients with serious and fatal prognoses could be cared for at home, if the family wished. No patient, however limited the care required, would be taken on the home care program if the family was unwilling. Sometimes there would be fear or reluctance, generated by awe of the disease or complicated equipment that might have to be used in the sick room. The patient and the family would be reassured that if it did not work out the patient would be admitted (or readmitted) promptly to the hospital. Patients or families would try this, call in for emergency care frequently in the beginning and, when finding prompt and friendly response, would relax.

The understanding among professionals and administrators of the Montefiore program that the patient had top priority in decision-making was the key to the success of the program. Patients would be brought back to the hospital for a weekend or a month in the summer to give the family a needed rest or vacation. Montefiore Home Care continues to be a paradigm of successful community response to a complex problem of care for the aged. It reduces nursing home and hospital inpatient care, by offering safe, satisfying, *happy* family care with professional support.

For those situations in which a home is simply not available (20 percent of all elderly people have no families and live alone) neighbors might be brought into the act to develop *foster homes* for old people requiring care. There are many low income families who would welcome the opportunity to augment their income by undertaking such responsibility. Again, if there were flexibility in the Welfare Department or in the Medicaid program, such arrangements could be made for a substitute "family" to aid in carrying out a home care program. Where neither their own family nor a substitute family is avi, the elderly could receive care in small scale institutions; the "cottage parents arrangement" might be established. At present this is only used for delinquent children, but it could easily be extended to handicapped old people.

There is a curious indignity and impersonality in large institutions. The opportunity for losing people "in the cracks" in a large institution is very great, and older people need supervised *personal* care. A "cottage parents" structure would provide the equivalent of a mother and father as a family surrogate, together with the associated routine help from a nurse or someone with modified nursing training; this system, caring for 12-24 elderly people, would augment the team program of a usual home care service. It would more than adequately substitute for nursing homes, providing better, more personal and more sympathetic care.

However, all of these depend on the creation of a community network of service. Until there is a general community medical care responsibility, so that everyone who needs care is guaranteed it, it will be very difficult to establish such a general pattern of home care services to replace the present inadequate and neglectful nursing home situation.

## YOUTH

Young people in our society are clearly recognized as the responsibility of parents. The courts rarely, and then only with reluctance, take children away from a mother or father except under circumstances of incapacity, neglect or cruelty. Since the parents' responsibility is recognized by law and custom, society tends to do very little on behalf of children, even in the cases of clear parental neglect and abuse. If the children are not immunized to protect them against preventable infectious diseases, and as a consequence they incur such a disease and perhaps even die from it, society does not punish the parent. If children are not taken to a physician when illness threatens and the child is therefore not seen until he is seriously ill, the parents are not punished. It is also true that except for the free clinics and emergency room services when they are available, physicians or other provider agencies do not seek out and look after sick children.

These facts may help explain the United States' surprisingly poor statistical record in child health. Despite our wealth, our infant mortality rate compares unfavorably with that of other developed, industrialized countries. To some extent this mirrors the poverty and deprivation of minority groups who suffer from the lack of adequately distributed medical services. But it is also true of a large segment of the reasonably affluent white population, where the record of infant mortality is still above that of the average in Scandinavia or Holland. Some people asscribe this to the meddlesomeness of obstetricians; that they intervene too much during pregnancy and labor: too many medicines, too much anesthesia to the mother, too much use of forceps. They point to the fact that in countries with better records midwifery with little intervention is the rule. Others simply see this as the result of poverty or malnutrition of the pregnant mothers; even middle-income American women do not concern themselves enough with adequate diet.

Although 100 percent of Danish children are immunized against smallpox, polio and a variety of other infectious diseases, 30 to 50 percent of American children are not, depending on family income level. In the chicano community in San Antonio, Texas, periodic epidemics of diphtheria have flared up since 1970. Diphtheria is absolutely preventable by immunization, yet a sizable proportion of the chicano population in that city have not been immunized. It is pointed out that when the medical society attempted to carry out a campaign for immunization education in that community, the educators could not speak Spanish. Texas spent some $20 million in combating an epidemic of encephalomyelitis among horses and about $1 million combating the diphtheria epidemic among the children in San Antonio.

We have no school health service worthy of the name. In some states children have to be examined by law; this often turns out to be a cursory look or simply a paper signed by the parent attesting that a local physician has taken care of the matter. In some instances the family doctor is expected to follow with a report and sometimes he does, with or without any real evidence that he has seen or examined the child. So the periodic examination of children is something of a joke. Furthermore, very little is done in the way of following up the findings of examination when they are made or reported.

A school nurse is in attendance in some school systems. However, she is usually preoccupied with small matters, looking after children who had been sent out from class for behavior problems, or children who claim symptoms of illness; she generally has very little to do in the way of establishing whether something is really wrong or not. Her role is to get hold of the the parent; to see that the child is removed from school if necessary; or to give the child an opportunity to rest in the doctor's office until school is over. Occasionally there may be nurse-teacher or nurse-parent conferences in which some of the problems will be discussed. There may even be situations in which the nurse will try to follow up by calling the parent to see whether suggested remedies for a condition found in the examination can be carried out, such as buying glasses, buying a hearing aid, or correcting a handicapping condition. But these situations are exceptional. A formal, intensive campaign for finding medical needs and arranging medical care of the children is rarely found in American schools.

Congress made an effort to lay a foundation for such a comprehensive program of children's medical care, but it has not worked out. In 1968, they passed legislation requiring the screening, diagnosing and treatment of children eligible for Medicaid. The cities, counties and states objected that this would add immeasurably to Medicaid costs (in which the states must participate financially); therefore, the HEW regulations as to the scope and procedures of these screening tests were not promulgated until 1970, and not mandatory until 1972. Even after that the states were not encouraged to follow through. There was little supervision or monitoring to be sure that it was carried out, and even where it was, the states tended to give only 5 or 10 percent of the children very limited examinations. The EPSDT program (Early Periodic Screening Diagnosis and Treatment) was weak from its inception. It was designed to try to examine children from poor families as early as possible after birth to find out what might be wrong early enough to provide treatment; to give the poor child maximum opportunity, at least from a health standpoint, to find its way in life.

We know that early childhood handicapping conditions can have much greater impact and consequences than handicaps developing later in life. The young child that does not see well — cannot see the blackboard, cannot follow reading in a book — might not learn to read or to write, lose interest, become bored and sullen: ultimately a school problem. The same is true of children who do not hear very well. To a lesser degree this is true of children with handicapping conditions which keep them from participating fully in the life of their classmates and peers. Aside from any *moral* responsibility to look after a child who is unable to look after himself, and the *parental* responsibility to be sure that a sick child is cared for, there is the *social* responsibility to ensure the integrity and quality of the next generation by avoiding and treating sickness, handicapping conditions and early disability. However, our society seems to be very reluctant to spend the money, organize the system or provide the service.

From a social standpoint, programs for medical care for infants and children should extend to all economic levels in our society. But more than medical care is needed. A whole range of social action should be carried out for all children. We still talk about day care, for example, as if it referred to only a small fraction of the children in the country, particularly the poor children. But better than a third of the married women in the United States are working; millions of children of all social classes and conditions could benefit from preschool and primary day care programs. More programs are needed after school, until one of the parents returns home. Inflation and declining education budgets reduce existing after-school school activities more and more, so there are not sufficient supervised play times, clubs and recreational activities. There is no appropriate supervision for study and guidance after school for those children whose parents are working. The absence of a significant social focus on assuring children adequate guidance, respect and support certainly aids in the distressing development of delinquency among children.

These matters of course apply with greater force to poor children and children of minority groups. For the adolescent, the social problems are further compounded by unemployment. Too many of the younger poor and minority children never get enough out of early education to want to finish high school or go on to college to prepare themselves suitably for jobs and participation in social activity. This, to some extent, results from our failures in early child care and child health services.

The social remedy would be far cheaper than disease treatment in long term social cost. The remedy should include active day care and head start programs for preschool children; active all day programs for children with working parents; the creation of educational as well as recreational activities after school; and a comprehensive health care service for all children. It might mean the difference between a generation bitterly hostile to society, and a society of young people eager and enthusiastic to participate in the advancement of social and cultural ideals.

Almost every country in the world except the United States has a children's health service and has trained large numbers of physicians and other health workers to be specialists in child welfare. Our lack of such a program is based in the traditional heritage of charging parents with child care responsibility and avoiding the appearance of allowing the state to take over parental responsibilities. There are things that parents cannot do and should not be expected to do. The state must intervene in health services in order to improve living conditions and even the life expectancy of many thousands of children.

For the fortunate children whose parents are in circumstances that allow them to obtain medical care, the United States provides very well trained physicians and pediatricians with a wide range of understanding and knowledge about children's physiology, pathology and mental health. The cost of care for children is not particularly great, with the exception of medical needs in the first year of life and for some of the illnesses suffered in the first four years. Except for accidents, they tend to be reasonably healthy once they enter school. An overall national program of child care would be far less expensive than medical care of adults and especially the elderly. This is evidenced in part in the distribution of Medicaid expenditures for the poor. AFDC mothers ("Aid for Dependent Children") represent the largest category of payments under welfare provisions of the Social Security Act.

Children represent 50 percent of all welfare recipients, but less than 20 percent of the money paid out for health services under Medicaid is for children. On the other hand, the federal government pays 65 percent of the health care expenditures of the elderly. Nursing home expenditures tip the balance; this is ironic since the care received is often poor. The imbalance of payment reflects the fact that we do not want to add tax funds to spend sufficient money for children.

In the 1974 fiscal year, out of the $12 billion spent on Medicaid, about $2 billion was for children; but less than half of low-income children received care under Medicaid payment procedures, because Medicaid is a *state* program and in the southern states, poor children's eligibility is severely restricted. Fewer than 10 percent of farm children receive services through Medicaid there; poor rural children receive a total benefit of only about $5 per capita from all Medicaid expenditures. (Karen Davis, *Setting National Priorities,* 1975.)

*Nutrition and Children*

Along with the other considerations of what has or has not been done in the schools and for children generally, there needs to be some mention of the fact that nutrition, an ultimate factor in medical care, has been badly neglected too. Advertising and promotional materials directed at children or their parents attempt to plant enthusiasm for packaged products that are profitable rather than substantial and useful foods needed for sound growth. More generally, harmful deficiencies are derived from the casual way in which Americans view their diets, paying little attention toward constructing regular service of essential food elements. Many children suffer from lack of supervision of what they get at breakfast, and certainly no supervision of what they get at lunch. It may be that only one meal a day is eaten under the thoughtful supervision of an adult.

For poor children, the defect is multiplied. Not only is there insufficient food at home, but the kind of food that is provided or prepared is often deficient in essentials. A child may come to school without breakfast, may not be able to afford to buy lunch, and will not get an after-school snack.

The evening meal will be equally impoverished. There is real question as to how much of a role the lack of adequate nutrition plays in the failure of many poor children to take appropriate advantage of the school system and to reach the same educational level as their better-fed classmates. I realize that many elements are involved here, but certainly lack of adequate nutrition cannot be ignored as one of the participating factors in the failure to learn. A hungry child cannot be expected to pay attention in class; and he may, by his lethargy and inattention, give the teacher a false impression of an unintelligent, passive or retarded child.

Just as we have very little in the way of a school health system or appropriate day care services in this country, we also have a shamefully inadequate child nutrition program. It's true that billions of dollars are being spent for food stamp programs, distribution of excess commodities, and school lunches, but in many instances the congressional intention behind the programs and the actual programs may be extremely discrepant. In many schools children are expected to pay a part of the school lunch cost because the federal funds are inadequate. Poor children cannot pay. Again, because the parents are expected to be responsible for the children, the distribution of commodities or food stamps supposed to benefit the children, may not. Parents may not give the children money for school lunches even if they have it. The school lunch may not be adequate; a school breakfast program may be necessary as well. Very few schools have school breakfast programs. Similarly, an after-school snack program may be important to those children who are not able to get adequate food at breakfast or lunch. Snack programs after school are almost completely lacking in this country.

The nutritional deficiency in our children can be compounded and carried on into future generations. Some statisticians and obstetricians believe that a good part of the prematurity rate (prematurity represents the largest cause of infant mortality in the United States) and the height of infant mortality here are related to what is called "interconceptional deficiencies," that is, inadequate nourishment of the mother prior to pregnancy. She cannot proceed to have a healthy child no matter what kind of nutrition she gets during pregnancy; that brief "normal" feeding is not sufficient if she has come to pregnancy inadequately fed.

### Funded Programs for Children

Because children played an important part in the labor pool in the early part of this century the Children's Bureau was created in 1912 and subsequently child labor laws were enacted. At first children were simply protected against the hazards of being treated as an adult worker. Gradually legislation raised the age at which children could be employed, and established special protective measures against their exploitation. At the same time agitation was begun to develop public measures for the protection of children's health.

In the early 1920's a tentative effort, the Sheppard-Towner Act, offered federal grants to the states as assistance in providing care for pregnant women and infants. Not all states took advantage of this. In the writing of the Social Security Act in the 1930's, when the bitter debate over the inclusion of a national health insurance program resulted in the elimination of national health insurance, the inclusion of a child health section was considered a reasonable substitute. This was Title V of the Social Security Act; it offered the states funds, largely on a matching basis, to help improve mother and child care particularly in rural areas. The funds made available by the federal government gradually increased, so that by 1973 almost half a billion dollars of federal and state funds were made available. In addition to the rather simple assistance to health departments that the early monies had provided, the more current bills provided more sophisticated approaches, including project grants for specially organized and staffed clinics in selected areas to look after population groups with higher than ordinary exposure to risk. One such project was the Maternity and Infancy Care project (M&C) which was to look after pregnant women considered high risks, primarily among poverty and minority groups, urban or rural. Eligible high risk situations included very young pregnant girls, older pregnant women and those who had had many children. Additionally, the Children and Youth (C&Y) project grants concerned themselves with children up to age 21 from impoverished and minority groups in urban and rural areas.

Despite the substantial sums of money involved, only a million women and children nationally actually benefit from all of these programs. Only 40,000 of the four million live births could be accounted for in the MIC program and, in the routine state programs, less than 10 percent of all women who had babies.

There is enough experience and sufficient information available to make it relatively easy to fashion a national health program for children. Some of the proposals for improved community service for old people could be equally well-applied to children: groups of health team specialists, composed of physicians and other health workers; and foster homes, patients' own homes, or cottage parent type settings for home and community care would result in infinitely more effective medical services.

First of all, it is clear that mother and child care can be carried out to a much greater degree without the current intervention of physicians. The use of pediatricians, family doctors and obstetricians can be minimized through the use of large numbers of paraprofessionals who would work in association with the physician specialists. They would provide the primary care, furnish "sorting centers" and provide most of the kinds of medical services that pregnant women and children need. A number of experimental programs of this kind are being carried out, such as the one at the University of Colorado under the leadership of Dr. Henry Silver, who has experimented for many years with different kinds of pediatric auxiliary workers. Dr. Henry Thiede at the University of Mississippi conducted interesting and exciting experimental programs using midwives. In both instances the effort was not to *replace* the physician but to use him more skillfully, sparingly, and economically: to supervise the work of associates and provide consultation and specialized services, rather than the totality of services which pediatricians are now expected to render. Services such as well-child examination and guidance, feeding advice, reassurance, attention to the variety of minor and inconsequential illnesses from which babies are wont to suffer, and immunizations on schedule should not require the mediation of a pediatrician with eight or ten years of specialized training.

## MALE AND FEMALE

In obtaining medical services, the male in our society suffers from certain socially-structured disadvantages. The male is supposed to be strong and dominant. He is not supposed to show signs of weakness or illness. The result of this is that he will hesitate before going to a physician and put off getting attention for important symptoms, until they are grave and sometimes less controllable. This may account for the fact that women use more medical services than men, show more minor illnesses, and yet have a greater life expectancy. The presumed weakness and lesser strength of the woman contribute to making it easier for her to see a physician or use medical services when her symptoms are earlier or lesser. Obviously her strength and durability must be greater than man or she wouldn't survive longer on average. Woman's life expectancy is five years greater than man's; there are more widows than there are widowers.

Other aspects of this "machismo" mystique against which the feminists are revolting also contribute to less male use of medical services and increase the male's chance of becoming ill and suffering more life-threatening diseases. The greater rate of male coronary and cardiovascular disease and death may be partially attributable to failure to look after himself adequately or to attend a physician when symptoms first appear. This has been pointed out in numerous texts and articles.

There is no "male physician" except for the urologist, who concerns himself with the urinary tract and the male genitalia. Although it is taken for granted that male mental processes and psychological difficulties are different from female, there is no psychiatrist who concentrates on male mental illnesses or emotional disturbances. Just as there is a place for a *pediatrician,* a physician who pays attention to the special problems of the very young; and a *geriatrician,* who pays attention to the special problems of the very old, there may be a place in our medical division of labor for someone to concentrate on the specific diseases of each sex. I do not intend to indulge in the pernicious habit of most professionals to divide and subdivide their profession into smaller and smaller units of activity. But I do feel that some specialized attention to the physiological, pathological and emotional problems of males might be beneficial to a better understanding of the striking difference in morbidity between males and females and in the increased mortality of males in their fifth and sixth decades.

Of course, the other side of this is that for all practical purposes, physicians consider the male the paradigm of study of human beings. Most reference points fail to take into account difference between males and females, except for the usual sexual patterns. It might be that a careful examination of supposed similarities might turn out to show significant variations.

Because of childbirth, the female has always had a specialized physician, but in a narrow sense. The historical midwife has been incorporated into the medical field and, in the United States particularly, midwifery gave way to obstetrical physicians. Most obstetricians understood themselves to be the woman's physician and merged this with gynecology, the morbidity and surgery related to the woman's genital tract. Obstetrics and gynecology became a joint specialty of medicine.

In the United States in the 19th century, when the first really new medical school was organized along modified European lines at John Hopkins University, an obstetrician, Howard Kelly, was one of the four founding fathers. Because he refused to associate himself with surgery, a separate specialty program of "female surgery" developed at Hopkins. Gynecologists did not perform obstetrics nor did obstetricians perform gynecology.

Actually the separation was not quite as sharp as that; there were obstetricians who had operating privileges and there were gynecologists who delivered babies. But there were separate departments of obstetrics and gynecology. It is no longer so; but maybe it should be, to focus more fully on women's needs rather than on organ specificity. The gynecology that women are interested in now is not mere surgery on the genital tract, but gynecology in the ancient Greek sense of the study of diseases of the woman and health care of the woman as a *female* human being; not, as a Philadelphia physician in the early 19th century described her, as "a uterus surrounded by a semblance of mankind."

The diagnosis and treatment of female diseases should be based on the specifics of the distinctly female context and not on some general ideas derived from male experiences. It is a logical extension of the idea that a woman's character begins and develops differently from the male and needs to be perceived as such. Some of the activities of feminists toward making changes in the way in which their medical services are provided will offer excellent opportunities for transforming all of medical practice. They are asking for individual treatment; for sympathetic understanding of what it is like to be sick and have to plead for care, to be exposed to the mercies of a stranger and to be afraid. That is merely what all patients want, regardless of sex, color, age or social condition. And it is one of the things missing from our system of practice. The emphasis on this request should be recognized not as an unreasonable demand from a radical social sect, but an expression of a universal plea.

So there are arguments for the development of medical specialists for the adult male and the adult female. Both kinds of specialties could have a beneficial effect on broadening health education for patients and basic medical education for doctors. Too little is taught currently of the physiology and psychology of sexuality except for sensational, pathological aspects and contrasts between "liberated" and old fashioned approaches. Everyone should be able to enter into adult responsibilities with a firm background of knowledge about these matters, including abortion and family planning. And health workers, doctors and others in the health professions ought to be knowledgeable enough to advise patients and understand their problems.

There are matters touching upon female health and female responsibility that deserve separate mention. Many of the problems relating to the provision of female health services derive from classical prejudices and discriminatory patterns of service for women generally; they need no further discussion here. Any number of books and articles have detailed the long history of oppression and secondary human status women have been forced to accept in a male dominated society. It may be that one important aspect that does need to be discussed in the health field has to do with that special capability of women, the ability to bear children. Whether or not a woman should have a child is heavily laden with myths, prejudices, traditional discrimination and outright male domination.

In many societies the submission of the female has historically been so complete that she has had no choice as to whether she would bear a child or not. Copulation has been the male prerogative, procreation the inevitable result. A woman might undertake to bring about an abortion on herself, but it could mean the risk of her life (from the abortion or as punishment from the dominant male); expert, if illegal, abortionists arose to meet this need. With time, too, methods of contraception were developed, and from the very earliest times we have evidence that men and women used them. In times of scarcity and in certain cultures, it was important to limit the numbers of children; therefore, contraception, abortion and infanticide were practiced. In one marginally impoverished society men even allowed themselves to be mutilated so that the semen could not be transmitted; it was ejaculated through an artificial wound at the base of the penis.

Efforts to make contraception easier, more satisfying and more efficient have resulted in a variety of methods; most of them involve *female* responsibility. With the complex nature of women's physiology, it would seem that a male contraceptive would be a more logical, safer course. A whole range of damage could ensue with internal female contraceptive devices, some possibly even dangerous or fatal to a child if it were born. However, probably as a result of unconscious bias, most of the emphasis has been in that direction. It may be that in the future, particularly with vasectomy, greater effort will be exerted in the area of male contraception. At the present time, however, discussions of family planning, contraception and abortion ought to be central to the education of women.

SPECIFIC HEALTH PROBLEMS OF MINORITY PEOPLE

We have already discussed in great detail the general disadvantage of minority groups in obtaining health care or medical services, which is largely a product of the poverty that minority groups disproportionately suffer. To some extent it is also because many among minority groups live in chronically underserved areas.

But there are sufficient unsettling data about the health of minority people indicating that there are special disadvantages entailed in that circumstance. Nonwhite people make up almost 12.5 percent of the United States population as of the 1970 census. Along with ethnic and racial minorities this totals almost 17 percent of the United States population. Because the census systematically undercounts minority groups, it is quite likely that a more accurate figure is 20 percent. The magnitude of this figure is ordinarily obscured because of the discriminatory residential arrangements in many communities. It is quite clearly evident that these groups suffer particular disadvantage when we note that infant and childhood mortality rates of the nonwhite are just about double that of whites; that the prevalence of chronic conditions is 20 percent higher in nonwhites than in whites; that blacks contract certain illnesses, such as anemia and hypertension, three times as much as whites.

The last point relates to the whole complex of poverty, which must play a role in the wider prevalence of malnutrition among minority groups. It is a truly vicious circle: minority status compounds poverty, which creates malnutrition, which is intensified by obstructed access to medical care.

Cultural factors unquestionably play a part, too. There may be strong elements of tradition and background that require a different educational approach in order to encourage nonwhites to make more use of available health services. But this only explains a part of the reason that existing services are not appropriately utilized. The larger reason is that the conditions under which services are rendered in impoverished, mostly minority communities are often confused and disorganized. Among the American Indians, particularly those still on the reservations, a good case can be made for the fact that the standard white European type of medical care is not what the Indians want, know how to use, or can use, given the difficulties of transportation, understanding the language, etc. The same may be true for the strong cultural enclaves of chicanos or Puerto Ricans in the large cities. Lack of familiarity with the language terminology would direct the minority patient toward some other type of care rather than the traditional majority model standard in the clinics. But the most deterring factor are the actual clinic conditions: the long waiting, humiliating conditions, and in rural areas the lack of physicians and other resources for medical care. The inability of minority groups to obtain or use health services and medical care is more ascribable to the system structure than to cultural conditions among the patients.

In recent years many efforts have been directed to correcting the deficiencies in approach and attitude. To mention a few, there was the OEO Neighborhood Health Centers and some independent, nonfederally funded units based on ethnic or racial composition of the community. These attempted to appeal to the particular expectations of the potential users as well as provide physicians, nurses and other people which would be standard in the white American community. They have had a moderate degree of success in various parts of the country. The outstanding OEO Centers of Mount Bayou, Mississippi; Martin Luther King Jr. Center in Bronx, New York; Mission District in San Francisco; Denver Clinic; and Mile Square in Chicago are examples of such large city efforts. East Kentucky; Selma, Alabama and other such rural experiments in California and Colorado are other federally funded models. Maria Varela's pioneering effort in the Cooperativa Agricolta in New Mexico is an outstanding example of such a privately funded enterprise.

The Indian Health Service's project that has brought medical care to the Navajo Reservation since 1955 has learned from the Navajos to deal with the tribal officials so as to encourage enrollment of Navajo nurses and family health workers. They now help train Navajo medicine men and encourage more young people from among the Navajo to attend college and medical school. These efforts have not been wholly successful, of course, but with continued support from the Congress there may be a most interesting and satisfactory model of cooperative action between federal officials and Navajo officials in the development of a Native American Health Service.

It should be pointed out that these experimental programs affect a total of only a few hundred thousand people out of the 30 to 40 million that we need to reach among minority groups. We cannot yet point with pride to very much success in the limited number of experimental and pilot models that exist. A great deal more will have to be done to test the models and assure that minority groups are able to get the benefit of good medical care. Whatever we may say about the defects of medical service delivery for many Americans, it is unquestionably a fact that the more intense examples of deficiencies and inadequacies are visible among those services required by minorities.

There are thoughtful medical care pioneers and reformers who believe the most effective response to the special needs of minority groups and the poor is social action to provide a better standard of living, integrated housing, education, neighborhoods, etc. It would be most interesting if, when sufficient numbers of minority group people are fully integrated into the majority community, they and their children obtain equivalent health services; and if so, whether their current statistics on longevity, infant mortality, prevalence of chronic disease and infectious disease are significantly different.

It is certainly true that the discriminatory housing patterns define disease incidence sharply. In the case of the diphtheria epidemic of San Antonio, for example, the lack of immunization among the impoverished chicanos made it possible for 12.5 times as many brown children to contract and die from the disease as white children. It must certainly be true that the malnutrition of Indian babies on the Navajo Reservation contributes to the excess of deaths from gastrointestinal and respiratory diseases. If social circumstance were equal to that of well-to-do white children, would so many Indian babies die?

One cannot leave a discussion of differential medical care among minority groups without saying something about the situation of Asian Americans. Of the 1.5 million Asian Americans in the United States, a little more than a third are Japanese Americans; a little less than a third are Chinese Americans; the remainder are about 20 percent Filipino (350,000), along with lesser numbers of Hawaiians, Koreans and others. The public health statistics on Asian Americans is markedly different from that of blacks or chicanos. Asian Americans have the lowest mortality rate (4.5 per thousand as compared with 9.5 for whites); the lowest infant mortality rate (8 per thousand live births as compared with 17 per thousand white or 30 per thousand black). This may be correlated with the very small number of families below the poverty level (8.8 percent); the highest mean family income ($12,420 per year as compared with white Americans' $11,348 and black Americans' $7,074); an infinitesimal unemployment rate and dependency ratio; and a very high percent who have attended or completed college. It is hard not to recognize the correlation between education, high income and improved health status in the comparison among the Asian Americans, white Americans and nonwhites. This gives added force to the argument for recognizing the importance of improving the standard of living, housing conditions, employment and nutrition, as *well* as health care facilities, if any significant impact is to be made on the poor health status of minority groups.

Improving medical care and distribution of health services is probably an easier route than waiting for the long-term effects of improved standards of living. Many government programs under conservative administrations tend to work for improvement of living conditions by improving production and employment. One often hears this philosophy referred to as "feeding the sparrows by way of the horses." They give the money to industry, under the theory that it will give work to the poor and enable them to buy the things that would otherwise have to be given through welfare or government handouts. This argument would apply only if we were starting from scratch, with a healthy population all eager and able to go to work. But they have suffered long years of inadequate services, food and housing; and the mental and emotional stress of unemployment and minority discrimination. It does not seem likely that simply giving industry capital investment opportunities is going to bring about a marked change in the poverty situation. Furthermore, even if it ultimately could, there is no excuse for holding back needed changes in the health care delivery system to make it more effective and efficient in meeting peoples' needs *immediately*. That in itself might make it possible for them to secure employment that they might not otherwise be able to do because of illness or chronic disability. It may be the lack of an effective medical care system that is holding up the cycle!

# Chapter 5
# The Doctor: His Role Expectations and His Job

To discuss medical care in our society and in most parts of the world is to talk about the doctor. He is admired, respected, and perhaps even idolized in the United States and in many European countries, perhaps in the world. It is the status to which many young people aspire and for which many give up a good part of their lives to intensive study and struggle to achieve. It is true that in some socialist countries efforts are made to reduce the doctor's status to that of just another worker, giving him fixed hours, salary and working conditions; and providing that his working conditions and salary are negotiated by the union. But in very interesting ways the sense of helplessness, fear and dependency that illness promotes, results in an extraordinary reaction of respect for the doctor and a somewhat pitiful appeal for his concern and tender services. After all, the terror that afflicted the great spiritual leaders *("Timor mortis conturbat me")* did not reflect only the imminence of God's justice, but the problematic unknown. To be sick is to fear death. The doctor with his knowledge and skills is a barrier to death and a hopeful warrior on behalf of the sick person. In that context the physician will probably always be respected above others.

On the other hand, there are the more mundane aspects of medical care. How well trained is the doctor? Does he really know what he is doing? How much does he care? Is he really listening and interested? What if he is so crassly human as to be more concerned with how much money you have than the nature of your disease? What if he fails to do what he should because you are not paying enough or he does not think you will? What if he does more than he needs to do in order to get a higher fee? What if he is the curious experimental sort who wants to try new and maybe dangerous treatments? What if he does not want to do *anything,* but prescribes a "placebo," making a mockery of your illness? Too much of modern psychology and Freudian psychiatry has crept into popular thinking to allow many people to avoid a conceptual feeling that the doctor is contemptuous of their symptoms, that they are not really "sick," that he thinks it is all "in their heads."

How much of this goes through the average person's mind and how much only through the head of the already uneasy, insecure, middle-class, middle-income, middle-educated man or woman?

When we think about doctors we have to think about money. It is expensive to be sick not only because one loses time from work but because one has to pay — doctors, hospitals, pharmacists, nursing homes, physical therapists, etc.

The doctor orders, the patient pays. The doctor commands, the hospital admits. The doctor refuses, the patient must go back to work. No emperor, king or judge held more control over care and cure with word and writ than the doctor does. As Shakespeare's Cassius said of Caesar: "Why, man, he doth bestride the narrow world like a Colossus. . . ." *(The Tragedy of Julius Caesar)*

## WHO THE DOCTOR IS

The doctor tends to be male (88 percent); white (95 percent); from relatively well-to-do families (40 percent from income groups representing 12 percent of the population); living in large cities and metropolitan areas (80 percent); and a specialist (70 percent). He has to be reasonably well-educated, because most of the 114 American medical schools, who admit about 15,000 students every year, have rather stiff requirements. The MCAT (Medical College Aptitude Test) is difficult enough so that only a third of the 45,000 who took it last year were able to make scores that medical schools considered acceptable.

Tables 5-1 and 5-2 illustrate the rise in physician specialism, and consequent decline in general practice, in the early 1970's. As of 1974, there were 366,379 physicians in the United States. Of these, 324,367 were active; 22,000 inactive; and another 19,000 not classified for one reason or another. Of the roughly 300,000 doctors involved in direct care of patients as their primary activity 200,000 were in office-based practice; 35,000 were physician staff in hospitals, as teachers or other; 6,000 were exclusively teaching; 60,000 were interns and residents (the "pipeline"); 12,000 were in administration; and 8,000 were in research.

Of those in general practice, 48,000 were in office-based practice; 78,000 in specialties; 88,000 in surgical specialties. This breaks down in percentages as follows: of the 200,000 physicians in office-based practice, 12.5 percent were general practitioners; 25 percent were medical specialists (less

TABLE 5-1:    Specialty Distribution of Physicians, 1963 and 1973

| Specialty Group | 1963 Number | 1963 Percent | 1973 Number | 1973 Percent | Change Number | Change Percent |
|---|---|---|---|---|---|---|
| Total Physicians............... | 276,475[1] | 100.0 | 366,379m | 100.0 | 89,904 | 32.5 |
| Anesthesiology ........................... | 7,639 | 2.8 | 12,196 | 3.3 | 4,557 | 59.7 |
| General Practice........................ | 73,489 | 26.6 | 53,946 | 14.7 | -19,543 | -26.6 |
| Internal Medicine...................... | 39,109 | 14.1 | 61,735 | 16.8 | 22,626 | 57.9 |
| Obstetrics and Gynecology ....... | 15,720 | 5.7 | 20,494 | 5.6 | 4,774 | 30.4 |
| Pathology.................................. | 7,347 | 2.7 | 11,498 | 3.1 | 4,151 | 56.5 |
| Pediatrics ................................. | 14,207 | 5.1 | 20,849 | 5.7 | 6,642 | 46.8 |
| Psychiatry ................................ | 16,581 | 6.0 | 25,063 | 6.8 | 8,482 | 51.2 |
| Radiology ................................. | 8,751 | 3.2 | 15,345 | 4.2 | 6,594 | 75.4 |
| Surgery..................................... | 54,776 | 19.8 | 71,055 | 19.4 | 16,279 | 29.7 |
| Other........................................ | 24,109 | 8.7 | 32,186 | 8.8 | 8,077 | 33.5 |

[1] Includes 14,747 physicians (13,412 inactive and 1,335 address unknown) who are not distributed throughout the table.

m Includes 42,012 physicians (13,744 not classified, 22,624 inactive, and 5,644 address unknown) who are not distributed throughout the table.

*Source: Socioeconomic Issues of Health 1974,* American Medical Association, p. 17.

TABLE 5-2:    Decline of General Practice

|  | 1965 | 1970 | Change |
|---|---|---|---|
| Total M.D.s in civilian practice.................. | 215,650 | 242,622 | + 13% |
| Private practice..................................... | 180,868 | 195,890 | + 8 |
| Specialists...................................... | 115,310 | 136,946 | + 19 |
| Full-time G.P.s.................................. | 43,621 | 40,770 | - 7 |
| Part-time G.P.s.................................. | 21,937 | 18,174 | -17 |
| Nonprivate practice.............................. | 34,782 | 46,731 | + 34 |
| Hospital staff................................... | 19,346 | 29,140 | + 51 |
| Medical school .................................. | 8,231 | 10,431 | + 27 |
| Research.......................................... | 3,440 | 3,904 | + 14 |
| Administration .................................. | 3,045 | 3,256 | + 7 |
| Unclassified...................................... | 720 | — | — |

Interns, residents, and M.D.s in military service are not included. Figures for 1965 adjusted to allow for changes since then in American Medical Association classifications of physicians.

*Source: Medical Economics,* September 28, 1970, p. 85.    Copyright © 1970 by Litton Industries, Inc.    Published by Medical Economics Company, a Litton division, at Oradell, N. J. 07649.    Reprinted by permission.

house staff, administrators and researchers); medical specialists are 43 percent of all specialists.*

---

* Specialists are all physicians who have had advanced training beyond internship and either qualify for or have passed examinations and been certified as practitioners in a particular specialty whether it is medical or surgical.    Medical specialists are those like cardiologists, neurologists, diabetologists, who do no surgery.

There are 12,973 women physicians in active practice in the United States at this time. Excepting interns, residents, administrators and researchers, 2,250 (17 percent) are in general practice, somewhat less than the proportion of male physicians in general practice. The distribution of female specialists is also a little different from male, in that fewer are in the surgical specialties.

However, not all of the physicians in practice in the United States were native born or trained in an American medical school; 34,703 were foreign medical graduates. Of these, 6,643 are general practitioners (about 20 percent), about the same proportion as their American colleagues. Of specialists, 8,700 are in medical specialties, 25 percent of the total; 8,764 in the surgical specialties, also 25 percent; and 50 percent in the other specialties, largely anesthesiology and psychiatry. It is significant that of the house staff (interns and residents) in the United States last year, 12 percent are women and 33 percent foreign medical graduates. We are apparently increasing the numbers of women and foreign medical graduates in the physician population. The following tables illustrate the rise of foreign medical graduates and their appearance in various areas of American practice in the early 1970's.

In 1930 we had 76 medical schools and 22,000 students altogether, graduating 4,700 physicians. In 1973 we had 112 medical schools with a total enrollment of 47,500, graduating 10,400 students. Women in American medical schools have increased in enrollment from 5 percent to 13 percent and the number in the entering class in 1974 rose even more spectacularly from 5 percent to 17 percent. Minority representation in medical schools has not increased spectacularly. First year class minority numbers have gone up in the past five years from 2 percent to 4 percent. The number of minority physicians has increased only slightly, so that there

TABLE 5-3:  Comparative Specialty Distributions of Male and Female Physicians and Achievement of Board Certification, by Specialty and Sex

| | Specialty Distribution | | Board Certification | |
|---|---|---|---|---|
| Specialty | Percent of male physicians in specialty | Percent of female physicians in specialty | Percent male physicians board certified | Percent female physicians board certified |
| All Specialties | 100.0% | 100.0% | 53.9% | 39.6% |
| General & Family practice | 22.9 | 15.8 | 13.4 | 7.9 |
| Internal Medicine | 16.3 | 9.7 | 49.9 | 22.6 |
| Pediatrics | 5.8 | 17.6 | 80.6 | 54.9 |
| Obstetrics-Gynecology | 7.3 | 9.0 | 74.3 | 39.7 |
| Surgery | 24.5 | 5.1 | 74.4 | 60.6 |
| Psychiatry | 5.8 | 18.3 | 53.4 | 33.3 |
| Radiology | 4.2 | 3.0 | 85.7 | 78.9 |
| Anesthesiology | 4.8 | 10.6 | 60.9 | 51.5 |
| Other Specialties | 8.4 | 10.9 | 56.0 | 54.3 |

Source: *Profile of Medical Practice*, American Medical Association, 1974, p. 40.

TABLE 5-4:    Foreign Physicians and Surgeons Admitted to the United States in Comparison with Number of U. S. Medical Graduates: 1962-73

| Fiscal year | U. S. medical graduates | Foreign physicians [1] | | | |
|---|---|---|---|---|---|
| | | Total | Immigrants | Nonimmigrants | |
| | | | | Exchange visitors | Other |
| Total | 97,809 | 101,066 | 43,089 | 55,360 | 2,617 |
| 1962 | 7,168 | 5,767 | 1,797 | 3,970 | N.A. |
| 1963 | 7,264 | 6,730 | 2,093 | 4,637 | N.A. |
| 1964 | 7,336 | 6,767 | 2,249 | 4,518 | N.A. |
| 1965 | 7,409 | 6,172 | 2,012 | 4,160 | N.A. |
| 1966 | 7,574 | 6,922 | 2,552 | 4,370 | N.A. |
| 1967 | 7,743 | 8,897 | 3,326 | 5,204 | 367 |
| 1968 | 7,973 | 9,125 | 3,128 | 5,701 | 296 |
| 1969 | 8,059 | 7,515 | 2,756 | 4,460 | 299 |
| 1970 | 8,367 | 8,523 | 3,158 | 5,008 | 357 |
| 1971 | 8,974 | 10,947 | 5,756 | 4,784 | 407 |
| 1972 | 9,551 | 11,416 | 7,143 | 3,935 | 338 |
| 1973 | 10,391 | 12,285 | 7,119 | 4,613 | 553 |

[1] Including Canadians.

*Source:* Reference 22.    Unpublished data from the U. S. Department of Justice, Immigration and Naturalization Service.

*Source: Foreign Medical Graduates and Physician Manpower in the U. S.,* Department of Health, Education and Welfare (HRA) 74-30, February 1974, p. 12.

TABLE 5-5:    Foreign Medical Graduates in Comparison with all Physicians in the United States, by Major Professional Activity and Country of Graduation: 1970

| Major professional activity | Total physicians | | U. S. medical graduates | | Foreign medical graduates [1] | |
|---|---|---|---|---|---|---|
| | Number | Percent | Number | Percent | Number | Percent |
| Total | 334,028 | 100.0 | 270,637 | 100.0 | 63,391 | 100.0 |
| Patient care | 278,535 | 83.4 | 225,622 | 83.4 | 52,913 | 83.4 |
| Office-based practice | 192,439 | 57.6 | 167,949 | 62.1 | 24,490 | 38.6 |
| Interns and residents | 51,228 | 15.3 | 33,969 | 12.6 | 17,259 | 27.2 |
| Full-time physician staff | 34,868 | 10.4 | 23,704 | 8.8 | 11,164 | 17.6 |
| Other professional activity | 32,310 | 9.7 | 25,542 | 9.4 | 6,768 | 10.7 |
| Medical teaching | 5,588 | 1.7 | 4,446 | 1.6 | 1,142 | 1.8 |
| Administration | 12,158 | 3.6 | 10,667 | 3.9 | 1,491 | 2.4 |
| Research | 11,929 | 3.6 | 8,321 | 3.1 | 3,608 | 5.7 |
| Other | 2,635 | 0.8 | 2,108 | 0.8 | 527 | 0.8 |
| Not classified | 358 | 0.1 | 73 | — [2] | 285 | — [2] |
| Inactive | 19,621 | 5.9 | 17,330 | 6.4 | 2,291 | 3.6 |
| Address unknown | 3,204 | 1.0 | 2,070 | 0.8 | 1,134 | 1.8 |

[1] Including Canadians.
[2] Less than 0.05 percent.

*Source: Foreign Medical Graduates and Physician Manpower in the U. S.,* Department of Health, Education and Welfare (HRA) 74-30, February 1974, p. 25.

are about 7,000 minority physicians in the United States out of a total of 200,000 in practice. There is some considerable bitterness in the fact that there are more native Philippine physicians in practice in the United States (over 9,000) than black physicians.

It might be added that while in 1968, 25 percent of the families in the United States had an income of less than $5,000 a year, only 9 percent of medical students came from that income segment. Forty percent came from the $10,000 to $25,000 income group, which represented 30 percent of American families at that time. From those families earning $25,000 or more, which represented about 5 percent of all American families, 20 percent of the medical students came.

## MEDICAL EDUCATION AND SOCIAL SERVICE

So we have a picture of the doctor in the United States: white male; upper income family; with an education that extends from college, medical school and four years of specialty training; before he enters practice he is about 30 years old. As a matter of fact, because of the special doctor draft law, many physicians had to put in an additional two years of military service, which would make them 32 before they became independent doctors.

In earlier times this was particularly difficult, because during medical school and the training period physicians earned little or no money. Since 1964 this has changed radically. Federal intervention provides scholarship aid for some and federally guaranteed loans for others; and federal work/school programs provide opportunities for earning money while attending school. There are also increasingly larger payments to house staff for the work performed; at recent count 3rd or 4th year residents in most large urban hospitals were paid between $15,000 and $20,000 a year for their services. At one time it was fashionable to excuse some of the evidences of greed or price gouging on the part of physicians with the argument that during the difficult and lengthy educational period they did not have the opportunity to earn money and sometimes went deeply into debt. The explanation was they had to attempt to make what they could while they could. There seems to be hardly any further excuse for this. In addition, it must also be recognized that the largest part of medical education costs is not carried by the student, however difficult it may be for him to support himself and pay the tuition. Tuition represents only ½ or ⅓ of the cost of medical education. It is difficult to accept the fact that the doctor must charge high fees or earn high salaries as a result of his investment. Society has a great investment in him as well, and in some fashion the balance between student and societal investment has to be rationalized for their mutual benefit.

Increasingly, students have come to recognize this paradox and have expressed willingness to repay society for its investment by undertaking to serve in socially useful programs. Unfortunately, federal policies currently operative mostly benefit the armed services, and only to a lesser degree the Public Health Service. Under these laws the student receives an effective commission and a respectable sum of money that supports him through medical school, paying his tuition, books and living expenses; and he returns services year-for-year for those years he has received support. Recent legislation does provide more loan forgiveness (a form of support) to students in return for service in the National Health Service Corps.

It has been suggested that this be made into a regular service for all students, whereby the student is supported in medical school throughout his training and returns year-for-year service to a disadvantaged or under-served community. Although one would have suspected that this form of "indentured servitude" might be objectionable, there seem to be very few students who object. It remains to be seen, however, whether such a plan in large scale operation might not work in the same way a volunteer army works; that is, to draw into it the poor, and have *them* pay society's debts while those from economically more advantaged families are able to escape the social obligation. The draft riots in New York in 1863 were a protest to the system that allowed the well-to-do to buy themselves out of the military draft. However, if the tuition is raised to express the true cost ($10 to $15 thousand a year), it may be beyond the capacity of even well-to-do families to support a student in medical school; therefore, all students would have to take advantage of the "earn and serve" provisions of the law. Of course, those with sufficient independent income would need it to a lesser degree.

## DOCTORS IN PRACTICE

As for the type of service in which most doctors find themselves today, more than half are still in solo practice. About 17 percent (40,000) of the physicians in the United States are in group practice, although a much larger number will be found in associated or partnership practice. But the American patient who goes to a doctor's office is generally seeing a solo physician.

Most physicians are paid on a fee-for-service basis. There are only about 385 prepaid groups in the United States, serving about seven million people. The average American citizen will expect to pay a fee each time he visits a private physician in his office; this is the standard pattern of

American medical practice, although some of the fee might be borne by an insurance company and some of the physicians may have partners.

The advantages and disadvantages of this system have been argued for generations.  It is not likely that they will be settled in this generation.  There are strong partisans on both sides.  There are good reasons for suspecting that solo practice has a disadvantage professionally: by eliminating the possibility of supervision and control, there is less incentive to the physician for providing better care.  He cannot share observations to defend his diagnosis or treatment.  On the other hand, clusters of physicians tend to facilitate bureaucracy.  The requirement of accepting personal responsibility and discharging it, which is more readily visible when one physician is interacting with one patient, becomes gradually diluted when more than one physician works on a patient's behalf; each one may feel that the other has the responsibility.

Solo practice has other rewards for the physician, too.  An entrepreneur in private, solo fee-for-service practice is his own master.  He establishes his relationship with the patient.  If his personality and character is such that the patient likes him and becomes confident in his care, although he may have no way of judging whether the physician is right or wrong, he trusts him.  The physician keeps as little or as much in the way of records as he chooses; he does as little or as much in the way of diagnosing and treating as he chooses; he feels the responsibility; it gives him emotional satisfaction and it gives the patient a feeling of security.

Group practice, on the other hand, may give the patient the feeling that he is just one of many.  He may not always see his own doctor, he may have to repeat his symptoms or recall the entire history, the chart may get lost; there are definitely bureaucratic problems and not every patient is prepared to tolerate them.  Just as there are dangers of abuse on the part of solo physicians who are not accountable, there may be dangers of abuse by group physicians who fail to take responsibility and accountability.  Like so many other things in our society, we are presented with choices in which there are benefits on both sides; the difficulty is in judging where the better or maximum benefits are.  It is for this reason probably that decisions at the legislative level on a national health service will probably leave more than one style of practice to be followed; and there will be "coexistence" of solo and group practice.

But there is very little excuse for the perpetuation of fee-for-service.  It has long been argued that the exchange of the fee between the doctor and the patient has both a sacred and therapeutic quality.  The English anthropologist Pitt-Rivers pointed out that among the African tribe of the Azande, the witch doctor proclaimed that without a fee there could be no treatment.  Freud is quoted to the same effect.  Many physicians in the official medical organizations subscribe to this notion passionately. If one were cynical enough, one could argue that the exchange of a fee has a much more important effect on the physician than on the patient; the patient's therapeutic value is less than the obvious value for the physician. It is certainly true that fee-for-service as a method of practice is a powerful incentive for multiplying services. The great fear of the physician seems to be that if there is no direct exchange of money, the patient will feel no hesitation in using services without regard to their need or priority.

There is no reason why other ways of reimbursing physicians cannot be devised that would satisfy the doctor so that he can feel that he is not being taken advantage of and that his services are appropriately reimbursed. But it is true that every alternative way devised also has defects. With the capitation system, where a physician receives payment for a period of time and the patient may claim any service during that period of time, the physician feels that he can be taken advantage of insofar as there is no barrier to the patient making as many claims and demands as he chooses. British physicians are arguing for a safety device in the form of a fee, however small, to be paid at the time of services rendered in addition to the capitation. Under salaried service, of course, it is obvious that the physician will resent any extra time that he has to put in or a multiplication of patients within that time. And the capitation argument applies again: there is no hindrance to overuse at the patient's whim. But the physician might do as much as possible to resist or obstruct the provision of services in order to achieve what must be the perfect goal: guaranteed salary and minimum service.

From my own experience with group practice and prepayment, I know that there are patients who take advantage of the system just as there are doctors who take advantage of the system. In my opinion, it is not the method of payment that *causes* people to take advantage of the system, but systems do *allow* people with a proclivity to overuse the system to indulge that proclivity. The hypochondriac who likes to see the doctor and can never be satisfied that he has been properly diagnosed or treated will make lots of visits to doctors whether he has to pay fee-for-service or if he is covered by capitation or salary plans. A physician who is lazy; who resents providing services; who has contempt for his patients and who sees his job as a business; is bound to take advantage of any situation in which he can do less for more money, whether it is fee-for-service, capitation or salary. And I believe that just as there are few patients who would milk the system or who are so hypochondriacal that they have to abuse it, so there are few physicians who are so unprofessional and unethical that they would abuse the system outrageously.

In my opinion, what is needed is collegial supervision, visible evidence of what is going on so that colleagues may be able to discipline one another;

and consumer participation, whereby the patient has access to information and an avenue for the expression of his grievance. So long as there is opportunity to express disapproval and punish those patients and doctors who are not dealing fairly with the system, it will work. I think that this sort of accountability, professional among colleagues and quasi-legal between consumers and doctors, along with some sort of arbitration mechanism would eliminate the abuse completely.

I can recall clearly, as a group practice director, an accountability situation involving doctors covering for one another on night call. If one would fail to take care of a patient adequately, the next day when the reports came around as to the night's activities, the physician responsible for the particular patient would take to task the colleague on call who had served inadequately. If the medical group is small enough so that the doctors know one another, and so that the doctors get to know one another's patients, the human relationship would forbid a great deal of abuse.

I do not believe that there is a perfect system any more than I believe that there is a perfect human being or a perfect life. But I do believe that some systems are better than others, and I think that a better system is one that has a built-in accountability mechanism. I do not believe that the accountability has to be entirely "after the fact," involving someone checking records every few months. I think that open discussions, between doctors and patients, of the ways in which cases and people were handled will make all the difference in the world in the way in which patients treat doctors and doctors treat patients.

I am reminded of the malpractice difficulties because in many ways malpractice is the only, albeit explosive, expression of dissatisfaction between patients and doctors. Unfortunately, there is no other current way for patients to deal with their dissatisfaction than by entering suit. I am sure that there are lots of malpractice suits that are not justifiable; in some cases patients do not understand that there is no such thing as a perfect cure; in some cases patients deliberately seek some financial award; in some cases they are egged on by lawyers. But in all probability, half or more of the malpractice cases may be justified in that the doctor did something wrong or failed to do something right.

If there were better information given to patients prior to medical service; if there were another way for them to express their grievance; and if there were collegial supervision among physicians, far fewer of the adverse things would happen. And far less litigation would result, because there could be settlements among the disputants along the lines of arbitration procedures and dispute settlements. A group practice with prepayment lends itself to full accountability and such relationships. But we will never have a good system as long as solo practice and fee-for-service without accountability is the mode.

## ROLE EXPECTATION VS. THE JOB

### DIFFERING DEFINITIONS OF THE DOCTOR

Some of the conflict situations between patients and doctors derive from the differing interpretation of what the doctor's job is supposed to be. The patients define the doctor's job in terms of *their* needs and what they think medicine is or ought to be. Their definition derives largely from traditional, historical relationships between physicians and patients; in other words, the way in which physicians have educated patients as to how doctors *ought* to behave. Anger can result from a kind of desperation on the patient's part, in that he feels he needs help because he has the classical symptoms of pain, bleeding, or fear, and he wants somebody to do something about it. To the best of his knowledge the person who is in charge of all those things relating to dysfunction of the body is the doctor.

The doctor, on the other hand, is constantly refining his conception of what he ought to be doing, based on the way in which he was trained and educated. The role models he has seen throughout his training determine his conception of role, perhaps more strongly than the demands of patients. As in so many things we do, there is an unconscious weighing of the varying forces at work; his ultimate attitudes reflect a resolution of the combined forces. If the doctor is more responsive to the patients' demands, he might do things that are not as acceptable to his colleagues, as defined in medical education. So he is less likely to accept responsibility just because a sick person says he wants or needs care. However, if the direction of his attitudinal scales tilts toward the *professional* side, so that respect for his teachers and role models is stronger and more important, he will tend to reject patients' demands that he feels are not consistent with the role model image.

### DIFFERING APPROACHES TO DISEASE AND TREATMENT

One can define a disease *professionally,* as a physician would; *popularly,* as a patient would; or *socially,* as an institution or government would; the definitions are not necessarily congruent.

There was a time when disease was thought to be a form of religious punishment: God did something to you because you had sinned. Under those circumstances not every disease was to be treated by a doctor; a priest was needed to intervene. Early physicians, therefore, were just as much priests as medical doctors; as a matter of fact, in very early times it was the priests who *became* physicians.  To this day in many primitive cultures, the shaman is a mixture of God's advocate and professional physician.  The Navajo medicine man is just such a mixture.  His diagnosis and treatment involves equal parts of religious ceremony and medical pre-scription — casting out devils, invoking God's help, praying, and per-forming mystical rites and ceremonies; as well as administering herbs, chemicals, poultices or surgery.

The belief of spiritual causation of illness was especially prevalent regarding mental and emotional illness.  In early times the mentally ill were considered possessed by the devil or other spirits.  For instance, in some countries the mentally ill were considered "touched by God," holy fools sacred to the Lord.  Mental or emotional disturbance easily lends itself to mystical interpretation because it usually manifests itself solely by behavior change and lacks obvious physical symptoms.

I remember an amusing incident, in my early training in public health, that brought this home to me with great force.  I was participating in a seminar at the London School of Hygiene in which a number of the students were asked to put on a play illustrating the difficulties and opportunities in health education.  A young African prince was a member of one team.  He chose to show health education as an aid to the control of tuberculosis in a developing country, comparing it to the utility of health education as an aid to the prevention of lung cancer in a developed county.  In the developing country, the mystical nature of tuberculosis (hemorrhage, weight loss, gradually increasing weakness and death) was ascribed by the native who suffered from it to evil spirits, a "hex" put upon him by neighbors who wished him ill.  He did not want to go to a sanitarium for fear that when he died his spirit would not rest in the ground where he had been born and be permitted to continue to live in the bodies of his descendants; he preferred to stay at home and die without treatment.  When the colonial physician attempted to explain to him about the bacteria in his lungs, the native nodded his head in agreement.  He understood about the tubercle bacillus; it was an invisible evil spirit that was destroying his lungs.  An intelligent and culture-wise health educator persuaded him to go to the sanitarium for treatment by assuring him that (a) if he took treatment he probably would not die in that place; and (b) if there were danger that he would die, his son would be brought there in order to receive the *mana* before he died and bring it back to the place of his birth.  Under those circumstances the health educator was able to persuade an otherwise reluctant patient to accept treatment.

On the other hand, in that same playlet, the health educator trying to prevent lung cancer was *not* able to persuade the developed country's hard-smoking intellectuals to give up their cigarettes, or at least respond in some measure to the increasing incidence of lung cancer, because he was not able to find the same kind of handle of persuasion. The developed country's smokers did not know why they were smoking and so could not be persuaded to give it up by being offered an adequate substitute.

DIFFICULTIES IN PATIENT/DOCTOR COMMUNICATION

There are other problems between patients and doctors related to contrasting definition of disease that are not related to ignorance, religious obsession or primitive culture. These differences may arise from contrasting interpretations of events; cultural incongruities concerning diet, rest, the taking of medicine and the convalescent procedure. In some cultures the person is sick only if he is not ambulatory. If a doctor says "come to my office," it is equivalent to telling the patient that he is not really sick. The patient cannot accept this. All patients require explanation in order to accept the fact of illness. A man may be told that he has to change his job because of the onset of physical disease, but if he does not recognize the importance or danger of not complying, the difficulty of making a job change — the impact on his income and family, etc. — will take greater precedence than concern for his life and health.

The doctor must explain fully to a patient what the condition is; what the consequences may be; what sorts of treatments are available; and what the consequences of each kind of treatment would be so that the patient can have intelligent input in the decision on a course of action. The difficulty is that physicians today are not given this conception in the role models provided in medical education. Spending a lot of time with the patient, offering a sympathetic interpretation and attempting to come to some democratic decision with the patient is not the way in which medicine is customarily practiced in the teaching hospitals of medical schools. Consequently, doctors do not carry away with them an impression of practice that resembles this. It might be what the textbook says that they should be doing, as many medical textbooks do, with glowing role models of historically great physicians who practiced this way. But what the student sees in the everyday work in the institution affects him much more than what he reads in a book; when he goes out into practice he will carry on what he has seen in his role models and not what he has been told he ought to do. I am reminded of Shakespeare's Ophelia's adjuration: "Do not, as some ungracious pastors do, show me the steep and thorny way to Heaven whilst, like some puffed and reckless libertine, thyself the primrose path of dalliance treads."

So there is much in the way in which doctors are educated and what they expect to do as physicians that differs markedly from what the patients think doctors ought to be.  Under such circumstances there is bound to be a range of conflict that doesn't have anything to do with methods of payment or organization, and only distantly with poverty, minority status and sex role conflict.  Reaching some decision as to how the doctor's job can be made congruent with both his and the patient's *image* of the job requires some change in the method of selection of doctors.  This is a first step, before one considers the way in which doctors are educated, how doctors should practice or how they should be paid.  It seems to me that to concentrate on changing the organization of medical care, the system of reimbursement, or the way in which medical care is financed altogether, will not be sufficient to make a difference in the degree in which patients and doctors are satisfied; unless some very strong additional efforts are made to modify the conditions and harmonize the understanding that create this clash of expectations.

### THE DOCTOR'S PROFESSIONAL/SOCIAL ROLE

There is another aspect of the physician's role in which the patient sees him not only as a professional, but as a personal friend, advisor and confidant who explains carefully, listens patiently and advises surely and gently.  This role is defined by Sigerist in "Trends in Medical Education" (from *The University as the Crossroads,* 1946) as:

> Scientist and social worker, ready to cooperate in team work, in close touch with the people he disinterestedly serves, friend and leader, he directs all his efforts toward the prevention of disease, and becomes a therapist where prevention has broken down — the social physician protecting the people and guiding them to a healthier and happier life.

The implication here is that the doctor sees himself as the protector of the patient against more than disease:  against difficulties such as the rape of the environment by industry or callous real estate developers, or employment-related poisoning and accidents.  This is more the vision that Virchow, a 19th century German pathologist, had of the physician's role in society: "the natural attorney of the poor," of those who were oppressed in whatever way and who required protection and help.  Today among physicians and the various scientists associated with health there are radical philosophers who feel that doctors should be even more than this; that they should be leaders toward social change generally and not simply antagonists of medical oppression.

# CHANGING MEDICAL EDUCATION
## TO HUMANIZE THE DOCTOR

### DIFFERENT MODELS

It is necessary to define exactly what changes in medical training of the physician are needed — what it is that will make the difference in the way in which he responds to the patients' social needs.   In the first place, we want to be sure that any alternative training procedure is not going to lessen the doctor's professional competence.   Perhaps we should concentrate first on which doctors are influencing medical students in their educational experience.   There are 20 or 30 thousand doctors working in medical schools and teaching hospitals in a full-time capacity, and an additional 20 or 30 thousand in a part-time capacity.   It seems to me that we have been putting our emphasis in the past on the wrong portion of the teaching equation.   Instead of trying to influence students, we should be trying to influence faculty and teaching staff.   This will require powerful changes within medical schools and teaching hospitals; surprisingly little attention has been given to this problem.   To the people of the United States generally who are upset about existing medical services, to the editorial writers and cartoonists in the newspapers, the enemy of progress and the villain in the deficiencies of medical care in the United States is the American Medical Association.   Now, I am hardly one to post a defense for the AMA, and certainly this would not be the place to do it, but I think it should be understood that it expresses the political, economic and social attitudes of a powerful interest group *within* the medical profession that has learned its professional role and attitude *in* the medical schools!   Without powerful change in the way in which medical schools influence their students, it is hardly likely that succeeding generations will be too far different.

The key development to improving medical practice, then, will have to be a transformation of the attitudes of the medical educators.   They ought to demonstrate the appropriate roles, ways of behavior, attitudes towards patients, and professional conceptualization that approximates what we hope the students will emulate.   This will mean, for example, that the method of treating ward and clinic patients in teaching hospitals will have to change; that the discriminatory patterns of admission and treatment that pervade teaching institutions will have to be modified.   The doctors and professors will have to show as much concern for these social values as for the professional values of microbiology, physiology, pathology, biochemistry and the scientific formulations that are preeminent in the concept of medical education at present.

## "WEDDING" OF SCIENTIST AND HEALER

All sorts of lip service has been paid to this in the past. The professors and dignitaries from the medical schools have written learned articles in all the journals and in popular magazines describing what they call the "wedding of scientist and healer," or in other such terms and phrases to that effect. Most of this has been window dressing, since those who are *healers* rarely get to carry out the scientific experiments upon which appointment and promotion depend. They get to write up or publish anything to give them the platform from which an academic career can be launched. The academic *scientists,* on the other hand, are the ones who do accumulate a substantial bibliography that results in appointment and promotion. Only through eventual restructuring of the departmental procedures responsible for organizing and carrying out the education of students can teaching be changed. A more ideal "wedding" would result in professors with a balanced concern for both healing and science, who would create within their students as much interest in and concern for methods and intricacies of practice as in arcane laboratory procedures and rare disease diagnoses.

Some of the medical school lions are beginning to see the light. The distinguished physician Paul Beeson, who ran a "tight ship" when he was professor of medicine at Yale, had the humility and perception to learn a different lesson when he served as Regius Professor of Medicine at Oxford. He saw then that it was possible to work in a different kind of system, for students to learn a different kind of medicine that was not *worse* than American medicine but in many ways *better.*

So there is something that has to be done with faculty. The money that is spent on changing the curriculum for students to learn different things is largely wasted. The people who are supposed to be *teaching* these things have to be convinced themselves. A great deal more money will need to be spent in providing seminars, educational opportunities and firm leadership in transforming the teachers before the students can learn anything. The well-known Spanish artist Goya published a set of etchings entitled "Los Caprichios" with a donkey as a representational type. In one of these etchings, the donkey is a doctor and he sits by the bedside taking the patient's pulse, saying "I wonder what he'll die of?" In another the donkey is a teacher and a smaller donkey sits in the corner wearing a dunce cap. The legend reads "Can the student learn more than the teacher knows?" Both of these have application to what needs to be done to improve medical education if we hope to change physicians and improve medical practice.

### BETTER CRITERIA IN STUDENT SELECTION

It is also important to change the cultural components of the student body if progress is to be made in eliminating the social distance between doctors and patients. If the largest number of physicians come out of the upper social and economic class that represents a small proportion of the American population, it stands to reason that there will be some degree of cultural dissonance in expectation and acceptance between doctor and patient. The discordance can be modified in one of two ways, or perhaps in both: more students can be brought into the medical schools from those social classes now disproportionately represented; or the medical education itself can change to include anthropological and sociological educational activities to modify the perceptions and cultural ignorance of the students. The latter has been tried in many guises over the years and has not been too successful by itself; I believe that both will have to be tried in order to be effective.

One of the problems of our time, of course, is that when such suggestions become implemented, it usually turns out that changing the ratio is accomplished not by introducing larger numbers of a minority group, or of women, or of different socioeconomic groups, but by reducing the numbers of those in the previously favored groups. Blacks are admitted at the expense of other ethnic groups; women are admitted at the expense of men; poor at the expense of the well-to-do. In some ways this form of retributive justice can be rationalized. But we are dealing with a social situation in which such a change in numbers should not be to the benefit of one at the expense of another; it should be instead a search for equity — equalizing benefits so that no one suffers. Improvement in the numbers of previously neglected groups should be accomplished through the enlargement of the total number taught.

### ALTERNATIVE APPROACHES TO MEDICAL EDUCATION

Enlarging the total number of doctors may also be counterproductive because it may only serve to increase the total amount of money spent without actually increasing the accessibility of services. We might want to look at some different ways of carrying on medical education that would not involve huge expenditures of money, while still attacking the problem of poor distribution and lack of accessibility. I have three such solutions.

One solution is that students should be selected for medical education not by the medical schools but by the communities themselves. This might produce certain problems if the community's decision were the sole contingency. But if the community recommends and the medical school selects it seems to me that both objectives could be served. This would make it more likely that those selected would return to where they are needed; perhaps this could be insured by seeing to it that the selecting communities also pay for the education. The student would then be obligated to return to the community and provide services for some agreed period of time.

Another solution might be to create large numbers of small medical schools associated with the larger community hospitals with no current medical school affiliation.    Many of the approximately 160 Veterans' Administration Hospitals are in such locations.    If this were combined with an organized exchange of house staff between the large urban centers and the more scattered hospitals in the areas away from these teaching centers, there could be a very significant leveling out of the distribution of doctors, the availability of medical education and the costs.

Perhaps a third solution would be a reintroduction of the apprenticeship method that was abandoned a few generations ago because the complexity and expense of the new kinds of medical equipment and teaching tools required centralization of medical education.    Modern developments now make it possible, through audio-visual mechanisms of one kind or another and development of new textures joined with computer simulation, to design mannequins that react for students the way human beings react; large pools of human "teaching material" may no longer be necessary. Individual doctors in group practices could sponsor students on their premises.    While some of the medical education could continue in centralized facilities, the rest could be done in the old fashioned, apprentice-type one-to-one relationship between a practicing physician and a student.    This would have the added great advantage that preceptors could be selected who would have the attitudes and values that we want to inculcate in the students.

The organizational attributes of group practice are discussed elsewhere; here I would like to discuss group practice as against solo practice from the standpoint of a doctor's training.    Solo practice is the mode for medical practice.    It encourages the doctor's independence of action.    It makes him fully responsible for each of his patient's care.    But unless he makes specific arrangements, there is no one to look after his patients when he cannot. And if he does make arrangements, it is bound to be *ad hoc,* because permanent arrangements presume permanent shifts in responsibilities. From a patient's standpoint, an organization that accepts and discharges responsibilities for patient care is to be greatly preferred; the patient is always covered.    The problem with group practice is organizational supervision; someone has to make sure the doctors are qualified and available, and that they carry out instructions and maintain communications.    What problems there may be are *managerial,* not professional, assuming the same kinds of doctors go into group as into solo practice.    One does not learn this, but should, in medical school.

## WHAT THE PATIENT WANTS AND NEEDS

### THE "GOOD OLD DAYS"

In Alexander Solzhenitsyn's novel *Cancer Ward,* he establishes a close relationship between a character's political attitudes and philosophy concerning the working of the medical care system.  Perhaps it is not so unusual that those who argue for more state involvement in general would also argue for more organization and control in medical practice.  It is easy to see how one's social attitudes would influence ideas about solo versus group practice, or fee-for-service versus salaries.  It is a little more difficult to see the effect in one's attitudes toward specialism and family doctoring.  Solzhenitsyn, a dissenter from Russian communism and a powerful exponent of individual freedom, has very strong feelings against technological mechanization of medical practice.  In *Cancer Ward,* he uses the figure of an elderly general practitioner to voice this:

> "Generally speaking," he remarked, "the family doctor is the most comforting figure in our lives, and now he's being pulled up by the roots.  The family doctor is a figure without whom the family cannot exist in a developed society. . . . There's no shame in taking to him some trivial complaint you'd never take to the outpatients' clinic, which entails getting an appointment card and waiting your turn, and where there's a quota of nine patients an hour.  And yet all neglected illnesses arise out of these trifling complaints.  How many adult human beings are there, now, at this minute, rushing about in mute panic wishing they could find a doctor, the kind of person to whom they could pour out the fears they have deeply concealed or even found shameful?  Looking for the right doctor is the sort of thing you can't always ask your friends for advice about."

He then argues along the same lines some economists do with respect to nationalizing health services.  Through the physician, Solzhenitsyn points out that that kind of family doctoring would not fit into a system of free universal national health service.  The old doctor continues:

> "What does 'free' mean?  The doctors don't work for nothing, you know.  It only means that they're paid out of the national

budget and the budget is supported by patients. It isn't free treatment, it's depersonalized treatment. If a patient kept the money that pays for his treatments, he would have turned the ten roubles he has spent at the doctor's over and over in his hands. He could go to the doctor five times over if he really needed to. . . . He would say, 'To hell with the new drapes and spare pair of shoes. What's the use of them if I'm not healthy?' Is it any better as things are now?"

And he goes into a long laudatory statement about how nice it was when there were free clinics, when the doctors gave things to patients, and he emphasizes that "the doctor should *depend* on the impression he makes on his patients, he should be dependent on his popularity." He makes a very interesting point:

"With the right kind of primary system," Oreshchenkov countered, "there'd be fewer cases altogether, and no neglected ones. The primary doctor should have no more patients than his memory and personal knowledge can cover. Then he could treat each patient as a subject on his own."

And he makes a strong pitch for eliminating specialists altogether:

"The patient gets tossed from 'specialist' to 'specialist' like a basketball. . . . If you wanted to understand the patient as a single subject, there'd be no room left in you for any other passion. . . . The doctor ought to be an all-rounder."

Finally, he attacks specialism in Voltaire's words: "Doctors prescribe medicines about which they know little for an organism about which they know less."

These are some of the very conceptions that Americans yearn for in terms of medical care: that they will be able to find a doctor who knows everything, who is prepared to deal with everything, who is kind and gentle, is not interested in money, and is very readily available. It may be that all of these objectives cannot be reached, but certainly every effort should be made to create a system in which they are encouraged. Perhaps we will have to have fewer specialists, although we can't do without them altogether. But can friendly, attentive, empathetic care be accomplished without different training of medical students; or different standards of candidate selection; or different organization of practice? Can we go back to Oreshchenkov's "good old days"?

### REESTABLISHING THE "GOOD OLD DAYS"

We have discussed possible changes in the selection of medical students and the teaching procedures and models that might be utilized to change a doctor's attitudes toward patients and practice, and his overall role conception. The location of the teaching might also be crucial; it ought to be as far from the hospital as possible, a setting that simulates the kind of setting where, hopefully, the young physician will practice when he completes his education and training. Therefore, group practices in a variety of locations — in well-to-do, suburban, ghetto, rural and urban areas — have to be constructed as part of the university program. They may continue to be run independently, but with the university's supervision. Students must also be encouraged to undertake a variety of medically related experiences, so that they will have a more comfortable feeling about the variety of things with which physicians have to deal. For example, it would not be amiss to expect young physicians to begin their training as nurses' assistants, emergency room technicians or laboratory technicians; they would therefore understand what is expected of those working with physicians. Perhaps during the first year or two of professional training, all of those who will be working in the medical field should take courses together. This would help to develop a mutual respect and understanding of one another's roles. The student physicians could also get experience with government at various levels — in administrative work, with welfare departments or in a variety of policy-making agencies — in order to get an understanding of patients in social settings, of all those who need to deal with doctors in whatever capacity.

In modifying the settings in which the students are taught their clinical subjects, it would be well to vary the organizational base of the units in which the teaching would take place, as well. For example, there could be some in which the university would actually control and administer; some in which the physicians would control and administer; some in which the community would construct the center and employ physicians to work there, such as the neighborhood health centers that were developed under OEO; and some in which there are even new types of administrative mechanisms — worker control as in Yugoslavia, or worker management control as was attempted here in the United States in a number of cooperative groups, etc. The more the student can learn; not just about the human body, but of the society in which human problems occur; the better he will be able to deal with the individual problems that are brought to him. If he understands more about families, he will be able to see physical disease symptoms within a larger framework of psychological and genealogical motivation — to see how it is connected with family problems;

the same is true of occupational and school activities. Unless the doctor is prepared to see the whole of society as within the patient and the whole of the patient as within society, he cannot make effective judgments about a particular condition, its cause and its treatment.

Everyone knows that a computer responds truly and accurately only on the basis of the information that is fed into it. A physician may be seen as a kind of computer. The accuracy of his diagnosis and the appropriateness of his treatment is only as accurate as the information that is fed in and only as knowledgeable as the memory with which it interacts. It may be only fair to point out at this time that the same is true of the patient, that his reaction and response will be only as good as the information that is transmitted to him. A good deal of the argument about "informed consent" needs to be put, not on the basis of the doctor's moral or legal obligation, but on the simple basis of giving the patient a clear, intelligible understanding of the illness and its treatment. What a patient does *not* know can hurt him.

## THE FOREIGN DOCTOR FLOW:
## KEEPING AN EYE ON QUALITY

To change American medical education is indeed a crucial step toward improving the social consciousness of our doctors; but there are many doctors who will not benefit from the enlarged or shifted educational emphasis. It may come as something of a shock to realize the increasing numbers of physicians practicing in the United States who are not influenced by the American medical education system at all.

Foreign medical graduates have always been a part of the American medical practice scene. Early in the century, while American medicine was just beginning to assume a scientific or technologically advanced model, many American physicians "finished off" their education by studying abroad for a year or two. The specialist with some European training and qualification was considered superior to any American specialist. In addition, as a result of the same factors that led to a torrent of immigration of all kinds of people, numbers of doctors emigrated to the United States and formed a portion of the practicing body of physicians here. Their numbers were small; the question of quality did not arise because by and large European schools were considered equal or superior to the American medical schools. Cultural and language differences made little difference, since the immigrant doctors tended to practice among their own people. My own doctor in my childhood was a Polish Jew who had been educated in Switzerland and who practiced among the Russian and Polish Jewish community in South Philadelphia.

The technological and scientific revolution that put American industry on top of world commerce and trade also affected American medical education. In part this was a result of the figurative expectations. That is, more science and technology in medicine was good, American science and technology was the best; therefore, American medicine had to be the best in the world. But in part it was an inescapable worldwide development, following the explosion of new knowledge in chemistry and physiology that changed the concepts of modern medicine, of health and disease, of diagnosis and treatment. The American medical educational system and American medical research did capture the high ground and did advance far beyond that of European colleagues, who seemed to remain somewhere in the late 19th century.

After World War II, the research, education and practice gap between Europe and America widened. Congress invested increasingly greater amounts of federal funds in biomedical research, resulting in the graduation of increasing numbers of specialists, raising the cost of medical care and the status of the practicing physician. Doctors from all over the world were drawn to the United States by the educational opportunities, the technological magnificence and the great sums of money that could be earned here. At the same time their own countries, damaged and impoverished by the War (or wars), and technologically backward if they were newly liberated developing countries, had very little to offer them. At the same time the shift in American medical education and practice made for increasing demands for doctors to fill hospital positions created by the increasing specialism. Our own medical schools were growing at a relatively slow rate and were unable to meet the increased demands, so that there was an added enticement on the part of institutions and communities in the United States to bring established doctors from other countries here to do increasingly demanded work. Between 1962 and 1972, of doctors entering the country, as many foreign medical graduates were immigrants as exchange visitors (many of whom ultimately stayed and became immigrants); and as many were licensed as were U. S. medical graduates. By December of 1973, there were over 70,000 foreign medical graduates in the United States, in a medical work force of only 350,000; just about 20 percent of all physicians. Of the 60,000 doctors in our "pipeline" (interns and residents), 20,000 were foreign medical graduates. In 1972, 46 percent of the physicians licensed in the United States were foreign medical graduates; 75 percent of these were licensed in only 12 states, so that there were regional differences, but the point remains an important one. Some people shrug and say, "If we need them and they want to come, where's the harm?"

Looking at it from the standpoint of the countries from which these immigrant physicians come, and the majority are from poor countries, the problem is really one of equity. It costs $50 to $75 thousand to train an American physician. If 10,000 foreign medical graduates enter the United States each year, it would cost us somewhere between $500 and $750 million to train them. In a sense, we're receiving "reverse lend lease" from poor countries who can ill afford to pay for the training of these doctors and ill afford to lose their services.

From the standpoint of the United States, there are some other problems as well. In the first place there is some question about their quality. This can be argued in many different ways and I hesitate to put too much emphasis upon it. But of the 1,000 medical schools in the world, very few of those outside the United States provide either the scientific experience or the bedside training of direct patient care that we consider the hallmark of good medical education. Many of the schools are poorly equipped and the teachers are either not full-time or, because of private commitments, pay little attention to the students. Textbooks may be out of date. There are usually so many students in a class (until recently in Madrid the entering class was 2,000) that the students get very little attention or supervision. Assuming that the best of the students are attracted to the United States, there is still some question as to their quality. We have evidence, for example, that they do not do as well in examinations as American medical students. And although American students who study in foreign schools do better than foreign graduates of the same class (which may have something to do with their knowledge and use of the English language), they still do not do as well as American students trained in American medical schools.

There are also important cultural and language barriers experienced by foreign medical graduates as physicians of American patients. The foreign doctors tend not to receive equitable treatment in terms of their intern or residency experience because of the competition among the "better" teaching institutions for American graduates. The foreign medical graduates therefore gravitate towards service in hospitals and communities where they may be taking care of mostly poor people and minorities, emphasizing and exaggerating the cultural differences.

Another question of equity raises itself in considering that if we do need more physicians, we should attempt to increase the numbers of minority group American physicians who are underrepresented here, rather than import more foreign doctors. How can we justify the fact that there are 9,500 Philippine doctors in practice in the United States, and only 5,800 American black physicians?

And from the standpoint of world need, world health and world peace, it would certainly seem fair and logical for the United States, a wealthy and powerful nation, to train *more* physicians than it needs, in order to export them; to help provide medical care in parts of the world where needs are desperate. It is cruel to bring in physicians from those very needy places to serve our own selfish needs. Currently, about 7,000 American students are studying medicine abroad, and it would seem fair that we should take steps to see to it that we train those students ourselves, in this country.

# Chapter 6
# Nonphysician Health Care Personnel

## PUTTING THE DOCTOR IN PERSPECTIVE

Almost invariably when one discusses or criticizes medical care, key consideration generally turns to the physician. But it is only fair to try to see the doctor in proper perspective. In order to recognize the total extent of medical care as it is in the United States, one has to realize that there are more than four million people concerned with the delivery of health services; and that less than 10 percent of these are physicians. This is not to say that good medical care is a matter of numbers; or that the fact that there are ten times as many people in the field who are not doctors makes the doctor unimportant; his part in the job is larger than the 10 percent would indicate. But it would be virtually impossible in our society for medical care to be delivered by doctors alone. Physicians and the rest of the health care manpower are so intricately interrelated that medical care can no longer be considered the responsibility of one profession alone.

Some people believe that health care can be accomplished without physicians altogether. And so a very strong self-care movement has grown up, claiming as a model the efforts of the Chinese government. They are aiming to modify and improve the medical care system in that country by circumventing the academic physician and creating large numbers of informally trained "barefoot doctors," who take care of the bulk of the people's medical care needs.

These movements do derive in part from the arrogant domination by physicians over medical practice for so many centuries. But there are other factors at work, too. America has learned to analyze jobs and make cost and motion analyses of who does what and how. We invented the assembly line; we think in terms of division of labor. And much of what doctors do can be considered inconsistent with their higher degree of training.  Also, because of the rapid inflation of costs seen largely as the responsibility of physicians, and perhaps even because of the incredibly high incomes that physicians earn, the doctor's job is being rethought. Doctors do make heavy financial demands on patients:  they require expensive tests, diagnostic and therapeutic procedures, and prescriptions of drugs and appliance; and most major services require very expensive hospitalization.  Doctors demand but they do not have to provide; they prescribe but they do not have to pay for the prescription; and they are in a supernatant way the creators of the phenomenal costs of the system.  In order to reduce these costs, managerial analysis is being applied to suggest ways of using less expensive people in the provision of services.

## THE HISTORY OF PARAMEDICAL PERSONNEL

Historically, the nontraditional physician was the person to whom a segment of the sick turned, particularly the poor.  Those things that we call "medicine" today were not the responsibility of the physician, the surgeon or the apothecary, but a large number of categorically specific practitioners of pieces of the diagnosis and treatment.  For example, there were midwives, bone setters and those with the special skill of crushing stones in the bladder.

It is certainly true that by the beginning of the 19th century the physician was already looked upon as the person who did all those things, for many of the separate categorical disciplines were folded into medicine and taken over by the physician.  At that time, for example, physicians rather than midwives were beginning to deliver babies, particularly in the United States; surgery became an integral part of their general training.  And the idea of licensing became of paramount concern.

However, only a hundred years later, the technological revolution and the resultant growth of science and medicine's dependence on science created a situation in which it became necessary for more and more people to become reinvolved in the medical care system.  Science had "slenderized" the system, reducing the multiplicity of practitioners, and then fattened it up again!

### NURSES

First there was growth in the number of nurses, those responsible for looking after the sick in a continuing way after the physician had made his diagnosis.  These nurses were not required to make a diagnosis or provide treatment; but they were trained to be observant of change and condition of the patient so as to be able to advise the doctor on his periodic visits as to what had happened and what else might be necessary. They were to insure that the treatment the doctor prescribed was given and taken. The nurse also had the responsibility of making the patient comfortable, of supplying the needs he could not supply for himself and of seeing that no harm came to him by virtue of his helplessness.

The function of nursing was enlarged with the growth of institutions for the care of the sick. In earlier societies those institutions were rare because they were rarely needed or wanted. With the industrialization of society, and the accumulation of people in urban tenements, a place for the sick outside the home became a necessity. In the 19th century, the community or a public organization built the hospitals in conjunction with workhouses and poor houses. Then fraternal organizations, religious organizations and the *bruderschaften* and *landsmannschaften,* corresponding with the influx of immigrants over time, built themselves hospitals to protect their own against the indignities and humiliation of public care at workhouse hospitals.

Attending nurses began to increase in response to the consequent demand. Furthermore, the impact of Florence Nightingale's recognition of the need for providing some sort of standard experience for those who were to be the nurses, resulted in the growth of nursing schools. As there always is, when there were more schools, there grew to be more demands for the product of the school. However, the growth of numbers of nurses was slow. By the end of the 19th century, when the explosive growth of medical education had resulted in a phenomenal number of physicians for the United States (some 150,000 of them for over 75,000,000 people), there were fewer than half that amount of trained nurses.

MEDICAL TECHNICIANS

From that low point, medical specialism and technological advances such as the creation of new kinds of machinery for diagnosis and treatment, resulted in a powerful efflorescence of medical technicians. The demand for nurses increased, as did the demand for technically trained people to work the instruments, and specially trained assistants for physicians. Physicians expanded their specialty and subspecialty services to meet demands of a populace enamored with the benefits of science; at the same time physicians were able to spend less time in hospitals, yet more and more people were needed there.

In the meantime, physicians had been exercising a form of birth control over the production of new physicians in a number of sophisticated ways relative to the scientific rationalism of the period. For example, the length of medical education was more than doubled, in response to the need for more accurate scientific training in specialism. Whereas in 1900 a high school graduate could enter a medical college and after three or four years receive a medical diploma, by 1970 he needed a college education in order to enter medical school and almost four years of specialized training beyond that. From a minimum of three years, medical education has gone to a minimum of ten years. Furthermore, the imposition of state licensing by examination was culling doctors with inferior credentials. The American Medical Association was moving to certify institutions, which made it necessary for these schools to equip themselves at great expense to meet the accreditation standards. This reduced the numbers of schools drastically between 1900 and 1930.

These pressures increased the demand for trained doctor substitutes or extenders to look after patients. There were doctors' office assistants, for example, without any training in school, who learned by experience how to deal with many medical situations, became quite expert and were given large leeway by the employing physician. Growing recognition and importance of mental health gave rise to a large-scale movement of people to take care of those who were emotionally or mentally disturbed. The movement was accelerated because until the 1960's very few physicians were trained or interested in the care of the mentally ill. Therapists and social workers began to take over the field.

The major contributions to the influx of increasing numbers of para-professionals into the field were by physicians themselves. From the turn of the century, they had looked about for workers who would assist them in giving better supervision to patients when they were too busy in the office or were not immediately available. In part it was an economic effort, to increase their income. The paraprofessionals could look after the routine and minor needs of more patients; giving the physician more time to take care of more people. The doctors took nonmedical professionals and gave them a medical role.

### MEDICAL SOCIAL WORKERS

Such activity may be seen in the development of the medical social worker as visualized by Dr. Richard Cabot at the Massachusetts General Hospital in Boston in 1910. Cabot wanted someone to work with him in the clinic who would be able to transmit information and translate his directions to the patients as well as bring back to *him* information about the patient's ability to comply, what the situation was at home or with the family; information he thought would be of help in the diagnosis or treatment of the disease. The medical social workers developed a sound and resolute disciplinary base for their activities, incorporating some knowledge of medicine, psychiatry and sociology.

As more and more evidence appeared of psychological or sociological components interfering with the capability of the patient to comply with the doctor's orders or contributing to the causation or maintenance of the patient's disease, these medical social workers began to concentrate on the mental and emotional side. They would devote more time to exploring and supporting their own discipline and relationship with the patients than to carrying out the physician's orders. The medical and psychiatric social workers became almost independent practitioners. With changing physician roles, tension developed; mutual dissatisfaction between physicians and social workers arose. Medicine was becoming "scientific," laboratory and research oriented. The personal problems of patient care were of less interest to doctors; rare and complex medical conditions of more interest. The physicians saw, resentfully, the medical social workers carrying on this independent role for "their" patients. Medical social workers saw, resentfully, physicians refusing to give sufficient attention and consideration to the findings and concerns of the medical social workers. They began to drift apart.

At the same time, concern about the mental and emotional health of people (not only as a disease entity in itself, but as an elaboration of physical illness) attracted more attention from physicians. There began to be more specialization in the field of psychiatry. From the 1950's on, more federal funds became available to divert physicians from other specialties and general practice into the field of psychiatry. The psychiatrists and the social workers found themselves in a much more congenial situation than the social workers and physicians had shared. Social workers began to become much more psychiatric social workers than medical social workers.

Ironically, as better understanding of mental and emotional illness penetrated society and medicine, they turned away from those desperately in need of emotional treatment, the *mentally* ill. They took under their wing the "walking wounded" — people with *emotional* disturbances. A special category of health workers in the field of psychiatry was now available and, for those with money, services could be purchased. The field of mental health is now so well-established that the question is how to open up psychiatric help and the kinds of services needed to the poor; it unfortunately remains largely elitist.

There are, of course, dissenting voices who feel that this kind of psychiatric help may preempt the valuable "self-healing process" by which individuals learn to come to grips with the reality of fate and adversity. These partisans object to emotional treatment because they believe people ought to deal with their own unhappiness, rather than submit to forms of treatment that subtly encourage continuing dependence. However, that may be a subject for another book. What is important to emphasize here is that, as medical progress resulted in the growth of large numbers of associated technicians and nurses to look after the physically sick, a parallel development took place in the field of mental and emotional health.

## EFFECTIVE USE OF THE PARAPROFESSIONAL

Over four million people other than physicians are engaged in various aspects of the health delivery system. While more than 300,000 are physicians' aides, almost 300,000 more are in dentistry; over 200,000 are engaged in the environmental health field. Two million people are engaged in nursing, although only half are R.N.'s. Licensed practical nurses, aides and assistants make up the other half. The following table provides a full breakdown of health industry personnel.

TABLE 6-1:   Health Industry Personnel

| Field | 4.4 million |
|---|---|
| (selected) | |
| 1. Administration | 50,000 |
| 2. Clinical lab. services | 160,000 |
| 3. Dentistry | 275,000 |
| 4. Sanitation | 100,000 |
| 5. Health education | 30,000 |
| 6. Medical records | 50,000 |
| 7. Physicians & osteopaths | 350,000 |
| 8. Nurses | 2.2 million |
| 9. Occupational therapists | 13,000 |
| 10. Optometrists | 25,000 |
| 11. Pharmacy | 135,000 |
| 12. Physical therapists | 25,000 |
| 13. Psychologist | 27,000 |
| 14. Radiological technician | 100,000 |
| 15. Secretarial | 300,000 |
| 16. Social work | 35,000 |
| 17. Rehabilitation and corrective | 50,000 |
| 18. Veterinary medicine | 27,000 |
| 19. Miscellaneous assistant | 260,000 |
| 20. Chiropractors | 14,000 |

Source: *Health Resources Statistics, 1974,* Department of Health, Education and Welfare (HRA) 75-1509, pp. 9-12.

These people are absolutely essential in making the health system work; given the specialism of physicians, it would be absolutely impossible for people to get modern medical care without this added professional staff. Their numbers continue to grow as technology advances and specialism increases in the medical profession.

## AN EFFICIENT WORK FORCE

The hope is that paraprofessionals will completely take over some of the jobs that physicians either do not want to do, or cannot do. There is also the hope that by providing physician assistants or associates, the lack of distribution of physicians can be corrected. Perhaps they could be used instead of physicians in underserved areas, or to relieve the pressure of physicians and so allow them to take care of more people in underserved areas. The movement to create a class of secondary medical practitioners in the United States is partly because of the shortage and partly in the hope of putting a ceiling on costs. Some people are somewhat cynical about this, believing that as long as the medical care system remains an open one in regard to reimbursement, the introduction of additional workers in the field will only multiply costs and only partially operate so as to reduce the number of underserved areas.

The likelihood is that more physicians will use these trained assistants in their offices, enabling them to reinforce their activity where they are. It will increase their income because charges will continue to be as they are, while the reimbursement of the assistant, who will be providing a good part of the service, will not be comparable to what the physician earns himself. And as a consequence more services will be provided, to the same people, at higher costs, and with significant augmentation of the physician's income.

Without a radical reorganization of the system, it is hard to see how paraprofessionals like the physician assistants will be used effectively, unless they are permitted to practice independently. If that does occur, there is considerable danger insofar as the physician assistant will not be trained to the same degree that the physician is, will not have the same grasp of the essentials of diagnosis and treatment, and will therefore be providing what is in essence a second-class medical service. It is to be hoped that if physician assistants are to be used in large numbers to improve medical practice, it will be done under suitable supervision and organization and with every effort at accountability, to be sure that quality of patient care does not suffer.

## UTILIZING SURPLUS PERSONNEL

There is no doubt that we have been very prodigal in the use of the associated health workers in the medical care system. Because of the cost-plus nature of hospital reimbursement, there has been no control over the increased use of health workers in hospitals. Our use of hospital workers, the so-called "staff-to-patient ratio," has increased by over 50 percent in the past 25 years. Comparable developments in European countries do not show such a great increase in the use of such personnel. The inefficiency created by hiring assistants carelessly, without regard to significant reform in either task distribution or job description, is very difficult to correct once it has become established. It is one thing to redefine a man's job with his understanding and acceptance, but it is quite another to try to reduce the numbers of people working in institutions once the jobs have become established and, of course, once the workers have become members of a union or part of a civil service organization. The elimination of jobs at that point becomes practically impossible. A saving grace is that reorganization of the system, with added emphasis on ambulatory services, would result in closing institutions; therefore, there may be some scurrying around to improve efficiency as institutions compete for the privilege of remaining open.

I hope that this discussion will not leave the impression that I have no concern for those thousands of people who are really surplus to the needs of the institutions as they are now operating, but who are soaked up into the system because of its inefficiencies, inconsistencies and casual mismanagement. I do believe that in the considerations required for reorganization, primary concern should be given to the fate of the people who will be designated as superfluous. Certainly, moving people from unnecessary inpatient to desperately needed outpatient services can be carried out intelligently, so as to use such people most productively, to provide better and more equitable service in places where services are now in short supply or inadequate.

The outstanding example of a field of effort needing enlargement is mental health. Too many patients (600,000) are now in institutions. Community ambulatory services, foster home care, cottage parent approaches, etc., would provide far more suitable, satisfactory, humane treatment, as well as socially desirable and useful activities for those who are mentally and emotionally disturbed. Those people who are now working in mental hospitals would be better employed supervising community health activities. At present, community mental health centers are inadequately staffed without sufficient outreach to provide the full range of mental health services required in the community. As a consequence, mental hospital patients who are discharged wander through the community, half dazed with the drugs which are supposed to keep them under control, but without the supervision, observation and social services they truly need. Organization of mental health care might very usefully put hospital personnel to work in community health services instead.

The same applies to the surplus of people now working in general hospitals. The surplus involved in in-patient activities ought to be used in the provision of extensive community services for ambulatory care.

## THE PHYSICIAN/PARAPROFESSIONAL
## RELATIONSHIP

The relationship of the paraprofessional and the physician in carrying out the necessary duties of patient care can present problems.  As long as the nonphysician is regarded by the doctor as ancillary, a mere hand maiden carrying out orders, there will be problems of personnel with regard to capability, performance and costs.  Until the time that the nonphysician health worker is accepted by physicians as a professional in a *colleague's* role and the job descriptions are modified accordingly, it is very doubtful that cost containment and quality control will be obtained.  As long as the physician is autocratically demanding, defining and directing the medical care system, it is not likely that much change can be made.

There are dangers, of course, in trying to create the sort of naive democratic format that so many passionately active health workers with a strong bias against physicians recommend.  The so-called "demystification" of medicine, whereby people are encouraged to take care of themselves without consulting a physician, is useful only if those people so encouraged have sufficient background and understanding of disease, diagnosis and treatment to be able to deal with the symptoms in a reasonable, truly beneficial way.

### THE MEDICAL TEAM

The most effective use of paraprofessionals will be obtained when the physician and the paraprofessional are conjointly educated to work as an effective health team.  It is interesting that the training process for specialists has evolved in just such a fashion, at least in the better training programs. The young man fresh from medical school begins to learn his specialty under supervision.  He is given very limited responsibility for independent action in terms of patient care at first, but is expected to spend a great deal of time working with a colleague who is further advanced and with those who have already achieved the level of independent action.  Over time he is given increasing responsibilities until eventually he is allowed independence.  Even then he reports to a supervisor from time to time.  This is a relic of the guild system of training from apprentice to journeyman to master.  It is a fine model.  It is in this fashion that paraprofessionals should be trained in conjunction with physicians.  With continuing supervision, the doctor in charge would be assured that his patients would never be in the position of being treated at a level below their needs.  At the same time, the democratic discussion opportunities between those who are learning and those who are teaching will make it possible for useful exchange of information.

It seems to me that this is what Sir Theodore Fox, the great editor of the *Lancet,* spoke about in a graduation address 20 years ago when he discussed "The Greater Medical Profession." He stated that the physician should not act like an autocrat, giving orders and expecting the lesser breed to carry them out; instead, he should be "first among equals" in medical situations, using his added knowledge and experience for the benefit of bringing about useful and satisfying performance from those of different and lesser training or experience.

### EDUCATIONAL INTERCHANGE

As we realize the necessity for a more dignified relationship between professionals and paraprofessionals, it is also easy to recognize that different ways of training and educating the paramedical, paraprofessional and intermediate level health practitioner will be required. It is popular in the United States today to utilize what is known as an "algorithm," a plan of action in which the student is taught to follow a pattern, a sort of branching mechanism of diagnosis and treatment. For example, if event "X" occurs, or symptom "Y" presents itself, the health worker is expected to follow procedure "Z." The difficulty with this, of course, is that human beings respond in fairly complex ways; the picture may not always be exactly as it is represented in this branching tree. Furthermore, the student is not encouraged to think or to respond automatically. There are advantages to this kind of behavior and expectation, of course. Whenever something arises in a situation in which the student has had no experience, and nothing in the algorithm tells him what to do, he is not supposed to do anything independently before calling the preceptor. The disadvantage is that the student never learns to take an intelligent overview of the situation and make comparisons or arrive at decisions based on his own experiences and capabilities. It would seem to be far better if the training experiences were visualized in a more dynamic way and that the various cadres of students were educated together with periodic stopping levels. For example, everyone starts year 1 of medicine; at year 3, those who cannot go further for one reason or another remain as "group 3 paraprofessionals." At year 5 another group falls out, until a cadre of the class goes on to become physicians and other specialists with advanced training.

### NONTRADITIONAL MEDICAL PRACTICES

I would like to make two more points with regard to the variety of professionals and paraprofessionals providing medically related services. One has to do with the kinds of health workers who are not included in the close-knit framework of medical care services as we ordinarily understand them, although they provide services we commonly associate with physicians.

OSTEOPATHY AND HOMEOPATHY

While they are growing closer to the orthodox medical profession, and in some places work together fairly closely with physicians, osteopaths are still not traditional medical practitioners. In some instances they prefer to retain their identity and keep themselves separate from orthodox medicine, but in some cases they are deliberately excluded by orthodox physicians as being inferior. It may be well to review the background of osteopathy in order to assess the position we are in now with regard to this professional group.

In the 19th century when medicine was becoming more scientific, careful physicians were encouraged not to offer any treatment that could not be established under the scientific umbrella. Consequently, doctors tended to tell patients that they knew what was wrong but that they really did not know what to do about it. Naturally, the sick patient, frightened and unhappy, would look for cure elsewhere.

Coupled with this is the observable fact that when revolutionary changes occur, all sorts of enthusiastic and ambitious people jump in with their own novel ideas, claiming new truth, since the old truth is being replaced. As scientific medicine was beginning to unsettle former established medical orthodoxy, questioning the values of the prescientific age with strange combinations of therapeutic chemicals, herbs and drugs, other forces also began to claim they had the *true* diagnostic and therapeutic knowledge.

In the United States, osteopathy developed around the idea of disease being caused by disturbances in the central nervous system. It was based on the theories of Andrew Taylor Still, who in the 1870's promulgated the doctrine of disease being the result of disorders around the nerve roots as they exit from the spinal cord. "Adjustments" directed at correcting these nerve root disorders would result in the cure of any illness. A fairly complex diagnostic and etiologic mechanism was devised as the basis for the theory and practice.

Over time, osteopaths adopted much of the formal structure of more traditional medicine and their schools attempted to develop standards of admission, education, and graduation not too different from that of medical schools. Their medicine was similar with the exception of this added "science" of causation and treatment. It was not an unfamiliar theory.

About 100 years before that, Samuel Hahnemann had introduced homeopathy as a form of disease therapy, using a Latin phrase *"similis similibus curantur"* ("like cures like"). If a certain herb produced a symptom similar to the symptom of a disease, it could be used to cure the disease, if applied in very small quantities.  For example, the redness of people who were flushed with illness ought to be treated with minute quantities of a substance that produced redness.  The dilution of the substances prescribed was so enormous that it seemed ludicrous to traditional physicians.  Oliver Wendell Holmes, in his polemic against homeopathy in the middle of the 19th century, talked about pouring a teaspoon of medicine into the Atlantic Ocean and then dipping a therapeutic dose out of the Pacific.

Over time homeopathy began to teach its students many of the same things that medical students were learning in the traditional medical schools, but with the addition of homeopathic theory.  Within the past 50 years, homeopathic schools have practically disappeared as such.

In California an osteopathic school has become absorbed into the California State Medical School system.  The title of "O.D." and the title of "M.D." are used synonymously in California.  The same event may take place in Michigan, where the state legislature has appropriated funds to build a new osteopathic school.  In some parts of the United States osteopaths may actually outnumber M.D.'s, as in the northern parts of Maine or Michigan.  It may not be too long before the 12 thousand osteopaths in the United States will be absorbed in the ranks of traditional physicians and their schools disappear as independent institutions.

The reason for this, as the reason for the disappearance of the homeopathic schools, is that science has made its way into the far corners of these formerly dissenting institutions, and overcome the irrational and unscientific aspects of their teaching.  What cannot be defended in the laboratory ceases to exist.  This has been the fate, for example, of phrenology, which was greatly popular in the 19th century.  It is said that in the 1840's the phrenologists missed by only one vote from having a chair of phrenology established at Harvard University.  The likelihood is that if it had been established at that time, there would still be such a profession today with graduate students receiving research grants from the National Institute of Health.  But phrenology has died out.  Similarly, astrology has been replaced to a very considerable degree by astronomy (although it has regained popularity lately), and alchemy has given way to modern chemistry.

Nevertheless, there is a residue of the unscientific or irrational that remains behind and to which many people return for treatment for a variety of reasons.  Some people do not trust science.  Others have diseases that traditional medicine has failed to cure or that their physician has not given enough attention to or offered appropriate treatment.  Some people are attracted to mystical and irrational beliefs.

## CHIROPRACTIC

The largest of the nonscientific groups that still provides diagnosis and therapy in place of traditional medicine is chiropractic. There are said to be 25,000 chiropractors in the United States; if each of them has in the neighborhood of 1,000 patients, which is probably accurate, the likelihood is that some 25,000,000 Americans consult a chiropractor on occasion for diagnosis and treatment.

Chiropractic considers disease to be caused by disorders of the arrangement of the vertebrae of the spine, a disorder which they characterize as "subluxation." This is a somewhat old fashioned medical term meaning displacement of one bone upon or to the side of another. In order to cure a disease, therefore, these "subluxations" have to be corrected. Chiropractors manipulate the spine in an effort to give relief and cure disease. Although no evidence has ever been presented that actual displacement of the vertebrae can be demonstrated, chiropractors verify their "diagnosis" with x rays. Radiologists have never been able to agree with the displacement theory or show that this actually exists in the x-ray pictures. However, many millions of people put their faith in chiropractors.

It is easy enough to say, as some people say of acupuncture, for example, that it is entirely a case of the individual persuading himself that he has been helped or that he was not really sick in the beginning. But this reaction is much too simple. The likelihood is, that in many instances manipulation, like massage, does have a beneficial effect and that many people are helped who were not helped by traditional methods. For those patients who have disorders in which muscles, ligaments or tendons would benefit from manipulation, as in the case of many athletes who strain or injure some part during athletic activities, the chiropractor may be of great and real benefit. Some athletic teams use chiropractors regularly and many athletes recommend them.

The fact is, however, that in some instances chiropractic can be dangerous, leading to damage or death. This has to be guarded against either by some sort of supervision and licensing or by the elimination of the practice as an independent entity. People with serious illnesses like pneumonia, diabetes or cancer will not benefit from chiropractic treatment, and the delay of traditional medicine may seriously prejudice their survival. Older people, and others with rather fragile bones, may suffer serious fractures as the result of chiropractic manipulation. A study has been undertaken by the National Institutes of Health to establish the value of chiropractic and to date the results are negative. However, under Medicaid, chiropractors can be paid; poor people who wish this kind of service or who are unable to obtain traditional medical services, can have their illnesses treated by a chiropractor who will then be reimbursed under the various state Medicaid plans as a "provider." There is a certain irony in the interpretation of the law, since it provides that if a diagnosis is made by a chiropractor, it has to be supported by an x ray read by a physician! The limitation of chiropractic activity in this way has been very sharp.

There are other nontraditional types of "medical care," including Christian Science, herbal medicine, naturopathy, hydropathy, spiritualism, the mystical practice of "spiritual surgery," and acupuncture. All have their devotees. I do not know that it is necessary to try to define or dispose of each of these nonscientific or antiscientific treatment areas, except to say that it is very likely that regardless of what society we live in, or to what degree of education the patient and the professional aspire, there will always be patients who seek help outside traditional channels. There will always be healers who will try to serve them. Since neither patient nor practitioner have been driven there by reason, reason will not serve to disestablish them.

# Chapter 7
# Education, Training and Licensing
# of Medical Personnel

---

## THE ACADEMIC APPROACH VS.
## THE TRAINING APPROACH

In order to have a better understanding of the procedures involved in patient health care, it is important to know how the personnel have been trained or educated for the job and what description they've been given of the role that they're expected to play. Everyone who becomes a specialist of any kind prepares in two ways: (1) he reads, studies and attends lectures; and (2) he is influenced by observations of the people already in the field.

If he does a lot of reading, studying and listening but doesn't have much chance to observe, then what he's told and what he reads creates an image in his mind of what is expected of him, and these built-in principles become the pattern of his behavior. This is essentially the *academic* approach.

If he doesn't read or isn't told anything at all, and he merely observes, usually he will behave according to his model. Apprentices learned this way. In most instances, this *training approach* is thought to be less desirable in professional education. If medicine as a profession and medical education require thought and judgment, unless one understands "how" and "why," one will not necessarily react suitably in complex situations. To do something without understanding *why* may not be only useless, but dangerous.

There are times, however, when it is terribly important to do just what one sees someone else doing, rather than to listen to someone describe it; doing something may be the best technique for learning how to do it. An athletic activity, for example, is much better learned by keen observation and practice than by reading about it. Learning the professional task of medical care should combine studying, observing, learning the meaning and reasons, as well as practicing for technical proficiency. Of course, the higher the level of professional skills demanded, the greater will be the

131

need for coming to an intellectual appreciation of what the intricate causes and relationships are that lead you to do one thing rather than another.

So observation and simulation are both important elements in the learning of medical procedure. In the days when the apprenticeship was the mode of medical education, for example, the apprentice learned what the doctor did and why, observed how he did it, and then went on to practice in that fashion. Of course he may have taken issue with his teacher later or put the conclusions of his observations together in some different way, but, in any case, he was doing substantially the same *things* that his teacher did. In modern medical schools, students have many role models in the ten-year period of medical school through residency training. In the beginning they may watch older students, then the interns and residents of the house staff, and ultimately the chiefs in the particular specialty, and leaders whom they choose to follow. Modeling themselves on other peoples' methods of diagnosis and treatment, and particularly on the way in which patients are treated, is an inescapable attribute of medical education. The same is undoubtedly true of nursing, if not to a greater degree. Since much more emphasis is placed on the way in which the nurse deals with the patient, the student's observations of the way in which the finished nurses deal with patients powerfully influence the way in which the student will eventually treat her patients.

In many of the technical fields, students may be taught very little about how they are to deal with patients because the major aim of the teaching program is to create technical skills. In those situations, the client, in a very subtle way, is not the patient who is receiving the technical care, but the physician who orders it. So technicians very often feel their responsibility is task-oriented rather than directly patient-related. A World War II army joke relates to this more directly: "Never mind if he's alive or dead, what does the field medical tag say?"

## TEAM TEACHING

It is often felt that if doctors, nurses, dentists, social workers and pharmacists would all take *some* of their training together, particularly when they are beginning to do the things that are necessary in dealing with patients, they would learn more through professional interchange than they are now learning from the specialized role models that they follow in carrying out their separate obligations. It is often said that good medical practice of the future will be team practice. This may or may not turn out to be true, but it seems terribly logical. So many different things have to be done to and with patients these days, by people with such a wide range of skills, that it stands to reason the work could be done much better and with a great deal more ease and simplicity if the people who were doing these things would do them cooperatively, not just sequentially.

A word might be said here about the special and growing value of the pharmacist as a member of the medical care team. Increasingly more complex medicines and chemical substances are being used for refined and delicate treatment. It is hardly possible for a physician, whether a member of the house staff or in practice, to become familiarized with all drug actions, the advances in chemistry and new drugs on the market, their side effects and contraindications. The physician is at the mercy of the drug manufacturers for what they tell him and what they concentrate on advertising to him. For the protection of the patient, the physician ought to be working more closely with the pharmacist, especially in the hospital. Educating physician and pharmacist in the same classrooms and laboratories would create a bond of understanding between them and a channel of communication later. It may rescue the doctor from unhealthy reliance on the drug manufacturers. And it may rescue the pharmacist from isolation and from becoming an instrument of the drug manufacturers.

However, some of the things that we've discussed earlier, such as the entrepreneurial philosophy of teachers; the weight of solo medical practice; the baleful influence of fee-for-service; and the autocratic, hierarchic methodology of medical practice with the doctor at the top put a fairly high price on cooperative relationships. It is very difficult to expect the doctors in training to work together with paraprofessionals on equal footing. On the other hand, one would think that in a prepaid group practice setting where fewer of these obstacles exist, a greater flow of students would be realized, and a democratic program of team practice education could be established. Too few medical schools use group practice even for teaching locations for medical students. It might offer a solution, but the powerful prejudices of the medical profession are really overwhelming. Even in prepaid group settings the various professional units will tend to work as separate enclaves, informing one another better, perhaps, but still not actually working cooperatively.

## THE PHYSICIAN'S EDUCATION

The medical school is really a forcing bed in which all kinds of pressures are applied to produce what the current profession considers to be the ideal modern physician. The expectation is that he will have a great deal of scientific background; be very much attached to the laboratory and use it extensively; will understand and use the available diagnostic tools; and be able to play rather complex games of adjusting body chemicals and physiology through medications and drugs. There is no doubt about the complexity of the doctor's task in many instances, considering the very complex and delicate procedures they must follow to cure and heal. All kinds of organs can now be removed and replaced, and chemical equilibrium reestablished through the use of various drugs and medications. Patients who once would have died as a result of pancreatic, pituitary or adrenal malfunction are now kept alive with combinations of hormones and chemicals. When organs are removed, like the stomach or intestines, replacement substances for the missing enzymes can be administered to assure normal continuation of physiological processes. The awesome nature of transplant therapy in which the patient has to be prepared with substances that will destroy his power to reject the transplant, yet not poison him, is a delicate balance.

This picture of crucial technical skills that require complex knowledge colors the whole of medical education. The medical graduate is expected to know enough to treat the most complicated conditions under the most difficult circumstances, even though the bulk of the things that he will see in his everyday practice, or even perhaps in all his lifetime of practice, may not demand it. "Readiness to serve" is one of the great distorting mirrors in medical education, practice and, consequently, medical costs. If anything can be said to be the single cause of the present dilemma in medical practice, it can be attributed to the distortion imposed by the almost religious worship of omniscience as the ultimate goal of medical education. To know more theoretically is to do better as a physician; and to know the *most* theoretically will be to do the best. A good deal of this philosophy derives from 20th century worship of science — scientific achievement and scientific potential — but some of it is inherent to medicine. Cognate with this is the concentration on technological development and production as a good unto itself for society. These are under attack now, as the danger of environmental poisoning and drying up of natural resources become issues. In medicine the worship of knowledge as the means to help people has gradually become the worship of knowledge for its own sake. Physicians are honored and rewarded with teaching positions, promotions, status, income, medals and commendations of all kinds, on the basis of what they contribute to knowledge. An Israeli Minister of Health, congratulated on the quality of the programs in one of the medical schools, grumbled, "yes, but they're all working in Sweden," a reference to their concentration on work they hoped would lead to a Nobel prize. A few achieve equivalent rewards on the basis of being "good physicians," capable of serving people well. Yet even those who are so recognized are generally in the forefront of some program for the treatment of rare, complex or difficult illnesses rather than doctors who serve "average" people in "average" need, and serve them diligently.

It is difficult to be critical of physicians for sharing what is a common American trait. Medical schools traditionally select the most talented and capable applicants in the various scientific fields; give them exceptionally fine scientific educations and magnificent laboratories in which to study and work; and reward them for producing and carrying on research activities as students. It would be foolish to expect that the product of this education would not be a laboratory-oriented, research-yearning, scientific practitioner who is somewhat impatient with the necessity of dealing with ordinary illnesses.

It is not surprising that when the great debate of the 1960's and 1970's began, as to who should be the family doctor and how and where he should be trained, very few physicians raised their voices and said with indignation, "but that's what we're all supposed to do!" For the most part they felt that creating a cadre of paraprofessionals who could carry on a great deal of what the physician didn't want to, or was overtrained for, would be a better solution than altering medical education.

## THE NURSE'S EDUCATION

When we come to nursing education and the difficulties of providing sufficient numbers of quality nurses, many of the same obstacles in doctors' medical education appear. In the first place, in addition to the scientific attitudes and requirements for more modern knowledge, there is a current necessity for putting a nurse on the same footing as a doctor. This need has several sources: resentment against doctor and general male domination, and a real need to come to terms with modern medical science, so that the nurse will understand what the doctor means or wants in order to fulfill his orders properly. More and more nurses now have to be trained or educated (or both) along some of the same lines as physicians. The effect has been to change the location, duration and status of their training. Until about 1940, the major location for nursing training was in the hospitals; it was a three-year program that took a girl out of high school and put her to work in a hospital setting where she lived a rigidly controlled existence. The student nurse worked part-time as assistant to the nurses on the ward and attended class part-time.

You will notice that we use the terms medical *education* and nurse *training;* Congress passed a "Health Professions Education Act" and a "Nurse Training Act." After the Second World War, we began to talk about nursing *education,* too. Actually the change had begun ten years earlier, led by a book by Esther Lucille Brown entitled *Nursing for the Future* that came out under the auspices of the Russell Sage Foundation. With their help and that of other foundations, the drive to collegiate education began; foundation money was used as leverage to change the pattern of nursing training, nursing education and nursing practice in the United States. If nurses were to achieve dignity and status, be "professionals" in an American degree-oriented society, they needed a degree, too.

First, the effort was made to move nursing education into the universities and establish degree programs, to augment hospital training with a college education. The early efforts were stumbling, a little complicated and expensive; and very few new programs began. Eventually, however, as a result of the many forces at work, the nursing schools in the hospitals began to be phased out and nursing *training* began to decline, while nursing *education,* college degree programs, began to increase. It was a slow process and there was a long period during which it was touch and go. The nurses who had taught in the three-year programs in the hospitals began to be phased out; hospitals who retained faculty found there were empty places for students. High school graduates didn't want to go for hospital training, which by now they considered mere indentured servitude; they wanted the freedom of college, the added status, and the greater probability of advancement in their profession.

The following tables illustrate the student populations of varying nurses' training programs, and the overall proportionate rise of registered nurses between 1960 and 1973.

TABLE 7-1: Schools of Nursing—R. N., and Number of Students and Graduates by Type of Program: Selected Years, 1960-61 through 1972-73

| | | | Graduates | | | |
|---|---|---|---|---|---|---|
| Academic year [1] | Schools | Students [2] | Total | Diploma | Associate degree | Bachelor's degree |
| 1972-73 | 1,363 | 213,127 | — | — | — | — |
| 1971-72 | 1,350 | 187,551 | 51,784 | 21,592 | 19,165 | 11,027 |
| 1970-71 | 1,343 | 164,545 | 47,001 | 22,334 | 14,754 | 9,913 |
| 1969-70 | 1,328 | 150,795 | 43,639 | 22,856 | 11,678 | 9,105 |
| 1968-69 | 1,287 | 145,588 | 42,196 | 25,114 | 8,701 | [3] 8,381 |
| 1967-68 | 2,262 | 141,948 | 41,555 | 28,197 | 6,213 | [3] 7,145 |
| 1966-67 | 1,219 | 139,070 | 38,237 | 27,452 | 4,654 | [3] 6,131 |
| 1965-66 | 1,191 | 135,702 | 35,125 | 26,278 | 3,349 | [3] 5,498 |
| 1964-65 | 1,153 | 129,269 | 34,686 | 26,795 | 2,510 | [3] 5,381 |
| 1962-63 | 1,128 | 123,861 | 32,398 | 26,438 | 1,479 | 4,481 |
| 1960-61 | 1,123 | 118,849 | 30,267 | 25,311 | 917 | 4,039 |

[1] Includes Puerto Rico for all years, the Virgin Islands for 1965-66 through 1972-73 and Guam for 1966-67 through 1972-73.
[2] Fall enrollment at beginning of academic year.
[3] Includes students in one basic program that gives a master's degree.

*Source:* National League for Nursing: *State-Approved Schools of Nursing—R.N.* New York, 1973. Published annually.
*Source: Health Resources Statistics, 1974,* Department of Health, Education and Welfare (HRA) 75-1509, p. 207.

TABLE 7-2: Registered Nurses in Relation to Population: Selected Years, 1960 through 1973

| Year [1] | Resident population in thousands [1] | Number of nurses in practice | | | Nurses per 100,000 population |
|---|---|---|---|---|---|
| | | Total | Full-time | Part-time | |
| 1973[2] | 209,118 | 815,000 | 578,000 | 237,000 | 390 |
| 1972[2] | 207,364 | 780,000 | 548,000 | 232,000 | 376 |
| 1971[2] | 205,056 | 750,000 | 534,000 | 216,000 | 366 |
| 1970[2] | 202,617 | 722,000 | 519,000 | 203,000 | 356 |
| 1969[2] | 200,985 | 694,000 | 503,000 | 191,000 | 345 |
| 1968[2] | 199,017 | 667,000 | 489,000 | 178,000 | 335 |
| 1967[2] | 196,858 | 643,000 | 476,000 | 167,000 | 327 |
| 1966 | 194,918 | 621,000 | 466,000 | 155,000 | 319 |
| 1964 | 190,169 | 582,000 | 450,050 | 131,950 | 306 |
| 1962 | 184,598 | 550,000 | 432,810 | 117,190 | 298 |
| 1960 | 178,729 | 504,000 | 413,300 | 90,700 | 282 |

[1] As of January 1.
[2] Revised preliminary estimates.

*Sources:* Interagency Conference on Nursing Statistics. U. S. Bureau of the Census: Population estimates. *Current Population Reports.* Series P-25, No. 496. Also, prior reports.

*Source: Health Resources Statistics, 1974,* Department of Health, Education and Welfare (HRA) 75-1509, p. 201.

In 1960, when there were almost 120,000 students in the various nursing training/education programs, 25,000 of the 30,000 graduating (80 percent) came from three-year hospital schools and only 4,000 (13 percent) from four-year colleges. In 1972, however, out of 52,000 graduates, only 22,000 (42 percent) were from three-year diploma schools; 11,000 (20 percent) were from four-year degree programs. The other 19,000 were a new breed called "associate degree" nurses, graduating from two-year schools of nursing based in community colleges generally. These were two-year schools, funded from both state sources and special funds from the federal government. The growth of the community college is related to the growing appetite for college degrees in an upwardly mobile society. Community colleges were generally free and near home. The rhetoric behind them was democratic — "to give every American youngster a chance to go to college" — but the practice was discriminatory, serving poor and minority students almost exclusively. Better-prepared and wealthier students went elsewhere.

Many of the technicians needed in the various hospital and health agency activities were being trained in these two-year schools — physical therapists; occupational therapists; clinical, laboratory and x-ray technicians. Two-year nursing programs were a natural addition.

There are, in addition to two-year schools for technicians, three- and four-year training programs, whose graduates are termed "technologists."

They can go on to a Ph.D. There are also one-year training programs and the graduates are usually called "certified" laboratory assistants. In the nursing field, to be granted an "R.N." one attends either a two-year school with an associate arts degree ("A.A."); a three-year hospital diploma school; or a four-year school with a bachelor of science degree in nursing. One-year nursing programs earn an "L.P.N." (Licensed Practical Nurse or, in some states, Licensed Vocational Nurse); there is also a category of "nurse's aide," who receives less training, if any at all.

All of these programs grew because we needed more nurses; graduate degrees meant fewer, particularly as the diploma schools closed. Therefore, a host of less trained and educated "para-nurses" flowed into the field. But in this movement to develop a satisfactory number of nursing personnel of various kinds, there was no accepted hierarchic arrangement; none of the people could move from one level to the next according to standard training or educational prerequisites. There was a conglomeration of different kinds of people; differently selected, differently educated, and working in different kinds of places, many of whom expected to do the same kind of work. As there were three different methods to earn an R.N. degree, as discussed in the previous paragraph, three nurses with completely different backgrounds could be given identical responsibilities and pay.

For the most part the various programs of study are not meshed together. The three-year diploma schools of nursing, for example, are generally not related to the associate arts degree schools. And these two- and three-year schools are not directly related to the four-year university programs. It is unfortunate that there cannot be more interchange between the programs; that the *practical* training of the hospital schools and the more *theoretical* four year programs of the colleges and universities cannot combine strengths. But the universities fail to take responsibility for associating themselves with the practical institutions.

An amalgamation of practice and theory would be ideal. As it is for physicians, for nurses practical skills are equally as important as the amount of theoretical knowledge. The attitude toward the practical aspect should be determined by theories learned and techniques observed.

Americans may have to learn to forgo some of their appetite for diplomas and credentials if the appropriate mix of experience, observation and theoretical education is to be adjusted for the most effective preparation of health professionals. As long as greater deference is paid to *academic* learning and the necessary *practical* aspects of patient care are relegated to second priority, there will be justified dissatisfaction by patients who find themselves in the situation of being cared for by people who understand perfectly what is being done, but have no real interest in the people for whom it is being done.

## LICENSING AND ACCREDITATION

Licensing and accreditation affect educational activities in several ways. Accreditation can mean a great deal to institutions; unaccredited institutions cannot obtain federal funds, for one thing. The power is so clear that one wonders why it hasn't been used to better effect. The licensing leverage could be used to buttress efforts to unite the various training and educational institutions so as to provide better training as well as educational opportunity.

### LICENSING THE INDIVIDUAL PROFESSIONAL

The licensing of professionals is a state responsibility. There is no national licensing agreement except in the case of individual states accepting the transfer of license on the basis of reciprocity. There is a National Board Examination which permits the doctor who passes it to qualify in *all* participating states; but this involves 46 states. This is almost the equivalent of a national licensing examination, except that it is recognized as only a substitute for the standard state examination. There is no equivalent national examination for nurses or dentists. In addition to the professional licensure there is a state "permit to practice," which is issued by a state agency; there are some 30 occupations in the health field which are so licensed. There are 13 such occupations for which all states and the District of Columbia require a license: physicians, dentists, nurses of all kinds, veterinarians, pharmacists, podiatrists, physical therapists, optometrists, dental hygienists, environmental health engineers, and embalmers. In addition, administrators of nursing homes, chiropractors, and psychologists need to be licensed in practically every state and jurisdiction.

Licensure examinations vary considerably and from time to time a state has a minor scandal involving the membership of the licensure board, with some indication that something other than qualification may allow a license to be issued. Furthermore, the licensure boards rarely take steps to monitor the quality of practitioners of medical care in the state. Revocation of a license is considered such an extraordinary step, practically the equivalent of a death sentence, that it is rarely imposed. Futhermore, even when imposed, it is rarely made a matter of public record; if it is, it will not be prominently featured in any public newspaper, but may be hidden somewhere in the administrative columns of the official organ of the local or state medical society. Clearly, the facts of licensure should not be kept as secret. When the work is carried on in such a quiet, self-effacing way, most people simply take it for granted that if someone calls himself a doctor, he is. As a consequence, many fraudulent M.D.'s have passed themselves off as true M.D.'s for many years without being caught. One recent amusing case was that of a fraudulent M.D. in New York who had passed himself off as a physician for over five years, satisfied his patients, and had even managed to admit patients to hospitals, where he enjoyed the same privileges as genuine doctors. But he made the mistake of charging Medicaid for house calls. Inasmuch as the clerks who work in the Medicaid offices are well aware of the fact that practically no physicians make house calls, they made a quick inspection of his qualifications. It turned out that he had no license and had never graduated from either college or medical school. But he did make all those house calls.

PROFESSIONAL MEMBERSHIPS

In addition to licensing, many occupations subtly require membership in the professional organization of that group. If not actually necessary, it may be advisable in order to participate fully and have the status to get an appropriate job, promotion or advancement in the profession. For example, being a member of a medical association is not an absolute requirement for a physician. But a physician will suffer certain dis-advantages if he fails to belong to his medical society. Some hospitals may bar him from staff appointment. In those states such as Oregon, where the physician is required to participate in continuing education programs in order to retain his state license, the state and local medical societies provide the courses, and it would be difficult for a physician not to be a member. Many nursing organizations actually represent nurses in bargaining with hospitals or state agencies, and nonmembership in the organization means nonrepresentation in the negotiation for better working conditions or wages.

CERTIFICATION AND BOARD QUALIFICATION

Finally, there is the matter of certification or registration for special qualifications within a profession. When one graduates from medical school and passes the licensing examination in his state, he has been licensed to "practice medicine and surgery" (as the certificate reads). But in most hospitals, unless he has the advanced qualifications to show that he is knowledgeable in surgery, for example, he will have difficulty obtaining an appointment that would allow him to practice surgery in an accredited hospital. Certification and board qualification make it possible for an individual to advance within the profession.

INSTITUTIONAL ACCREDITATION

The licensing of programs and institutions is called accreditation. Accreditation is customarily defined as the process by which an agency or organization evaluates and recognizes a program of study or an institution as meeting certain "predetermined qualifications or standards." For example, the Council of Medical Education of the American Medical Association collaborates with 28 different allied health and medical specialty organizations in the accreditation of health educational programs in schools, colleges, universities and clinical facilities, in addition to medical schools. A great deal of argument goes on among those who do the training and education as to what constitutes "institutional accreditation" as opposed to "program accreditation." Institutional accreditation means that the whole institution or university is considered to meet standards established by some accrediting agency, such as the National Accrediting Association or a regional accrediting agency. Then, any programs carried on within the university are within the accreditation. Under program accreditation, however, particular parts of an educational institution have met criteria which are usually developed by a particular profession. The profession will fight doggedly to retain the idea of program accreditation, whereas institutions and very often state agencies resist program accreditation and prefer institutional accreditation. Physicians have been powerful enough to retain program accreditation; therefore, no medical school can select or graduate students without satisfying the program accreditation standards of the Council on Medical Education.

For a long time nursing programs were accredited through the National League for Nursing, and their effort in raising standards of nursing education played a very great influence in the decline of the diploma schools and the growth of the university schools of nursing. However, when it came to the two-year associate degree programs for nursing, the program directors resisted allowing the National League for Nursing to control the content and educational activities. The states, too, resisted acknowledgment of nursing program accreditation; many states provided licensing for the graduates of associate degree programs whether or not they were accredited by the National League for Nursing. The National League retaliated by imposing national regulatory barriers, so that nurses graduated from unaccredited schools might not be able to get licensed in another state. The war still goes on, but it seems that the National League may have lost a good deal of its power in determining the accreditation of nursing schools. It may not be long before nursing education will be covered by the institutional accreditation process.

The AMA still has powerful influence in determining the accreditation of the school where medical technicians and technologists are trained. Institutional accreditation, which is fostered very stongly by the National Commission on Accrediting, has not been able to reach those professional training areas or educational activities that are still under the dominance of the medical and dental professions.

A national standard of program accreditation may make many professional skills more portable. Briefly, state licensure of graduates is so varied and complex for many occupations, that graduates of some technical programs may not be able to practice in other states. Five states have already licensed physician assistants so differently that none of them can practice in any other licensing jurisdiction.

Hospital accreditation will be discussed fully in the next chapter. Briefly, accreditation is extremely important because patient care in unaccredited institutions is not covered by Medicare. The accrediting agency, however, in the hospital field, is a private agency controlled by professional interests. Many people think that the government should play a much more important role than simply to accept the accreditation by a private agency; but to date the procedure remains.

In closing we might say that the education of those working in the health profession, regardless of overall quality, essentially suffers from two things: (1) insufficient attention to the overall goal of patient satisfaction, and (2) lack of effort to form a cohesive interchange of individual approaches and strengths.

# Chapter 8
# Hospitals and Other Institutions
# of Patient Care

The various types of facilities for the medical care of people who are sick or injured range widely in size and complexity. The best known is the hospital. Hospitals are usually divided into categories by size, type of service, ownership or sponsorship.

## HOSPITAL SIZE, SCOPE AND OWNERSHIP

Tables 8-1 and 8-2 illustrate size and type of American hospitals from 1963 to 1970. As of 1972, there were about 7500 hospitals in the United States. Of these, 6500 were general medical and surgical hospitals; about 1000 were specialty hospitals: 500 were psychiatric; and the others covered chronic disease, tuberculosis or another specialty. This classification is by type of service. The beds in these institutions were rather unevenly distributed. In that year, in those 7500 hospitals, there were 1.5 million beds. One million of them were in the 6600 general hospitals, and a half million in the 1000 specialty hospitals; of the half million beds in specialty hospitals, the greatest number (372,603) were concentrated in psychiatric hospitals. Interestingly enough, ten years ago there were almost 600,000 psychiatric hospital beds. This has been cut so dramatically because of the introduction of drug treatment, enabling patients to leave hospitals and be cared for on an ambulatory basis. This will be discussed more fully later.

Also, general hospitals vary rather widely in size. About 30 percent, or about 2,000 hospitals, have a capacity of 50 beds or less; only 3 percent have a capacity of more than a thousand. The median size is just under 100 beds. This is a rather interesting and even striking fact in a country where size is usually the measure of institutional quality. When we look at hospitals in respect to the ratio to population, there were nearly 7 beds per thousand people in North Dakota and just about 3.6 per thousand in Maryland.

From the standpoint of sponsorship, there are public hospitals, private voluntary hospitals (nonprofit), and proprietary, profit-making hospitals.

TABLE 8-1:   Hospitals and Hospital Beds: Selected Years 1963 through 1972

| Year | Total hospitals | General medical and surgical | Specialty | | | | |
| | | | Total | Psychi-atric | Chronic disease | Tubercu-losis | Other [1] |
| --- | --- | --- | --- | --- | --- | --- | --- |
| | | | Facilities | | | | |
| 1972.............. | [2] 7,481 | 6,491 | 990 | 497 | 78 | 75 | 340 |
| 1971.............. | [3] 7,678 | 6,607 | 1,071 | 533 | 90 | 99 | 349 |
| 1970.............. | 7,638 | 6,574 | 1,064 | 494 | 126 | 108 | 336 |
| 1969.............. | 7,845 | 6,715 | 1,130 | 506 | 189 | 116 | 319 |
| 1968.............. | 7,991 | 6,539 | 1,452 | 494 | 291 | 129 | 538 |
| 1967.............. | 8,147 | 6,685 | 1,462 | 573 | 333 | 169 | 387 |
| 1963.............. | 8,183 | 6,710 | 1,473 | 581 | 211 | 258 | 423 |
| | | | Beds | | | | |
| 1972.............. | [2] 1,467,040 | 1,014,064 | 452,976 | 372,603 | 23,962 | 12,351 | 44,060 |
| 1971.............. | [3] 1,507,988 | 1,004,799 | 503,189 | 418,487 | 24,614 | 17,806 | 42,282 |
| 1970.............. | 1,534,779 | 1,004,415 | 530,364 | 437,969 | 38,144 | 19,836 | 34,415 |
| 1969.............. | 1,565,908 | 989,733 | 576,175 | 477,309 | 40,790 | 20,960 | 37,116 |
| 1968.............. | 1,564,444 | 934,297 | 630,147 | 503,042 | 43,921 | 25,381 | 57,803 |
| 1967.............. | 1,631,101 | 958,729 | 672,372 | 545,913 | 61,211 | 33,335 | 31,913 |
| 1963.............. | 1,549,952 | 811,876 | 738,076 | 614,104 | 38,213 | 50,074 | 35,685 |
| | | | Beds per 1,000 population | | | | |
| 1972.............. | [2] 7.0 | 4.9 | 2.2 | 1.8 | 0.1 | 0.1 | 0.2 |
| 1971.............. | [3] 7.4 | 4.9 | 2.5 | 2.0 | 0.1 | 0.1 | 0.2 |
| 1970.............. | 7.6 | 5.0 | 2.6 | 2.2 | 0.2 | 0.1 | 0.2 |
| 1969.............. | 7.8 | 5.0 | 2.9 | 2.4 | 0.2 | 0.1 | 0.2 |
| 1968.............. | 7.9 | 4.7 | 3.2 | 2.5 | 0.2 | 0.1 | 0.3 |
| 1967.............. | 8.3 | 4.9 | 3.4 | 2.8 | 0.3 | 0.2 | 0.2 |
| 1963.............. | 8.3 | 4.3 | 4.0 | 3.3 | 0.2 | 0.3 | 0.2 |

[1] Includes eye, ear, nose, and throat hospitals; epileptic hospitals; alcoholism hospitals; narcotic hospitals; maternity hospitals; orthopedic hospitals; physical rehabilitation hospitals; and other hospitals.
[2] Preliminary data.
[3] Revised.

*Sources:* Unpublished data from the National Center for Health Statistics Master Facility Census. U. S. Bureau of the Census: *Current Population Reports.* Series P-25, No. 500, May 1973.

*Source: Health Resources Statistics, 1974,* Department of Health, Education and Welfare (HRA) 75-1509, p. 350.

More than half of all the beds in general hospitals (880,000) are in non-profit establishments; a little under half of all hospital beds (600,000) are in federal, state or local government hospitals. There are only 70,000 beds in proprietary hospitals. State and local hospitals represent 75 percent of the government-owned hospitals; only 140,000 beds are in 400 federal hospitals. And local urban public hospitals represent 214,000 beds in the United States. (See Table 8-3.)

TABLE 8-2: Bed Size of Hospitals: 1972

| Bed size | Total hospitals[1] | General medical and surgical | Specialty | | | | |
|---|---|---|---|---|---|---|---|
| | | | Total | Psychi-atric | Chronic disease | Tuber-culosis | Other[2] |
| Total ........................ | 7,481 | 6,491 | 990 | 497 | 78 | 75 | 340 |
| 6-24 ................................. | 571 | 483 | 88 | 13 | 2 | 3 | 70 |
| 25-49 ............................... | 1,561 | 1,441 | 120 | 48 | 4 | 5 | 63 |
| 50-74 ............................... | 1,036 | 913 | 123 | 42 | 10 | 13 | 58 |
| 75-99 ............................... | 766 | 676 | 90 | 39 | 3 | 11 | 37 |
| 100-199 ........................... | 1,506 | 1,335 | 171 | 72 | 21 | 19 | 59 |
| 200-299 ........................... | 753 | 674 | 79 | 33 | 15 | 12 | 19 |
| 300-499 ........................... | 707 | 633 | 74 | 38 | 12 | 11 | 13 |
| 500-999 ........................... | 378 | 288 | 90 | 67 | 6 | 1 | 16 |
| 1,000 beds or more ........... | 203 | 48 | 155 | 145 | 5 | — | 5 |

[1] Preliminary data.

[2] Includes eye, ear, nose, and throat hospitals; epileptic hospitals; alcoholism hospitals; narcotic hospitals; maternity hospitals; orthopedic hospitals; physical rehabilitation hospitals; and other hospitals.

*Source:* Unpublished data from the National Center for Health Statistics Master Facility Census.

*Source: Health Resources Statistics, 1974,* Department of Health, Education and Welfare (HRA) 75-1509, p. 357.

TABLE 8-3: Ownership of Hospitals: 1972

| Ownership | Total hospitals[1] | General medical and surgical | Specialty | | | | |
|---|---|---|---|---|---|---|---|
| | | | Total | Psychi-atric | Chronic disease | Tubercu-losis | Other[2] |
| Total ........................ | 7,481 | 6,491 | 990 | 497 | 78 | 75 | 340 |
| Government .................... | 2,770 | 2,248 | 522 | 328 | 49 | 70 | 75 |
| Federal .......................... | 405 | 369 | 36 | 29 | — | — | 7 |
| State-local .................... | 2,365 | 1,879 | 486 | 299 | 49 | 70 | 68 |
| Proprietary .................... | 986 | 811 | 175 | 88 | 8 | — | 79 |
| Nonprofit ...................... | 3,725 | 3,432 | 293 | 81 | 21 | 5 | 186 |
| Church .......................... | 854 | 797 | 57 | 14 | 5 | 1 | 37 |
| Other ............................ | 2,871 | 2,635 | 236 | 67 | 16 | 4 | 149 |

[1] Preliminary data.

[2] Includes eye, ear, nose, and throat hospitals; epileptic hospitals; alcoholism hospitals; narcotic hospitals; maternity hospitals; orthopedic hospitals; physical rehabilitation hospitals; and other hospitals.

*Source:* Unpublished data from the National Center for Health Statistics Master Facility Census.

*Source: Health Resources Statistics, 1974,* Department of Health, Education and Welfare (HRA) 75-1509, p. 365.

About 33 million people were admitted to general hospitals in 1973 (the last year for which complete data are available), or about 158 admissions per 1,000 population.  On any day there would be just under 800,000 people in hospitals in the United States.  Figures for short-term stays in general hospitals are more important because they indicate the scope of general medical and surgical care.  People stay in those hospitals on an average of seven to ten days.  In the 500 psychiatric hospitals, very largely state hospitals, there are about 370,000 patients on any day.

## HOSPITAL COSTS

Hospitals represent the largest single element of medical care costs, almost 40 percent of the total medical care bill, about 40 billion dollars a year.  In addition, hospitals represent the fastest growing and largest inflationary element in medical care costs, per-patient-day expenses having gone up from $15/day in 1950 to $105/day in 1972 in the community (nonprofit) hospitals.  Present annual rate of hospital cost increase is better than 14 percent; this leads other medical care costs, which are rising at a rate of less than 10 percent, and doubles the rate of rise of the whole cost of living index.

The major reason for this is thought to be the fact that hospitals are reimbursed on a cost-plus basis; that is, they are reimbursed on what they have spent; either by the private insurance company, the government or the individual patient; based on accounting reports of expenditures.  It is not considered appropriate to allow hospitals to go bankrupt, nor is it possible for hospitals to operate at a deficit; quality of care might have to be compromised and services fail to be of a level necessary for adequate patient care.

Because cost of hospital operations is such a very large element of medical care costs, hospital beds per thousand population of each state will vary according to state capability or willingness to meet costs.  Again, poor and rural people will necessarily have less access to general medical and surgical, psychiatric and chronic disease hospital beds.  It may be less important to have easy access to the psychiatric, chronic disease and tuberculosis hospitals, so they need not necessarily be allocated by region; but general hospital beds certainly need to be readily accessible. One of the serious problems of funding hospitals at present is the need for hospitals in diverse locations accompanied by the inability to staff them.

Why are hospitals so expensive, and why are hospital costs rising at an extraordinarily greater rate than the general rate of inflation? Many explanations are offered, ranging from corruption (deals between board members and administration), simple mismanagement, skewed insurance benefits driving people into hospitals for unnecessary care, professional negligence in appropriate admission and discharge and careless supervision of reimbursement.

## PERSONNEL COSTS

About 66 percent of hospital costs relate to personnel; much emphasis on exploring cost controls is directed at this. There is a peculiar, even unique, quality to American hospitals, quite different from that of hospitals in other countries, in the extraordinary numbers of people employed. More than half of the total American health labor force (2.6 million people) is employed in general hospitals, as is illustrated in the following table.

TABLE 8-4: Employees in General Hospitals, 1972

|  | Total employees | Full-time employees (35 hours or more) | Part-time employees (less than 35 hours) | Full-time employees per average daily patient | Full-time equivalents per average daily patient |
|---|---|---|---|---|---|
| United States[1]........... | 2,621,558 | 2,108,325 | 513,233 | 2.8 | 3.1 |

*Source:* Unpublished data from the National Center for Health Statistics Master Facility Census.
*Source: Health Resources Statistics, 1974,* Department of Health, Education and Welfare (HRA) 75-1509, p. 371.

And this number has grown over the past ten years so that in full-time equivalents in 1972 there were 3.1 persons working per hospital bed! Some of the rationalization is that recurring introduction of new and complex equipment for diagnosis and treatment multiplies need for new people. But some of this undoubtedly has to do with the fact that as long as there will be cost-plus reimbursement, there will be no incentive for hospital administrators to devise novel and skillful ways of dealing with management problems, except by hiring more people. Then, as unions and civil service become the mode, it becomes impossible to introduce management efficiency by reducing staff. Without appropriate management controls and the reduction of the full-time equivalents for daily patient care, it is highly unlikely that there will be any significant change in the rapidly rising cost of hospitalization. Salvation may come through the reduction of patient admissions, by improving ambulatory and more comprehensive outpatient activity, but it is hardly likely that it will be improved by reduction in the numbers of people employed in the institutions.

## THE EFFECT OF HOSPITALIZATION INSURANCE

About 65 percent of all hospital costs are paid by third-party payers: private insurance companies, Medicaid, Medicare and Blue Cross. The patient doesn't have a real feel for what costs are because he isn't involved in paying for the whole of the specific elements. It is very much like the kind of automatic steering in which the driver doesn't feel the road. He doesn't really know what is going on and it is hard for him to be able to exercise full control. That is why some economists have urged that patients should pay their bills and then be reimbursed. At least the institutions would have to itemize the charges. Under the current system, charges are arbitrarily assigned and the costs that have to be paid bear no relationship to what the actual costs are to the institution. The insurance companies have agreed to these quasi-fraudulent methods of preparing bills in order to simplify record keeping and create a more uniform way of developing payment mechanisms. If there is to be effective hospital management, it will have to be on the basis of the assignment of real costs and real charges. Insurance companies have no incentive to institute rigid controls on institutions to prevent duplication of extravagance. The cost and charging mechanisms hide rather than reveal the ways in which duplications and extravagances exaggerate the inflationary trend in hospital costs.

This lack of effective control is demonstrated in many ways. For instance, it was pointed out that staff to patient ratio in hospitals has risen by 25 percent, from 2.3:1 to 3.1:1 over the past 20 years, while the number of beds has increased in the same period by less than 15 percent; even more interestingly, daily bed use has *declined* by almost 15 percent! No one attempts to rationalize these matters, or to create interhospital communication systems so that patients could be placed in available beds as they need them, wherever empty beds exist. In part this is because hospitals are unequally supplied and staffed, so that people may have good reason to want to be hospitalized in one hospital rather than in another. It is also because physicians don't have privileges in all institutions; if you want *your* physician you have to go to the hospital where he works. Popular hospitals have to increase the number of their beds, regardless of what the bed situation is in the rest of the city. Unpopular hospitals can't be taken out of circulation, because the community might demand that the hospital remain and, more powerfully, because the workers in them don't want to lose their employment. There will continue to be very serious problems of these kinds, no matter what the national health insurance program will be, unless rigid control is undertaken of hospital costs and charges, staff and admission. The great benefit of a unified federal program of hospital insurance would be the possibility of applying effective pressure to these management matters.

There is a wide variation in the full-time equivalents per average daily patient from state to state. The lowest number, 2.6, is in West Virginia; and other poor states, like Maine, Alabama, South Carolina and South Dakota, also have a low ratio. A few other states that are not as poor (Minnesota, New Jersey, Nebraska) also have a low ratio. Studies of staffing policies and patterns of administrative action in these states might be useful for other states to follow.

There is no doubt that the extremely high personnel costs and associated poor management policies are the leading causative factors of high costs, but the other factors mentioned all contribute to the maintenance of the high daily costs; attention to them might keep the costs down significantly. If the insurance companies and Blue Cross, in their direct role as insurors and as intermediaries for the federal government in Medicare reimbursement, were to demand meticulous cost accounting, the lax charging and easy hiring and salary practices might be controlled. Some New York hospital administrators, for example, receive $100,000 or more per year in income, plus prerequisites equal to nearly 50 percent more and have staffs of 30 to 40 assistants.

## PROFESSIONAL IRRESPONSIBILITY — PHYSICIAN AND HOSPITAL ADMINISTRATOR

Professional irresponsibility is also to blame in no small part. Physicians admit patients who do not require hospitalization for many reasons, some of them quasi-honorable, as in sparing the patient outpatient costs that customary health insurance does not cover. But it is easier to look after ten patients in the hospital than to look after them in the office: laboratory, x ray, house staff supervision and nursing services substitute for the doctor's office overhead. Teaching and research activities that occupy a portion of the time create added hospital personnel costs, as do various diagnostic and therapeutic activities; patient care costs are thus inflated, sometimes unnecessarily. And manpower doesn't try to separate out costs when billing, particularly when the intermediary payers do not look too closely at the charges. Bitter disputes with government agencies over methods of reimbursement and charges for teaching staff in clinical work are constant.

The "Friday to Monday" holiday schedule in hospital operating rooms is a contributing factor to extra costs. Informed management may help that. But also contributing is the duplication of facilities occasioned by hospital rivalry and competition. Some of this derives from neighborhood demands and lack of effective transportation, but the rest is from the pressures of hospital staff physicians who want everything possible concentrated in the hospital in which *they* work, because they might lose income otherwise. Since the physician cannot admit his patient to every hospital, and since the physician's income depends on the payment made by the patient (or his intermediary), this type of "empire building" is understandable, but not to be condoned. Duplication of expensive facilities and large numbers of specially trained personnel for rarely performed procedures is unconscionably extravagant. Perhaps more important is the fact that rarely performed procedures are rarely performed well; it is in the patient's interest that highly specialized providers be concentrated rather than dispersed to assure continued expertise of one *central* specialty team rather than dispersed mediocrity.

Aside from lack of effective supervision, the matter of hospital management inefficiency has sociological ramifications. I don't believe the conflict of interest pattern is a terribly important cause of hospital cost inflation. It is probably true that the items sold, legal services and interest free bank accounts, from which hospital board members benefit personally, add up to millions of dollars in excess costs. But *billions* are drained off in the other ways mentioned. Public hospitals suffer from bureaucratic inertia and underfunding. Proprietary hospitals share costs and inflate charges to make profits. Community hospitals are largely the victims of tension from professional pressures: doctors' demands for equipment, supplies and a service personnel; clinical overhead for laboratory and x-ray services and expensive medications; research use of facilities, personnel, equipment, and supplies; salaries for physicians who do not perform necessarily clinical activities. And these pressures are added to the management inefficiencies mentioned previously.

COSTS AND COMMUNITY ACCOUNTABILITY

The basic problem of costs in community hospitals is the lack of community accountability. The boards of these hospitals are self-perpetuating, their seats handed down from the days when wealthy members of the community philanthropically donated to keep hospitals going, before the federal government came in to pay all residual debts of nonpaying patients. Without accountability, management is bound to be loose, if not careless. Very few people, in this case very few administrators, are so driven by their conscience that they will do everything necessary, in rigid compliance with the rules, if they are unattended and unaccountable. And if the accountability is represented *only* by a few wealthy board members, who might be good friends or patients remote from the day-to-day operations of the institution, the accountability can be ludicrously inadequate. I have seen situations in which the board member-hospital administrator relationship is not one of employer-employee, but of indulgent father-ambitious son, and even worshipper-deity! The public needs open and full accounting by objective and knowledgeable representatives. "Informed consent" is probably as important here as in research on human subjects.

## THE EFFECTS OF SPONSORSHIP

We should now make an effort to sort out what differences there are in the way institutions react as a result of sponsorship, to community responsibility, for example; and how this affects these institutions in terms of funding, staffing, quality, and community support.

### FEDERAL

The federal hospitals, small in number and relatively few in beds compared to other hospitals, discharge the nation's responsibility toward particular groups; for example, the 169 veterans' hospitals discharge our obligation to those who suffer in consequence of having served in the armed forces. We still have patients being looked after who served in the Spanish-American War in 1898. There are periods of neglect and periods of intense absorption in the problem, but by and large since the Civil War, the United States has attempted to carry out this obligation.

There was a brief period of close attention to veterans' problems after World War I, but this soon faded and veterans' hospitals became seedy boarding homes of inferior care and attention. After World War II the veterans' hospitals gave the United States a model of how a public hospital could deliver good medical care, with a different way of organizing services, administration and even research. As a result of President Truman's concern, General Bradley's wisdom, and Dr. Paul Magnusson's energy, enthusiasm and intelligence, a magnificent system of veterans' hospitals was created in the late 1940's and early 1950's. The quality and intensity of care was raised not only through a massive building program, but through associations with teaching hospitals and medical schools ("Deans Committees") for staffing. For a long time the veterans' hospitals continued to provide model medical care. But there has been a recent perceptible decrease in quality, concern and professionalism, partly because of the way in which teaching hospitals and medical schools have tended to turn their attention away from matters of direct patient care concern, and partly because Congress has reduced its funding and concern to pay attention to other things, like the Vietnam War. There may be a recurrence of interest as a result of stimulus from the veterans of the Vietnam War; the end of that war; and a change in the composition of Congress. The outlook is not good. The Vietnam War was unpopular and the veterans have exhibited a radically reformist attitude toward the benevolence of government. An economic depression, inflation and preoccupation with other matters may jeopardize congressional actions toward improvement of veterans' care.

STATE

State hospitals tend to be almost entirely psychiatric institutions. These have been pest houses for hundreds of years, although periodically reformers attack the inhumane conditions. As early as 1848, Dorothea Dix (19th century reformer of prisons, hospitals, and mental institutions) tried to reform the "snake pits" with some modest success. There were similar periodic movements of reform after that. "Moral treatment" was a slogan of the 1880's. In the 1950's we attempted again to transform mental hospitals into humane institutions, but currently they are sinking back into their former desuetude. Fortunately, fewer people are remaining in the mental hospitals. Unfortunately, we are not doing enough to aid those who are discharged or those who are never admitted, but need care.

The major problem is that most people are afraid of mental illness; since we know so little of its cause, the fear is like that of leprosy in ancient times. The mentally sick are distortions of the norm or the ideal, and the average person doesn't even want to look at them. Some mental hospitals are built as far away as possible from the rest of society. Even if they are in the centers of cities, they have barred entrances and windows. Relatives cease visiting; city officials tend not to check what's going on; doctors and nurses don't want to work there. The attendants and orderlies who do take jobs there tend to become callous. The physicians who gravitate into the institutions tend to be foreign medical graduates, by and large, who cannot get by the state licensing examinations because their credentials are inferior or they are not competent in the English language. The language and cultural difficulties increase and exaggerate the distance between the doctor and the patient. The state legislatures appropriate proportionately less money as inflation mounts; so the institutions decay, the living situation deteriorates, patients are lost and hopeless. The major contribution of drug therapy has been to reduce the numbers of people left in these institutions; however, the condition for those who remain there is very bad.

PUBLIC

The urban public hospitals, which represent the general institutions for care to which the minorities and poor must go, at one time were important contributors to medical care. They began as alms houses, and were converted into organized institutions for the care of the sick poor in the 19th century. Local physicians once took pride in providing services as part of their contribution to social betterment and discharge of their Hippocratic obligation.

As medicine began to become a more scientific profession in the 20th century, the public hospitals became the featured setting for teaching and research in disease. Young physicians clamored to be associated with public hospitals. Despite the fact that these hospitals were inadequately funded by the city, physicians were so eager to play their part in the scientific revolution of medicine that they served without pay, giving much of their time to patient care, to study and to teaching. The students preferred to take their internship or residency training there, because of the educational opportunities, and were pleased to serve with little pay or compensation. All that has changed.

The urban public hospital today is as sick as its patients. Students tend to take their internships and residencies in voluntary and teaching hospitals, because the great teachers and research opportunities are there; or at federal hospitals to fulfill military or federal loan obligations. Practicing physicians don't have the time, or won't spend the time, to work in public hospitals. More and more foreign medical graduates are employed there under salary, to provide the needed services. As inflation boosts the costs, and as the sickest and poorest gravitate to these institutions, the city fathers find themselves strangled by mounting debts and consequently decrease the budgets for the institutions. By a variety of devices the city fathers either sequester or divert the Medicare and Medicaid reimbursements, so that the city hospitals are deprived of legitimate income that might salvage them; soon they deteriorate. In the meantime the sickest and the poorest patients continue to be admitted. Despite the large numbers of personnel associated with these institutions, the care that is given tends to be less than optimal.

The role of the city hospital needs to be reexamined, but the solution often put forth by the voluntary hospitals, that the city hospitals should be abolished, would be to throw the poor patients on the mercy of the well-to-do hospitals that have long neglected and scorned them. There is little hope that poor people will receive any better care or consideration when they come to be cared for as part of the voluntary hospital system. As the Medicaid program has now caused some physicians to create two levels of medical care, setting up so-called "Medicaid Clinics" to see Medicaid clients at different times than their regular patients, voluntary hospitals will probably do the same. Simply to abandon the urban public hospital is to abandon the poor.

On the other hand, those who claim that we should give up the voluntary hospital system and make all hospitals public hospitals, have to come to grips with realities. When the city is responsible, the lack of an adequate tax base that is destroying cities in the United States will destroy the city hospitals, too. If there is to be public control, it cannot be on the city tax base. There will have to be strong federal and state support. Under such a federal hospital system as the Canadians adopted in the 1960's, in which inhospital charges were all that were funded, there is the danger of gathering in even the sick in need of ambulatory care. The pump effect will be to inflate the system enormously in size and cost. However, it may be a most effective step in the direction of a national health service (as it was in Canada), and so it should be seriously considered. Certainly the urban public hospital is not serving its constituency well enough; and it will *not* serve them well so long as it is in competition with the voluntary sector for staff and funds, and has to rely on a city tax base for support.

It should be noted that in some parts of the South the public hospitals rely on a county tax base or a hospital tax base, similar to the school tax base. However, since the well-to-do live in counties outside the urban area, the public hospital tax districts in states like Louisiana and Texas are unable to support the hospitals any more adequately than urban communities. Rural poor under such circumstances suffer the same disadvantages the urban poor do. If there is a solution to this dilemma it may be found in the large and basic solution to the overall medical care dilemma — a constructive effort to obtain equity in the delivery of medical care.

Once adequate national resources are put to work in a unified hospital medical care system, the need to juggle priorities for veterans' hospitals, urban public hospitals, rural county or district hospitals and psychiatric hospitals will evaporate. And at the same time, the reduction in administrative and professional staff time to maintain medical records, insurance cross references and billings may cut the overhead greatly. We can't even guess how much more a disorganized, multiple system with its multiple staffs and record keeping amounts to in- inefficiency and administrative costs.

## NURSING INSTITUTIONS FOR THE ELDERLY

### SIZE AND SCOPE

Beyond the 1.6 million beds in 7,500 hospitals in the United States, there are 22,000 institutions and related "homes" for elderly nursing care. This represents about 64 percent of the inpatient health facilities in the United States. These 22,000 facilities had 1.2 million beds in 1972, and the variation in their quality is far greater than the variation in hospital quality. Although nursing home quality and scope of operation was discussed at length in Chapter 4, some details are worth repeating in a general discussion on health care facilities, particularly as a comparison to public and private hospital care, and the other alternative, supervised home care.

With the passage of the Social Security Act Amendments of 1965, providing Medicare and Medicaid, the nursing home industry boomed. The total number of all kinds of these institutions went from 16,000 to more than 22,000 between 1963 and 1971; *nursing care institutions* grew from 8,000 to 13,000, *personal care homes* (without nursing) from 3,000 to 5,300. The total number of beds in these institutions doubled from 568,000 to 1,200,000. This is illustrated in Table 8-5.

TABLE 8-5:   Number and Beds in Nursing Care and Related Homes: Selected Years 1963 through 1971

| Type of nursing care | Number of homes | | | Number of beds | | |
|---|---|---|---|---|---|---|
| | 1963 | 1969 | ¹1971 | 1963 | 1969 | ¹1971 |
| Total.................... | 16,701 | 18,910 | 22,004 | 568,560 | 943,876 | 1,201,598 |
| Nursing care.............. | 8,128 | 11,484 | 12,871 | 319,224 | 704,217 | 917,707 |
| Personal care homes with nursing........... | 4,958 | 3,514 | 3,568 | 188,306 | 174,874 | 192,347 |
| Personal care homes without nursing ...... | 2,927 | 3,792 | 5,369 | 48,962 | 63,532 | 88,317 |
| Domiciliary care......... | 688 | 120 | 196 | 12,068 | 1,253 | 3,227 |

¹ Revised.

*Source:* Unpublished data from the National Center for Health Statistics Master Facility Census.

*Source: Health Resources Statistics, 1974,* Department of Health, Education and Welfare (HRA) 75-1509, p. 383.

However, there are variations by state and region. Out of the 5,700 "skilled nursing homes" (eligible for Medicare reimbursement), California has the largest amount (1,200). In the United States there are approximately 58 nursing home beds for every thousand in the population aged 65 or over; Minnesota has about 100, West Virginia has about 20.

Homes vary in size. Sixty percent have fewer than 60 beds. Whereas only 12 percent of hospitals are proprietary and 5 percent of hospital beds are in proprietary institutions, 78 percent of nursing homes and 67 percent of all their beds are privately owned and operated for profit. Only 16 percent of all homes are voluntary and nonprofit.

THE PROFIT MOTIVE

This has created many difficulties; operation for profit in the health field usually means either the patient overpays in order to guarantee the profit, or the provider undercuts the services. As a consequence, there have been many scandals concerning the nursing home business during the past 20 years. Mary Adelaide Mendelson's *Tender Loving Greed* relates a web of sad, shocking and horrifying stories about what takes place in nursing homes as a result of the corruption, greed and inhumanity of proprietary nursing home operators. They multiply their profits and amass fortunes over the suffering bodies of the sick and helpless, dying old people who are in their "care." In many instances they starve them by supplying insufficient food of miserable quality, often tainted and discarded by the processors. They fail to provide them with adequate supervision, so that they may fall out of bed, fail to get their medication and develop bed sores from lack of being moved, cleaned or treated. They lie in their own filth, fall down closed stair wells where they're not found for weeks until the odor drives people to look for them. Unsafe homes are the rule, without elevators or safety precautions; home after home has burned down, incinerating the occupants. Why the American people tolerate this is difficult to understand. The media exposés of the scandals last a few days and then are forgotten, to be rediscovered by new investigators the following year.

### THE LICENSING PROCESS

It is true that through state licensing programs nursing homes are presumably inspected and licensed. In some instances, however, licensure is only a very superficial action and concerns itself with attending physicians and not to the quality of the overall care. In other instances, as a result of collusion between the nursing home administrator, the owner and the presumed licensing supervisor, many of the unsafe characteristics that would fail to meet criteria are waived and the institutions continue to operate long after they should have been disqualified. Because court cases are so long in being tried, in some instances when state health departments try to close inadequate or unsafe institutions, court orders restrain implementation and closures are held in abeyance. Justice delayed is obviously justice denied. Further, in many instances state regulations are inconsistent or contradictory because they come from different agencies, such as the Veterans' Administration, Medicare and Medicaid. Because they have different definitions of care, they exercise different degrees of control.

Until people are truly concerned as to what is happening to their relatives in these institutions, and until the profit motive is removed, it is hardly likely that the situation will be improved. It also would seem, in a nation that supposedly worships the work ethic, that these old people who have spent their lives at work deserve some dignity and respect in the care they get in their last years. Failure to look after the old appropriately in these nursing homes is really the shame of the states.

It should be pointed out in connection with this that 567,000 people are employed full-time in providing care to the million people in nursing homes. This is slightly less than one attendant for every two people, as compared with more than three per patient in hospitals. It is perfectly reasonable that there should be more people looking after the much sicker people in hospitals, but it is unlikely that a ratio of one attendant to every two patients in nursing homes is satisfactory.

### HOME CARE AS AN ALTERNATIVE

While the effort to improve nursing homes is as important as it is in mental hospitals, as much effort should be devoted to keeping people *out* of nursing homes as out of mental hospitals. Programs of home care are beginning to replace some of these inadequate and inappropraite institutional facilities. For a long time it has been known that the development of comprehensive supervised community programs of care in the home could provide highly adequate alternatives to institutional care. In many instances, it was not the *patient's* needs that mandated institutional admission. Many families, however reluctantly, would have to place an aged relative in an institution such as a nursing home or hospital ward because no one at home could or would look after the patient. In other instances, because of the kind of illness, it would not be possible for someone without medical training to give proper care. However, if there were some community resource, whereby some of the skills needed could be brought to the family from time to time; if nurses could come to give bed baths and injections, doctors could pay visits, social workers add counseling, and some central records be kept; it might not be necessary to keep a patient in a hospital or nursing home. Such home care activities at the Montefiore Hospital in New York City from the 1940's on (discussed in Chapter 4) demonstrated conclusively that this was both feasible and totally adequate. The patients did as well, if not better, at home and all the needed care was provided at far less cost than in hospitals.

However, the solo fee-for-service system; general lack of a team operation in ambulatory care; and the cost-plus reimbursement of hospitals have made it impossible to provide the incentives for introducing home care on a large scale in the United States. The Medicare provision, which allowed for at least 100 days of home health services after hospitalization did offer some incentive. The visiting nurse and various other nursing agencies throughout the country began to gear up to try to provide some of the needed services. However, because services even under Medicare were reimbursed fee-for-service, the incentive for a team operation was lacking; consequently, the true comprehensive type of home care never really got going. In 1973, there were about 2500 home care programs in the United States; but they varied all the way from comprehensive services to some rather simple basic combinations of health supervision and nursing. Only 230 were hospital-based programs that provided the entire spectrum of care required.

Current estimates show that home care costs about 25 percent of what hospital or nursing home care costs. This may vary from one part of the country to another, but it stands to reason that when a good deal of the hospital housekeeping overhead can be met by the family, costs will reduce considerably. Another cost sharing element provided is that those who are engaged professionally in home visiting are spending only a part of the time on any patient and can therefore see many more patients during the day than they would if they were taking care of one patient all day in an institution. The greatest objection or fear on the part of families in considering home care is that the patient may be abandoned to them. In some bureaucratic programs, such as some state psychiatric services, the patients are discharged from hospitals presumably to community care facilities, but no effort has been made to develop these facilities. The poor patient is lost without supervision. Some people see this happening in large-scale comprehensive home care programs for the elderly. It is possible, of course, but not likely if comprehensive home care programs would be restricted to small units of limited numbers of people in clearly designated geographic areas.

The patients like home care better than hospital care, the families lose the guilt that they usually feel for having hospitalized or institutionalized relatives, and the community benefits from the lower costs. There hardly seems to be any excuse for not introducing home care on a large scale all over the country. Many congressmen have become aware of the capabilities of home care as a substitute for institutional care. It is not unlikely that future legislation will include special incentives for the development of comprehensive home care services, to make it possible to create combined team care to relieve institutions and possibly to eliminate the need for proprietary nursing homes altogether.

## SUMMARY

Many of the issues raised about hospitals and nursing homes are really generic issues relating to the way in which the system now operates and the philosophy of medical care as it is now constituted. As long as the elements of the system — hospitals, physicians, the variety of other medical manpower, nursing homes, mental institutions — all see themselves as competing entities, operating almost independently and grumbling about the lack of social responsibility or priority for *other* elements, the system will fail to operate efficiently or effectively. Hospital administrators and hospital boards see themselves as responsible for the maintenance of their individual institution. Under such circumstances they will do whatever has to be done to maintain the integrity of that institution without regard to what happens to the rest of the hospitals or the rest of the system. What we see as bad *social* management in the larger view, may be from the short-sighted viewpoint of the particular hospital administration: "good business," "excellent management" or "sensible behavior." Despite the fact that hospitals are built with public money and have overall public responsibility, their basic response in most instances is to their individual requirements.

In a very comprehensive and thoughtful series of essays in the *Washington Post* in 1972, Ronald Kessler, an investigator-reporter, laid out a series of problems as they affected hospitals in the Washington, D. C. area. The headlines of his articles were undoubtedly purposely sensational, but they do offer a litany on the nature of this individualistic defect in social concern which lies at the heart of much of our medical care system problems:

> "Abuses Pad Costs of Hospital Center Care"
> "Hospital Quietly Raised Rates Before Announcing Cost Cuts"
> "Conflicts of Interest Mark Hospital Center Management"
> "Hospital Center Officials Use Connection to Reap Profits"
> "Pathologists Paid a Percentage of the Profit in Departments — making $200,000 a Year"
> "Some Hospital Center Anesthesiologists are Criticized — Accidents in Anesthesia"
> "Children's New Building Most Costly"
> "Experts Question $50 Million Cost of Children's Building"
> "Too Many Empty Beds Cause Children's Hospital Deficit"
> "System Lacks Public Control"
> "Lack of Controls Leads to Nepotism in Hospital Contracts."

The story of the Washington hospitals is one that might be repeated in any large city in the United States; it may not be true of the small cities in which one or two hospitals serve a population. But even there some of the accusations would undoubtedly apply. And as Kessler points out in his essays, there aren't any laws to compel an institution to make its dealings or finances public. As a consequence, it becomes very difficult to sort out what would be good for the community, the medical care system and the hospital to balance constructively what needs to be done. It is hard to find out whether institutions suffer from bad management, whether they deliberately refuse to take advantage of cost-cutting ways of delivering services, and why as institutions they fail to promote extramural services that would spare heavy institutional costs and provide equal or better patient services. A case can certainly be eloquently made for out-of-hospital care through three-dimensional community service networks to replace or augment mental hospitals and nursing homes.

Those dark secret fears within most human beings that I mentioned as a barrier to understanding and sympathy for the mentally ill probably apply as well to the elderly. Only by bringing them back into the community and providing satisfactory care can we overcome the fear and the quiet. And we have to do it through our lawmakers. We can't rely on administrators or professionals, with their special interests, to initiate the changes. The poor care of the nursing homes that seems to indicate that no one pays any attention to what goes on "inside" occurs partly because people are fearful of inevitable death; we'd like to avoid seeing it and having anything to do with it. We must undertake to make changes as an objective community; unlike mental illness and the fears associated with it, old age is a human inevitability that will come to us all; changes in elderly care must be initiated now.

Our hospital dilemma derives from a social philosophy that fails to distinguish between public purpose and private rights. Once hospitals are subordinated to public purpose they would not be able to exercise individual initiative to duplicate facilities, avoid provision of ambulatory care, and hire or expand at will, etc. It is this aspect of the hospital system that is most destructive. Yet it seems to be this aspect of the system that our society cherishes. We will overcome it only through acceptance of responsibility for equity in society.

# Chapter 9
# Other Critical Areas in Care

---

Everett Hughes in *Men and Their Work* states that in most instances the average citizen's emergency is the professional's daily fare. There may be situations in which the professional recognizes the emergent nature to a much greater degree than the patient, but in most instances there is common agreement as to what constitutes an emergency — coronary attacks; strokes; hemorrhage; broken bones; very high fevers or croup in children. These are the *disease emergencies.* Then there are *accident emergencies:* automobile or machinery accidents, wounds, falls, drowning, suffocation, etc. In any of these instances, it is obvious that immediate, efficient attention is mandatory.

## EMERGENCY CARE

### COMMUNICATION DEFICIENCIES IN EMERGENCY CARE

When an emergency occurs, there is always a need for telephone communication to a responsive center of help. In recent years, determined efforts have been made to introduce a simple single call telephone signal that can be used without having to find ten or fifteen cents at a highway telephone booth. This has not yet been accomplished.

When accidents happen on the road, even if a telephone is available, very often the individual who has suffered the accident or the person attempting to report it doesn't know how to specify the location for the response center. There is no systematic arrangement of numbered communication boxes along highways; with this system, the response center would automatically know the accident location by identifying the numbered location on the center's master chart. There are many such highways in the United States, but they are hardly the majority.

## EMERGENCY CREWS AND FACILITIES

The emergency responding system is equally uneven and inadequate. There is no national system, and most states do not have a state-wide system. Most cities do not even have a system. In some communities the responding agency is a hospital, but not every hospital has an ambulance to send out; not every hospital has an emergency ward. Very often ambulance systems depend upon volunteer services. There is no uniform training for those who man the emergency system; therefore, there is no guarantee of uniform quality of care throughout the United States. Travelers have no way of knowing what care they will find, should they be injured or seek emergency care far from home. The kind of ambulance or whether it will respond to a call without consideration of cost or payment is uncertain and, for most people caught in an emergency situation, unknown. In some places it is the responsibility of funeral parlors (ambulances and hearses are very similar)! Racial discrimination presents a problem in many communities. Certain hospitals do not want patients brought to their emergency room from certain other parts of the city. Efforts are made to localize the transport of the sick or injured, particularly if they are poor or minority people, to specific hospitals. The well-to-do may also try to localize emergency care of the sick or injured for fear they may find themselves in one of the hospitals or emergency rooms reserved for the poor, on the assumption that there must be poor medical care there.

Disparity in availability of facilities magnifies the inequality of a pluralistic and disorganized system, and not always for the benefit of the well-to-do or white. The grandchild of a wealthy white family brought to the circus on the other side of the town may be accidently injured and rushed to the nearby hospital emergency room. Here they may find an inadequately supported unit, staffed by physicians of questionable competence and language ability. They will be compelled to wait because of the absence of sufficient personnel. These are certainly far less than optimal conditions for anyone's emergency care. Health may be as indivisible as peace.

The deficiencies of American emergency medical care reflect the inattention to this area specifically and also to the larger overall inadequacy and disorganization of general American medical care service, within which a more efficient and effective emergency care service could be provided. It may very well be that effective emergency care will not be obtained until there is a national health service or at the very least a national health insurance program through which effective medical services can be developed, supplied and funded.

Appropriate staffing of emergency rooms is deficient today because it is so dependent on the ability of institutions to obtain house staff, and because most practicing physicians have neither the time nor the inclination to spend time in the emergency room. In a few areas, hospitals have begun to purchase packaged emergency room services in the same way they would purchase packaged services of other kinds. This is carried out by offering salaries or "concessions" to groups of physicians who undertake to staff the emergency room 24 hours a day and provide the services required. However, this is at best temporizing, insofar as the emergency service may or may not be related to other services required by the patient to supplement or support the emergency room care. It may be that we will have to develop a separate emergency service, separately staffed and operated, for major cities and large communities. If so, it should be with full realization that this will have to be accomplished through additional organization of hospital activities, so that there will be a more general pattern of progression of care for patients, from the emergency rooms through the wards, on to rehabilitation, home care and discharge.

## EMERGENCY SITUATIONS NEEDING ATTENTION

### HUNGER

It is important to discuss hunger as a part of the health picture because it is obvious that regular intake of improper and inadequate food for any length of time must result in disease, disability and eventual death. Every grade school child knows that the human body requires carbohydrates, fats, protein, vitamins and minerals. We also know that not all sources of nutrients are equal or adequate. In any case, one can be "hungry" in the sense of starving the cells disproportionately, even though eating substantial amounts of food. This is the subtle hunger; the body hunger for substances that are not supplied, despite adequate quantitative intake.

For a long time in the United States we thought that obesity, too much fat in our food and adolescent mismanagement of diet were our only real nutritional problems. About 10 years ago, when we rediscovered American poverty, we rediscovered our very real nutritional problem: starvation and malnutrition. We discovered that there were infants dying of diseases — marasmus and kwashiorkor — never thought to be seen in the United States, and considered a peculiar problem of primitive, impoverished developing countries. We found these diseases in the children of minority and isolated rural families, of course, where poverty has been an inescapable fact of daily life. But it was also found in the heart of great cities; a case of kwashiorkor was described in Baltimore. It took several years of intensive activity on the part of determined interest groups concerned about the poor, about children, about the condition of minority families, to move Congress to make some studies of the situation.

There is a curious irony in the fact that the Defense Department had American specialists do nutrition surveys in about 35 different countries for the purpose of establishing their "military capability." So we had a pretty good idea about the nutritional status of children and adults in places like Afghanistan, but had no idea at all about the nutritional status of Americans, or if and where there were hunger and malnutrition. After 1968, however, a number of such survey studies were carried out. They were of uneven quality and not too much can be said on their behalf as scientific research efforts. But they gave us a fairly good idea of what we should have known anyway: that poverty is ineluctably associated with relatively poor diet. As a consequence, poor children have low iron levels in their blood, they are of smaller size; and this may be related to higher prematurity rates among the poor and minority groups, which is further related to their higher infant mortality rates.

Some of these facts are used as arguments against doing anything to modify the health system. Some people insist that poor people are not unhealthy because they can't get to medical care; they reason that the high infant mortality among the poor is due more to diet, and has nothing to do with access to pediatricians, obstetricians or hospitals, or to the fact that poor women don't receive adequate or early enough prenatal care. The blame, they argue, rests in the fact that poor people don't get enough to eat; and once we initiate an adequate nutrition policy there will not be any need to fool around with a perfectly good medical care system.

This argument has a number of holes in it, of course; and it is quite self-serving. It is an argument that is put forth mostly by people who have the most to lose if the medical care system changes — the physicians and the providers in general. One has to look with some suspicion at any argument that serves its proponents so well. And, of course, we hardly ever see the American Medical Association lobbying in Congress to demand that something be done about food for poor people; or that there be better programs for feeding children in school. Frankly, I think that there is probably merit in the idea that if there were more abundant feeding of children and better diets for older people, there probably would be less need to see doctors. But that wouldn't make it any easier for the people who do have to see a doctor if he is still unaccessible or too expensive. It is frustrating and overwhelming that our society is so reluctant to establish food and nutrition programs that will benefit our children, especially since it is so often said we are a "child-oriented society." We don't have adequate health services in the schools, and we certainly don't have any better system for getting children to medical care than we do for adults; it is all one system. Most of the food programs, whether distribution of surplus commodities or food stamps, are not aimed specifically at children. There has been for a few years a special program called "Women, Infants and

Children Feeding Program" (WIC). Through this program, the Department of Agriculture supplies a variety of food stuffs — milk and eggs for mothers, special allotments of milk and foods for children — but these are very limited programs that only serve a few thousand people in a few selected places. As a matter of fact, the program remains in constant threat of elimination.

If we aren't going to do anything effective about health services, the least that we could do is encourage programs to keep as many people as possible from needing health services! Of course the best ways of preventing disease would be to ensure immunizations against specific diseases for as many children as possible and elimination of environmental hazards that kill, wound or injure people. But among the cheapest ways is to see to it that people are fed properly. And these programs ought not to be constructed with economic barriers such as means tests to keep people out. Of course there should be programs for the destitute, but total needs programs, not soup kitchens, and distribution centers in the neighborhoods to make it possible for poor people to get an adequate supply of what they need. This means food programs in the schools — breakfast and lunch and afternoon snacks — for children whose parents are working and who have no way of coming home to an adequate dinner. And if it turns out that there are some children fed at this table who don't really come from poor families, it should not be the basis for a scandal or a congressional investigation about abuses of the system. An adequate system for feeding children in the schools might cost a couple of billion dollars, which is a cheap way to fight potential health problems, particularly if we know that only a fraction of the costs have to be charged to misuse.

Feeding programs for old people are equally necessary for the same reasons and for additional ones. Old people tend to lose some of the zest for caring for themselves and too often fix simple, inadequate meals for their daily diets. If a common feeding program, or meals delivered to the homes for those with restriction of activity, were part of every community's social services, it would be a life-saving measure for many old people. It is not uncommon that many old people admitted to hospitals as "emergencies" are really suffering from malnutrition.

## HOUSING

When we are out to combat hunger and malnutrition, it is fairly easy to discern the physical symptoms. We can recognize the skinny legs and arms, the swollen belly, the distortion of the whole body structure. We can see how feeble and sick-looking the starved are and, of course, with certain kinds of malnutrition the special visible symptoms will appear: the reddish hair of kwashiorkor; the pigmented sloughing skin of pellagra; the ulcers at the corners of the mouth from Vitamin B deficiency; the bleeding gums of scurvy; rickets from Vitamin D deficiency, etc. These are all plainly visible evidences of malnutrition.

It is much harder to discern the symptoms of inadequate housing. The housing itself may have very little influence on the person, except in the case of utterly *unsafe* housing where the accidents happen that cause injuries, disease and death. We recognize housing problems when children are burned by the open flame of space heaters in improperly heated homes; when people are killed by improperly protected wiring of electrical appliances; burned to death in fires where there are no fire escapes; and hurt when elevators collapse, or staircases are broken and steps missing. Slum housing gives us the graphic, nauseating pictures of rats nibbling away at children's faces and extremities; of choked toilets with their backflow of sewage; of the garbage piled up in the backyards and front lawns where flies and rats breed, and the diseases are carried to the inhabitants of the homes. We must also think of the psychological and emotional damage that is done when people have to grow up or live together without any privacy, without any of the feelings of belonging, without the pleasant surroundings that allow human beings to feel at ease with themselves and society.

For most of us who live in relative luxury, whether it is in private homes or apartments, in the city or in the country, the desperation of living in a slum environment and under slum conditions cannot be grasped. Nor are we able to grasp the true meaning of desperate poverty, in a literally cashless economy, with no assurance of a "next penny" to buy food; with the hopelessness of joblessness; with no food day after day, and a gnawing, nagging feeling of hunger. No matter how much sympathy and empathy we may have, these things have to be experienced to be truly understood. The physical and psychological impact of bad housing is one of the things that must be dealt with in dealing with health in the larger sense.

Again, those who want to argue that nothing really needs to be done to improve our medical care system will say that it is living conditions that ought to be improved, and hunger eliminated. Everyone agrees that changes should be made, but in someone else's area of responsibility. If we improve nutrition and housing, and give people a better life, we supposedly won't have to worry about the medical care system. There may be as much truth in that argument as there is in saying that changing the medical care system will also improve other things in society. One cannot really do one thing without doing the others and expect to get complete turnover in the health situation or medical care needs of people. If we continue to let people starve, continue to keep them in hopelessly inadequate housing situations, it will do very little good to give them access to the best modern medical care. We will simply be running on a treadmill trying to catch up with the illnesses that result from these things. We have to do some of everything.

It hardly seems worthwhile to have the most skillful plastic surgeons patch up the torn cheeks of rat-bitten youngsters when it would be easier (and cheaper!) to keep the rats from biting the children in the first place. Conversely, the best housing situation remains inadequate if good medical care is not locally available. Effective action would be to correct both situations equally; to create a symbiotic environment, and not lopsided relief.

Among the economic problems raised by the attempt to equalize the delivery of good modern medical care are such questions as those addressed by Victor Fuchs in *Who Shall Live?* Society and social decisions are the base for economic theory. You can't have all the housing you need, or all the medical care you need, or all the education you need, or all the food you need, because there are priorities other than social welfare priorities. For example, no matter how much we detest great expenditures in the defense establishment, foreign policy priorities must concern themselves with the safety of the country through military strength. Herman Biggs, the great New York state health officer and one of the statesmen of modern public health, said, "Any community can have the death rate it is willing to afford." This applied in his day to public health measures. Today, a statement to this effect is very popular with conservatives, physicians and other providers and economists who want to emphasize the finite character of our resources. Unfortunately, the partisans of defense generally promote their priorities with implied threats of hidden dangers and shadows of doom if the maximum amounts demanded for guns, ships, planes and missiles are not forthcoming. They want *their* priority to be *the* priority.

I like to think that Congress represents all the people of the United States and that the priorities they establish are essentially the priorities of the American people. But in that case, do we want aircraft carriers, moonshots, financial salvage of Lockheed and Penn Central in preference to food programs for our children and medical care and decent housing for everyone? I hope the decisions are being made in full knowledge of the facts of *constituents'* priorities.

I'm not sure that the options are posed appropriately. It may turn out that nationalization of the defense industry and the subsequent elimination of defense profits might reduce the expenditures in that area without endangering the nation's safety. It may also be that nationalizing health services; setting limits to the income of the providers; and rationalizing the distribution of services by eliminating duplication, wasteful frills and mismanagement may go a long way toward enabling us to have *both* priorities.

The Spaniards have a proverb, " 'Take what you want,' says God, 'take it and pay for it.' " It may be that limiting the income of doctors and regionalizing hospitals may change the motivation of young people and reduce the influx into the health professions that we are seeing today. Maybe not as many people will want to be doctors or spend as much time practicing at it. It may be that we'll have to get a better transportation system to take us to and from hospitals that won't be as locally situated. We may have to be satisfied with less of something else in order to set priorities for good medical care and for everybody.

It is important for us to recognize that the kinds of choices we have been faced with until now aren't necessarily the only kinds of choices that there are. We might choose to provide a family allowance, for example, whereby families would receive additional funds for each child, to be able to supply children with better food and better housing. Even though we may be very strongly motivated these days to keep the population down, we shouldn't do it at the expense of the living. Every child born should be at least allowed to thrive and grow to proper strength, dignity and intellectual capacity so as to be able to serve himself and succeeding generations. We may mortgage the future with money but we shouldn't mortgage the future through the health of our children. Civilized countries are judged by their treatment of the sick, the poor and the helpless, which includes the old and the young.

### INDUSTRIAL ACCIDENTS AND POISONING

When I look back in history at earlier civilizations, one of the things I find hardest to understand about our ancestors is the extreme cruelty with which they treated one another and the blithe insouciance with which they killed one another. There were human sacrifices at religious festivals and legal executions for even the most trivial criminal acts. Every once in a while modern man seems to revert to these callous, primitive ways, as in our most recent wars when we firebombed great cities, gassed and burned millions of people in concentration camps and bombed and incinerated innocent villages in peaceful Asian countries. But to my mind nothing is more striking evidence of the persistence of the profound human killer instinct than the way in which we tolerate unnecessary deaths on the highways and in places of employment.

It would seem almost axiomatic that an employer would have to arrange for the safety of the work force so that they wouldn't have to risk their lives to earn their livelihood. Or if they did so risk their lives, at least it should be with full knowledge of the risks involved and they should be paid commensurately. This is clearly not the case. Approximately 15 to 25 thousand American workers lose their lives in industrial accidents each year; and perhaps 100,000 more die as a result of exposure to industrial diseases. Perhaps more horrifying, even than the deaths, is the fact that ten million injuries occur, disabling over two million workers, and the Department of Labor has reported that if all work accidents were reported the figure would be 25 million injuries. Technology is making the situation worse. Between 1960 and 1970, the injury frequency rate increased 30 percent: more production led to more health hazard; more technology, more injury; more sophistication in manufacturing, more industrial poisoning and disease.

What is even more interesting is that despite a long history of dreadful industrial accidents in inadequately protected working situations, it wasn't until the 1930's that the Department of Labor began to attempt to set and enforce occupational safety and health standards through the Walsh-Healy Act. But it was enforced in such a weak and gingerly way that it hardly had any effect on the work place. Coal miners, of course, have been exceptionally victimized because of the dangerous and unhealthy quality of the mines. A coal mine disaster precipitated an important additional law, The Coal Mine Health and Safety Act of 1969, which was followed by The Occupational Safety and Health Act of 1970. These two laws provided for the first time for participation by the workers in the inspection mechanism, with the possibility of closing down an unsafe place; and improved medical services, rehabilitation and compensation for affected workers. However, the problem is that some fine print takes away much of what the bold print gives; and inadequate appropriations from Congress reduce the number of inspectors able to make the investigations and inspections. However, even with these defects the laws go a long way toward improving the situation. Successive Congresses may be expected to strengthen and improve the legislation.

At the same time it has to be recognized that little enough is being done to protect workers or to compel industry to operate in such a way as to protect the community. One still sees headlines in the papers about powder plant blasts; explosions of trains and chemical plants; and poisons released from sinking ships, gasoline tank cars, etc.

It is almost as if having given up religion as the medium for human sacrifice, we now sacrifice our fellow citizens and children to the great god of industry, and we hesitate to prevent these sacrifices by improving the safety of the work places. Productivity and profit are important touchstones of America's leadership as the world's industrial giant. The American coal mining technique, for example, allows us to produce 20 tons of coal per man while the British produce only three, and the Russians two. We are still increasing the amount of tonnage produced per worker. Perhaps we need to review our priorities in that regard.

Poisons in the work place, such as asbestos or beryllium, which produce cancer to those exposed, are more insidious than accidents or other health hazards. Cancer is also a hazard for uranium and nickel miners; and there are literally thousands of materials in use with unknown effects, that may produce even more deaths from cancer or other diseases.

Any good occupational health program has to take into consideration a safe, poison-free and disease-free environment. It will not be easy. If a national health insurance act provides only for payment for health care or medical services, and still leaves the worker and his family to find that medical care, the worker's complex disadvantages will not be mitigated. It will still take special workers to identify causes of illness; to prove that it was related to the work; to assess the damage and its future effects; to compel the employer to improve the working situation to eliminate the hazards; and to obtain adequate compensation for the injured or sick worker and his family. Any good medical care system will require special attention to the work situation; the workers' health needs will not be satisfied simply by a national health insurance scheme.

Workmen's Compensation laws do nothing to challenge the employer to improve the work site situation or to compensate the worker for more than his disability. These laws are inadequate for modern technology. A good health law will take into consideration the hazards involved where 80,000,000 Americans work as well as where they live. The diseases to which man is exposed as a natural consequence of living are only a part of the diseases for which society should provide medical services.

It is well to remember that where one works and where one lives may be very closely related. Some of the things that go on in the factory will be carried over into the community in which the factory exists. We have learned that some of the poisons and pathogens (like asbestos) are carried home in the worker's clothes to sicken members of his family. We have seen the poisoning of community water supply from factory effluent. We have seen the consequence of the discharge of asbestos into lakes. What will happen in those communities in which drilling for oil or gas has resulted in disruption of the home sites, or where the sands from uranium mines were used as fill so that houses were built on radioactive plots? Occupational health and environmental health are related, and both of these are related to the personal health needs and personal medical care service requirements of every family.

What we have said of the "work places" applies equally to the "schools." A good medical care system must take into account the fact that 80 million Americans are gathered together in work places; that some 40 million Americans are gathered together in the schools. Provision of medical care can be more effectively and efficiently accomplished through concentrating some medical services at work and school as well as in the neighborhoods. Since we know that who pays the piper calls the tune, it will be important that the medical services — the providers, the physicians and the various health workers concerned — be paid *not* by the factories or the industrial complexes within which the services are given; but instead, paid out of community resources, public funds to which workers and their families contribute, and can therefore share in the decision concerning type and quality of the services provided. Just as it is important that there be community participation in the development of community medical services, there needs to be the same participation in school and occupational health services.

# Chapter 10
# Quality: Its Presence or Absence
# and How to Test for It

---

## INDICATORS OF LACK OF QUALITY

For middle income people, the problem in the medical care system today is very largely one of cost. There is also some emphasis on access; for example, Wednesday afternoons and Sundays, when so many doctors take time off. For lower income people the problem is *both* cost and access, and among the poorest the greatest emphasis is on access. For all Americans there is a growing concern about the *quality* of medical care. Sometimes it is reflected in dissatisfaction with the way in which the medical service is administered: haughtiness, impersonality or contempt by those providing the service, a gross lack of concern for the individual by the "system." Sometimes it is evidenced by the physician as he talks about the patient's illness to a group of students or other health workers in front of the patient, without seeming to recognize what effect this might have on the patient; how humiliating it is to be treated as an object. Or it may be the way in which research workers fail to observe human, ethical and even constitutional considerations when it comes to patient care. They may or may not concern themselves with informed consent; they might try out new, dangerous or even unnecessary diagnostic or treatment measures without explaining to the patient the consequences of the procedure, giving him an opportunity for intelligent choice. In some instances patients are used for experimental purposes in which the drug or treatment is not one that would benefit them at all. This may not be the place to discuss ethical matters related to medical practice and research, but certainly ethical principles enter into any consideration of quality because the lack of observance of appropriate ethical principles is by its very nature poor quality. This lack of concern as evidenced in failure to observe the need for informed consent has penetrated the consciousness of enough people so that many of us have considerable suspicion about medical practice and its bureaucratic nature.

The thought that we may be "guinea pigs," despite our own wishes and without our knowledge, can poison patients' attitudes and interfere with acceptance of treatment.

### MALPRACTICE SUITS

The increasing number of malpractice suits and the increasing sizes of the awards made is some evidence of physician carelessness and indifferent attitude that lead to real damage.   Many say that there are far more malpractice cases than actual suits would indicate.   While it is true that only a fraction of the malpractice suits are actually brought to court and while a good many are settled out of court in the patient's favor, those tried are rarely resolved in the patient's favor.   We will discuss elsewhere malpractice, malpractice insurance and the problems and consequences for physicians; at the moment it may be enough to say that the existence of a large-scale malpractice problem is evidence of some deficiency of quality.

### UNNECESSARY SURGERY

Some observers, like Herbert Denenberg, a former Commissioner of Insurance in the State of Pennsylvania, and Sidney Wolfe, who heads the Health Research Group in Washington, have made efforts to estimate the volume of unnecessary surgery carried out in the United States.   If only 10 percent of the 10 million surgical procedures carried out in the United States were of questionable necessity, and 1 percent truly unnecessary, it would give us 100,000 surgical procedures carried on needlessly each year.   But the Health Research Group estimates 3.2 million unnecessary operations each year!

The excess surgery performed has interesting associations, aside from the obvious lucrative aspects.   Obviously fee-for-service is more remunerative than a salaried surgical job, so one must expect more surgical procedures in a fee-for-service setting.   This is strikingly evident in the differences in numbers of routine surgical procedures in the two settings.   According to Health Research Group's statistics, almost 50 percent of women are at risk for a hysterectomy during their lifetime, but in prepaid group practice settings only a third as many (16 percent) are at such risk.   Children are at a 30 percent risk in the general population for tonsillectomies, but only a 10 percent risk in prepaid group practice; and there is a 17.5 percent risk for men for prostatectomies, as against 7.5 percent in prepaid group practice.   It would seem that fee-for-service leads to three times as much surgery as is necessary, according to the standards of the group practice settings.   In 1970, a California physician, John Bunker, studied British and American data on surgery and reported that we had twice as many surgeons as Britain, proportionate to the population, and performed twice as many surgical procedures!

Fee-for-service is apparently not good for your removable parts and hardly conducive to quality. A measure of patient control here would appear to be to get a second opinion in every case where surgery is recommended, with the second opinion perhaps from a doctor in prepaid group practice.

## MEASURING QUALITY

Quality is measurable in terms of physician behavior: satisfaction of the patient, suitable performance, appropriate outcome. This is not to say that everything a doctor does *must* result in the patient's improving, getting well or even surviving, inasmuch as there are diseases that cannot be treated appropriately as yet; and life has left scars on some people, which makes it impossible for them to cope with illnesses that would otherwise be fairly simple to treat.

However, we should be asking ourselves certain questions in the light of what doctors do:

(1)  Is what was done necessary?
(2)  Is what was necessary done?
(3)  Was it done properly?
(4)  Was it done in time?
(5)  Was it done with skill?

### PROCESS VS. OUTCOME QUALITY

There are also instances in which the physician may have done everything wrong or the hospital failed to fulfill its role appropriately, and yet the patient recovers normally! Not only is it impossible for physicians and the medical care system to cure everything, it is also obvious that nature is a very durable guardian of human beings. Sometimes no matter what the doctor does the patient will recover. When it comes to measuring whether quality existed in the medical procedure, precision becomes increasingly difficult. For example, if the patient survives and has no lasting disability from the medical procedure, the *outcome* must be judged to be good. If we then concern ourselves with quality of *process,* we can determine whether the things done were necessary and whether the necessary things were done. It would seem reasonable that, in order to establish whether good quality medicine is being practiced, one should look at *both* of these factors.

In courts of law, doctors' appropriateness of action is usually based on what is considered the common practice in that community. This is a rough rule of thumb, but it does allow for regional differences in the way in which certain kinds of diseases are handled. For example, in some parts of the country or in some institutions, radical surgery may be the mode for treatment of cancer of the breast, including widespread removal of the lesion along with much surrounding tissue. If the patient gets a bad result from a surgical procedure in which less than that was done, a court in that area might find that doctor at fault. The same doctor in another area, following a local pattern of much less radical surgery, would not be found at fault at all.

The reason for this kind of discrepancy is that without statistical evidence of the value of one procedure against another, there can be no evidence as to which is better. For much of medicine we do not have "field trial" tests, proving one method superior to another. Over the centuries, doctors learned to do, and continued to practice, methods that seemed to benefit their patients. In types of treatment where life is at stake, it is very hard for a doctor to say, "this procedure will save lives, but I am not going to use it on all my patients who need it, because I want to test it statistically." His conscience, or society, may not let him. That is why the Food and Drug Administration insists upon tests to determine the efficacy and safety of a new drug before they allow it to be sold commercially. Field trials on medical procedure are now standard, with similar conditions, but patients are treated in different ways without the investigator knowing which treatment is used on which patient (the "double blind" approach); this is the most reliable way of deciding what is good and what is unnecessary treatment. However, for many procedures we do not have such ex-perimental evidence of any value. Consequently, the rule or habit of local practice has to remain as the guide to decision.

In other circumstances, *process* is also a good measure for determining overall medical quality. For example, we know that many patients with diabetes are prone to develop significant changes in the eyegrounds as part of the natural progression of the disease. The doctor treating a diabetic who does not look at the eyeground periodically cannot be considered to be giving very good supervision. The patient's condition or *outcome* is not the gauge; it is the *process.*

Then also, skill is maintained by practice. A surgeon in a particularly delicate area, such as the brain or the heart, who is only rarely occupied in that process, cannot be considered as skilled as one who does these operations frequently. Here again, *process* is the measure of quality.

### PROFESSIONAL QUALITY

Less automatic, but still considered evidence of quality in this regard, is whether or not a particular physician has received the approval of his peers in terms of having passed a written or practical examination, or become a member of a "Board." "Board" members are groups of specialists in a particular field whose knowledge and skill are used to test newcomers' ability to decide whether or not they should be allowed to join their professional rank.  Naturally it is expected that those who acquire that rank will be better practitioners than those who do not.  Oddly enough two-thirds of the surgery in the United States is still carried on by *nonboard* surgeons; that is, they have not been sanctioned by the American Board of Surgery.

Most states hold to the 19th century view that if a physician is licensed in medicine and surgery, he is permitted to do *anything* in that field.  Although he might be a generalist, he is entitled to practice his skill on any patient who selects him and in any way he sees fit.  The courts are beginning to narrow down his privilege, but state licensing laws remain.  Hospitals have narrowed the privileges too, in that they are refusing to allow physicians to carry out complex procedures within their walls if they do not have the imprimatur of Board certification.  To some extent this is the "guild" protecting its own, but to some extent it is a measure of quality protection for the patient.  It is also a direct protection for the hospital against malpractice judgments, because the dissatisfied patient operated on by an incompetent or untrained physician would get cheerful support in court if he sued the hospital for allowing an incompetent physician to practice there.

The fact that one does have Board certification does not necessarily mean that one's competence is beyond question.  Unfortunately some Board physicians are as incompetent as the unsanctioned.  It goes without saying that in this measure of *process* as a standard of quality, the better trained, more "certificated" and busier the physician is in his specialty the more likely he is to be judged of better quality.  It is only a supposition, of course, but it is taken to be fact by both patient and the law.

In the past, the standards and control of quality have theoretically been left to the profession itself.  By definition, a profession is a group that sets its own standards, observes them, trains its own members accordingly and establishes the content of the discipline.  In this way medicine has always controlled the standards of education and practice.  However, control involves judging and punishing those who violate the standards.  Over time, the medical profession has been rather remiss in giving adequate supervision, bringing malpractice to trial and imposing suitable punishment. For this reason, and as concern about quality in medical services increases, the medical profession comes under great pressure to give more and better supervision to weed out the incompetent. At the present time this is under great public discussion. More and more laws regulating the use of federal money in paying doctors have requirements attached for "review," "standards," and "controls."

Medicine grew up historically out of many different branches, each of which grew into different guilds during the Middle Ages. The practicing physician was a member of the Artists' Guild; the dispenser or apothecary (the modern druggist) was a member of the Grocers' Guild; and the surgeons, interestingly, were members of the Barbers' Guild. The guild spirit remains very strong among physicians. A professional reprimand for inappropriate behavior is considered severe enough punishment in most instances. The reason for this, of course, goes back to the fact that in the selection process, those who became members of the guild were like members of one large family. The assumption was that the same ethical principles inspired them all; that there would be a sense of *noblesse oblige* among them, and they could be trusted to behave correctly once their error was defined.

Even in guild times this did not always work; and now that guilds no longer exist and medicine has become a competitive business, inbred with the ethics of the 20th century, these factors really do not work at all. A reprimand in the corridor of the hospital is hardly sufficient to control greed, restore competence, or create missing skills. George Bernard Shaw expressed these faults cynically and somewhat humorously in his introduction to *The Doctors' Dilemma*. He pointed out that a surgeon looking at a man with two legs could assure himself that the patient would be just as well off with one of them; and since to remove one would be extraordinarily beneficial to the surgeon financially, why not remove it?

The kind of ethical principle of "good business," typified by the slogan *caveat emptor* ("let the buyer beware"), should only be applicable when the buyer is competent to judge the quality of the product. In medicine, where the guild ethics have impressed everyone with the belief that only the *doctor* can judge quality, it is the duty and responsibility of the doctor to *guarantee* quality. This is particularly true in a fee-for-service system with insurance coverage, in which the patient need not hesitate to use a service since the insurance company will pay for it. This is bound to lead, in some instances, to excess services, and in some instances even to fraudulent practice. It will certainly do nothing to reduce unnecessary procedures, visits or services. The doctor must be the guardian of the patient's interests.

In addition, the competitive nature of modern medical practice discourages physicians from donning the appropriate robe of humility, accepting friendly censure, or yielding to the superior quality of a colleague. After all, his very livelihood is at stake; he cannot let patients know his defects or deficiencies. Conversely, the colleague may be unwilling to criticize his fellow doctor publicly, or undertake to see that he is removed from the possibility of injuring patients because, again, he is in competition and cannot afford to allow the profession to be endangered in this way. Given this method of practice and the atmosphere of our society, which does nothing to instill a cooperative of socially responsible attitudes among practitioners, how can the profession police itself?

In a word, internal professional supervision of medical practice has been almost entirely unsuccessful. Most medical societies have not had even a single case per year brought by one member against another.

### INSTITUTIONAL QUALITY

In hospital practice, one method of control is institutional accreditation. Measurements are made to determine whether the hospital has suitable facilities, properly maintained; whether it provides adequate delivery of these services, etc. This is hardly enough to protect the patient against poor quality, but it is better than nothing. It is unfortunate, however, that this accreditation process has been under the wing of the hospitals and doctors, with no representation from the patients or society at large. The Joint Commission on Accreditation is a four-legged stool, comprised of the American Hospital Association, the American Medical Association, the American College of Physicians and the American College of Surgeons. Whether or not important issues are thereby compromised due to "conflict of interest" is a question. American tradition veers away from government accreditation; but a possible solution is to add public members to the accrediting team.

Some hospitals voluntarily purchase a service whereby periodic investigations are made of certain aspects of hospital behavior. This large-scale participating study has been carried on over many years by a private, nonprofit organization called The Hospital Administration Services, directed by Virgil Slee in Ann Arbor, Michigan. Participating hospitals report on their diagnoses and kinds of treatment; from these data, tables are constructed of "normal" behavior and hospitals can measure their behavior against that of others. The assumption here is that a hospital or its board of managers will respond to signals from these reports as to what needs to be corrected.

Physicians have also created some mechanisms for the observation and control of the quality of hospital practice. For over 50 years there have been surgical mortality conferences in which the cases of those patients who die after surgery are reviewed by the surgical staff. Again, there is presumption that the physician who has behaved improperly or incompetently will benefit and change. If he does not and the improper behavior is repeated too many times, he may be dropped from the staff and not permitted to operate. He thereby loses his professional base, unless he can find another hospital in which to work. Such mortality conferences concerning maternal and infant care grew up out of health department activities and have been very helpful in maintaining levels of quality in hospitals. These are generally "peer" review; that is, a review of fatal circumstances surrounding hospital patient care by the members and colleagues of one's own group. The results of these conferences remain within the confines of the particular group or of a slightly larger group, including perhaps the hospital administrator and the executive committee of the medical staff. But the facts never become matters of public knowledge, although at the present time there is increasing pressure for these matters to be dealt with publicly.

In large part this pressure has developed out of financial and economic considerations, and has grown more persistent as the federal investment in medical care has grown larger. Congress has become concerned as to whether the funds being spent are spent prudently. So quality seems to be a major concern only because it influences cost.

In 1972, Congress legislated a Professional Standards Review Organization in an effort to reduce the number of persons in medical institutions and the numbers of days of stay of those admitted. This effort was based primarily at cutting government costs in individual medical payments. The institutions involved were not only hospitals, but also nursing homes of all kinds. The Professional Standards Review idea grew out of earlier legislation that required that every patient admitted to a hospital or nursing home had to have his record reviewed at the end of 14 days to be sure that he still needed to be there or should have been admitted at all. This was called "Utilization Review." The Professional Standards Review Organization has generated bitter discussion in the profession. Although it is to be composed entirely of representatives of the community's physicians, the fact that a physician's hospital practice will be visible to colleagues, in all the processes and circumstances, disturbs doctors sufficiently; many of them are taking court action and resisting participation in every way possible. It is hard to determine at present what will ultimately happen, but the law provides that if physicians do not participate in the Professional Standards Review, the Secretary of HEW can appoint groups of nonphysicians to do the job for them. This may create even greater tension and conflict!

A great many other types of controls have been set up to reduce federal costs in the hospital. These measures also contain some *quality* control items, but largely they concern themselves with matters such as over-building or duplicating facilities and equipment. For instance, a hospital must be "certificate passed" or it will not be able to obtain federal funds or be reimbursed the costs of construction or loans in per diem payments.

## CONSUMER REPRESENTATION
## FOR QUALITY CONTROL

An ideal board of measurement and inquiry regarding quality of medical care would involve large-scale consumer representation and control. During the 1960's, most of the OEO legislation and eventually HEW legislation and regulations required consumer "participation." The great planning acts of the 1960's and 1970's provided that there had to be consumer groups on the boards. Later the language was changed so that the boards had to be 51 percent consumers, implying an actual *domination* by the consumer of the advisory boards. But "advisory" is not necessarily control. And when it came to operation, the agencies behind the legislation and the regulations usually did not enforce the 51 percent requirement; while they might still insist that consumers should be there, they usually arranged it so that consumers would be a minority.

The problems raised concerning consumer "participation" and consumer "representation" are very real and ought not to be ignored. Not only radical, antiestablishment individuals and groups now feel that the patient should be involved in medical decision making and that it cannot all be left to the professionals. But defining the terms is difficult. Accepting consumer representation requires, for example, that we define who the consumer is. For many of the agency boards that were set up, the consumer tended to be somebody like a dentist's wife, a doctor's wife or a druggist's wife; someone who was closely related to the professional people and who had a very strong stake in the consequences. For all practical purposes the providers themselves were represented. There were other kinds of discrepancies in the way "consumers" are placed on boards.

In some instances the lack of true consumer representation in supposedly public organizations is not only denying and defying the rights of the members; it is also deceitful and corrupt. For instance, Blue Cross is purported to be a public, nonprofit corporation, claiming tax exemption under the rules of the Internal Revenue Service. The national organization claims that almost 70 percent of its more than 1000 board members in the various plans are "consumer representatives." But if the qualifications of these "consumer representatives" are examined more closely, it turns out that a sizable number are hospital trustees, hardly ordinary "consumers," and the rest are largely corporate executives, bankers and lawyers. A labor union delegate and a minority figure appear occasionally, but are also usually far from typical of the middle- or lower-income patients the plans are supposed to serve.

These boards are self-perpetuating, too, so that change has to come from within. Medical societies and hospital associations usually make the selections of the members or their replacements as the "consumer representatives." And recently, the AMA was revealed as keeping a list of "safe" candidates, association members who could be counted on to vote the "right" way, for membership on just such boards and similar committees. And in some cases the presence of bankers on boards, whose plan handles millions of dollars on deposit in those banks, leads to suspicion of conflict of interest. In some instances large sums of board funds are left in checking accounts, not earning interest; this is a windfall for the banks, of course. And the consumer's role is important enough for the current consumer representatives not to want to see their corporation changed.

In the ghettos and other areas where minorities are heavily represented, it is difficult to decide on a mechanism for consumer selection or election. Should those providing the funds or supervising the expenditures of the funds pick a community representative, or should the community elect their own? In those areas where elections were held, very few people actually voted. The vociferous individuals among the minority groups tended to be the ones who got the attention of the selecting group, and would therefore obtain the place of representative. Maybe they did best represent the aspirations of the community, but it was not clear, due to the superficial selection process.

We need to keep in mind that although consumer participation has been legislated in Congress for the past ten years, there is still only grudging acceptance of the presence of consumers in the various advisory groups and planning agencies. The advisory groups for the supervision of medical services, the various state commissions on costs and the boards of hospitals and medical groups are still poorly supplied with average patient representatives. And the people who are least served and most discriminated against by the medical care system, the isolated rural people and the minorities, are *least* represented on such boards. Only when there is effective and realistic consumer and citizen participation in the medical care system will the lack of effective service be resolved.

As you know, since former President Nixon made his trip to China, there has been a spate of articles about the operation of the Chinese system. The outstanding characteristic of the Chinese system evidently, as compared with our own system, is the dominance of the consumer as represented by the ruling groups in the Chinese community. The physicians, practitioners and educators take their cue from the public, from the communes and the regional bodies. Even the medical students are selected and recommended to the medical schools by community groups. It is hard to believe that anything like that could happen in the United States. The solution may be different in different places, but the contest of provider versus consumer, in establishing quality standards, monitoring supervision and controlling quality of medical services, is a universal problem.

# Chapter 11
# Organization of Health Services

---

## THEORETICAL OBSTACLES TO ORGANIZATION:
## BUREAUCRACY AND SOCIALISM

One of the greatest obstacles to improvement of the U. S. medical care system has been the resistance of most Americans to organization of the health care components; we have traditionally feared "bureaucratization."

For years the American Medical Association argued emotionally against even group practice and any kind of national medical care system by insisting that it would turn out to be just like the Army: patients lining up at sick call to receive only one of two standard treatments — either aspirin or foot powder. And the argument always worked; no one wanted a medical care system that resembled in any way a military bureaucracy or the indefensible, impersonal kind of medical care the average soldier or sailor remembered getting on sick call. I do not want to be understood as saying that the Army or the Navy in their hospital services for the sick and for those who required front line surgery or intensive medical services were impersonal or inhumane in their treatment. The contrary is the case. Once in hospital wards, under the care of physicians and nurses as a result of accident or war injury, the soldier or sailor received more than adequate care, in a friendly, humane, dignified professional way. The fact is, though, that most of the people serving in the armed forces were young people without many physical illnesses, and medical officers who were assigned to sick call were usually unhappy and frustrated in this kind of assignment. Most of the people who came to see them were either not very sick, suffering from minor complaints or actually trying to get out of onerous duty. As a consequence sick call was probably as bad as the sailor or soldier remembered after the war; the sort of thing that he did not want to see again.

So the medical establishment had a good case when they attacked "socialized medicine." This term was used to describe any effort at putting medical practice into some kind of reasonably organized form. And any talk of socialized medicine raised the hackles of the American people. For a generation we had been raised on an anticommunist, anti-Bolshevik diet; anything that came out of the Soviet Union had to be bad! Although the Russians had an organized, efficient socialist medical care system, the idea that an *American* medical system should be based on some sort of socialized, federal approach was an anathema. Therefore, the idea of an organized medical care system simply could not catch on and could not obtain very much public or congressional sponsorship.

## GROUP PRACTICE AS A FORM OF ORGANIZATION

At the same time, various factors were working on society: science and broadening medical knowledge; the changing age composition of the population, which meant that larger numbers of people were getting older and demanding more in the way of medical care services; and increasing specialism with its associated fragmentation, which made it very difficult for people who required a variety of different kinds of medical services. One urgent and logical demand seemed to be to combine the specialists in one place so that patients would not have to go from one doctor's office to another, sometimes to different parts of the city. It seemed reasonable at the very least to put the fragments together in a central location.

### HISTORY OF AMERICAN GROUP PRACTICE

Putting clusters of doctors together to serve patients in a unified center and calling it "group practice" was not a new idea for the United States, nor one imported from a socialist country. This actually began toward the end of the 19th century to serve the people who were building the American transcontinental railroads; the first American group practice was created by the Northern Pacific Railroad in the 1870's. Not too long after that (in 1899), Charles and William Mayo developed their group practice in Rochester, Minnesota, in an effort to provide the best of modern specialist capabilities.

From then on group practice was considered respectable but largely unpopular by the physicians. For most physicians the idea of having to share responsibilities for patient care with another physician was out of character. Students were selected for medical school because they displayed individualistic and entrepreneurial personality traits. The idea of medical teamwork was not attractive. While progressive medical reformers saw it as a way to restructure medical practice to serve social ends, the doctors themselves were very reluctant to join groups. Although the first

American group practice was created in the 1870's, by 1950, when the Pacific Health Service made its first study of American group practice, less than 5 percent of American doctors were involved.

We have discussed the advantages fully in an earlier chapter. Briefly, there were economic advantages for doctors: a group did not have to duplicate staff and equipment — they could share receptionists, technicians, x ray machines and other laboratory equipment, making overhead cheaper. It was also advantageous for patients because they did not have to go to a lot of different places; they could go to one place and get the variety of necessary services. And it was advantageous from the standpoint of overall quality. After all, the doctors would be looking over each others' shoulders, the records would be open to all of them and some degree of collegial supervision could be possible. This would lead to informal conferences and "curbstone consultations," creating better patient care and more alert doctors. Doctors could take time off without neglecting their patients; they could take holidays and, even more important, they could take courses to keep up with advances in medical education, and not lose time or money in the process. From any standpoint it would appear that doctors, patients, insurance companies and the welfare department would all benefit from group practice.

Why, then, was it unpopular?

It was unpopular mostly because entrepreneurial doctors disliked the sharing of responsibility and the insurance companies were unwilling to underwrite the costs of ambulatory care, as explained earlier. Doctors, of course, would not consider taking their pay in any other form than fee-for-service; flat rates were out. It was a kind of standoff. They felt that group practice did not offer the doctor anything better in the way of making a living. Even if group practice were more economical, only patients were to benefit; doctors were sharing costs on overhead anyway.

From the patient's point of view, group practice was unpopular because it made it difficult for patients to exercise choice, since they would have to take the doctor to whom they were referred within the group, and doctors could only recommend the doctors in their group. If for one reason or another the group contained an incompetent, the rest of the doctors would be stuck with him. Honorable doctors would be reluctant to refer patients to the bad apple. If a patient wanted to go outside the group for a particular specialist, that would be equally as cumbersome as it would be without the group practice. In addition, the opportunity and incentive for unscrupulous doctors to refer back and forth might generate unnecessary patient expense, and the temptation might be hard to resist. And although an independent doctor might well be able to diagnose or treat on his own, if he were in group practice he might feel under pressure to ask for a consultation with a specialist.

### HOW GROUP PRACTICE WORKS

Perhaps we should spend a little time discussing group practice and how it operates.  Everything called "group practice" is not the same, and the different kinds appeal to different constituencies.  Group practice can be classified by *sponsorship:* doctor-owned, community-owned, cooperative or industry-owned; or by *function:* general practice, specialty, mixed or diagnostic.  They may be *prepaid:* an annual premium covers membership, without or with a very small additional charge at the time of service.

*Most* groups are:

- Doctor-owned
- Fee-for-service
- Mixed general service
- Located in the middle or far west

### ASSOCIATE PRACTICE AND COOPERATIVES

For a long time group doctors were actually persecuted by their independent colleagues; they were kept out of medical societies and hospitals and more or less blackballed in the professional community.  At one time doctors in group practice had to go to court to fight for their rights to practice in local hospitals or join the medical society.  This is all changing now.  A bitter antitrust case in the District of Columbia, settled by Supreme Court action in 1943, took off some of the heat.  A prepaid medical plan of government workers, Group Health, Inc., with the help of the Department of Justice, was able to carry that off.

Today many doctors graduating from medical school want to have the professional advantages of association and the personal advantages of time off for study, vacation and family life.  More and more doctors are taking up some form of *associate* practice, such as partnerships.  More than half the doctors in the United States are now in some form of associate practice, although only 15 to 20 percent may be in group practice.

In the 19th century, Europe was firmly attached to the idea of *cooperatives.* America had a few cooperative communities, and they were primarily agricultural, involving cooperative purchasing, selling, storage and distribution of equipment and produce.  There are still some giant cooperatives among grain and dairy farmers.  But the medical cooperatives, although sporadically tested, did not thrive.

"Medical cooperatives" were of two kinds — cooperatives in the usual sense, but purchasing medical care as one of the benefits in the common purchasing scheme for their members; or specifically organized for the purpose of purchasing medical care for members whose only relationship to the cooperative was in sharing the cost of medical care.

The latter were distinguished in this purchasing of medical care in that they organized a group practice, employed the doctors, and designated the conditions of work and scope of coverage of the medical plan. The consumers, the cooperative members, were in control. The doctors were employed by the patients.

The only large-scale American medical cooperative today is the Group Health Cooperative of Puget Sound. It is a test of consumer control and it works effectively for both doctors and patients.

### GROUP PRACTICE AND THE FEDERAL GOVERNMENT

In the past 50 years group practice has increasingly become the symbol of the American way of "putting the pieces together" — insurance payment, family practice, specialist availability, quality control. As long ago as 1932, the Committee on the Costs of Medical Care urged this as an important segment of the solution to America's medical care delivery problems. As the federal government became more and more involved in medical care expenditures, the idea of organizing the medical system appealed to them as well. It seemed reasonable to suppose that if the system were better organized, it might be less expensive; furthermore, costs could be controlled easier if there were a single medical care unit that could be held responsible. As a consequence, in the 1960's much official pressure was applied to try to foster group practice. The Johnson administration, for example, promoted legislation that allowed for government guaranteed loans for the construction of group practice facilities, and various federal agencies engaged in assisting government supported health programs were encouraged to develop group practice. OEO neighborhood health centers were also encouraged to become group practices.

However, the government pressures were offset by the natural reluctance of doctors to yield any of their autonomy, and the opportunities for increasing or augmenting their salaries, as well as a natural reluctance on the part of patients to put themselves in the hands of a group with little choice of attending physician. Therefore, group practice grew not much more rapidly than it had grown during the previous 75 or 80 years.

The Nixon Administration showed little interest or concern about medical practice other than costs. Periodically, medical organizations received a sharp stimulus to organizational change, because the politicians and officials concerned with HEW's role in paying for medical services under Medicare, Medicaid or Children's Bureau Neighborhood Health Centers, etc. were anxious to see that the services were paid for most economically. Out of this came the package known as the "Health Maintenance Organization" (HMO). It included emphasis on *preventive* services, presumably to cut back on medical care needs; and on *integrated* services like group practice, associated with a hospital, to offer a more economical approach in the spending of billions of government dollars for medical care.

The HMO would be an insured package: the patient was guaranteed office, hospital and home medical services for an inclusive fee. If the doctors practiced in a group, such an arrangement would be basically a *prepaid group practice,* and the HMO actually would be nothing new. But the HMO proved to be more flexible. Groups of doctors or hospitals could arrange among themselves to guarantee the services, without necessarily establishing a classical group arrangement. The medical society, for example, could undertake to guarantee that the associated doctors would give the services. The society would receive the funds from the insurance company or federal agency, and then divide it according to some internal contractual arrangement among the doctors — fee-for-service according to a fee schedule, for example. And the doctors would continue to practice in their own offices.

### INDUSTRIAL AND COMMUNITY PREPAID PLANS

The earliest prepaid group practices stemmed from employer or welfare fund insurance contracts, efforts to establish fixed budget medical care responsibilities. A number of large industries attempted this. The first community-based prepaid group practice was the Elk City Program that Dr. Michael Shadid began in the 1920's in Elk City, Oklahoma. Prepaid group practice was even less attractive than group practice itself. But World War II gave it a boost. What is currently the largest, most influential group and a model for the United States is the Permanente Medical Group, serving a large part of California, Oregon, and parts of Arizona and even Ohio. Permanete began with the need of an industrialist, Henry Kaiser, to guarantee medical services to workers employed in areas where medical service was either absent or very expensive. It was similar to the needs of the Northern Pacific Railroad in the 1870's, who had to bring in salaried doctors to provide needed medical services to the transcontinental railroad workers cutting through wilderness. Kaiser was building aluminum plants, steel plants and shipyards during World War II, and he needed large numbers of workers in many areas. With the aid of a physician relative, Kaiser developed a prepaid scheme whereby, for minimal sums of money deducted from their pay checks, the workers were guaranteed the services of physicians, specialists and hospitalization. The doctors employed were given attractive salaries.

It was, in many respects, an extension of the Blue Cross idea that had captured the imagination of medical planners in the 1930's; but instead of guaranteeing just hospital services, it guaranteed services in and out of hospital. The Permanente Plan was a great success. It continued to grow after the War and now covers several million people on the West Coast. It is not a nonprofit plan; it is company-owned and operates as an industrial enterprise without public members.

Following World War II, another type of prepaid group practice developed under the aegis of New York City government and community sponsors. During the 1930's, Mayor Fiorello LaGuardia uncovered periodic corruption scandals; he found that the people who had been taking the bribes were heavily in debt, largely due to medical expenses. As a consequence, he agitated for and eventually created the first credit union among city employees. This enabled them to borrow money at reasonable rates of interest, and helped to keep them out of the hands of loan sharks. He also moved to develop a prepaid insurance scheme to keep them from debt caused by illness and associated expense. His advisors included people who had been in the progressive wing of development of New York City health services for many years, and they were convinced that the only way to establish an effective health insurance program was through group practice.

It is the organizational capability of group practice that gives it powerful leverage on improving accessibility and controlling costs of medical care. This is particularly true of prepaid group practice. An organized ambulatory care team can use more of the new, less expensive paramedic personnel in team practice; it can do more out-of-hospital surgery and give attention to postoperative patients at home instead of in the hospital. The "Surgicenter," a specially designed out-patient surgery center is growing more popular for that reason. Group practice can make more efficient use of all local institutional resources.

## INTERHOSPITAL COORDINATION

Another organizational problem relating to the delivery of medical services derives from the difficulty of adjusting in hospital care to appropriate range of care and duration of stay, allowing for the type of disease and actual patient need. Hospitals must achieve a coordinated, cooperative attitude in order to remain flexible in response to those needs.

Hospital services can be either short- or long-term (long-term: three months or more of institutional care), whatever may be necessary for the treatment of acute chronic diseases or mental illness. Something on the order of 80 percent of the 850,000 short-term hospital beds in the United States are "voluntary" beds, belonging to hospitals that are nonprofit and community-controlled.   About 10 to 12 percent of short-term beds are "proprietary" beds (for profit).  The majority of these are physician-owned and controlled.  A few short-term beds belong to the local, state or federal government; these are largely for specially designated elements of the population, such as Public Health Service hospital beds for merchant seamen.  Because of the cost of maintenance, long-term beds in the United States have historically been public beds.  There are about 2 million of these beds, almost equally divided between mental hospitals and nursing homes.  Almost all mental hospital beds are state controlled, a few by the federal government.  The bulk of the beds in nursing homes (80 percent) are proprietary.

For the most part, hospital beds are not integrated into any system.  Each institution and staff controls its own pattern of admission, discharge and kind of treatment.  Most often it also decides who shall be on their staff.  Governmental, proprietary and voluntary institution administrations do not interact as patient care providers, although they may belong to common organizations (like the AHA or ANHA).  However, they should; the kinds of needs that the patients have, over time, relate to all the aspects of institutional care.  On occasion the individual may require acute, short-term hospitalization; as he gets older or acquires a chronic illness, he may require nursing home care; if he develops a mental illness he may require institutionalization in a government-sponsored mental hospital.  Further, it might be advantageous for hospitals to divide some responsibilities; one could specialize in obstetrics, for example, because this is expensive care and should be done at capacity, rather than keeping separate, half-capacity maternity units at several hospitals.

### REGIONALIZATION

It was recognized in the Report of the Committee on the Costs of Medical Care,* that regionalization was an important component of an efficient medical care delivery system, particularly as a cost control factor to avoid duplication and foster efficiency and economy.  People had to be able to move from one institution to another without having to go through separate admitting procedures and various standards and criteria that might be

---

* In 1928, a foundation sponsored public group, the Committee on the Costs of Medical Care, sponsored a five-year study of American medical practice.  Their report, in 1932, covered the entire field in 11 volumes.  The "Final Report," which was reprinted in 1970 by HEW, contains a majority report and several minority reports.  It is the majority report that is referred to here.

imposed: Does your physician have hospital privileges here? Are you prepared to pay $400 in advance in order to offset the possibility of falling into debt as a result of your stay? Do you have the proper insurance that covers this care? Because of the variety of institutional beds, access was different in each one and related to different components of the system. The patient was very often deprived of access to some particular institution, regardless of his professional, medical or personal need, because he failed to meet a particular standard of admission to that institution.

A number of efforts were made at regionalization in the 1930's. But because of the proud independence of individual members of the hospital care system, regionalization could not be imposed professionally in the early days. These early efforts at regionalization stayed away from integrating specific patient care activities. They tended to include non-clinical background elements such as common laundry and common auditing and purchasing systems; much later and cautiously, this was extended to the sharing of interns and residents.

But the principal need for regionalization, that of being able to put patients in the beds best suited to their needs at the time of need, could not be accomplished very easily. Eliminating duplication of facilities to accomplish this was stubbornly resisted by the medical staffs of the independent institutions. Such integration of service would require, among other things, common admitting privileges for all doctors; most hospitals and their medical staffs wanted to preserve the independent right of staff selection and appointment. In a competitive medical system, the competition among the various specialists was hardly likely to tolerate this. So that while some management efficiencies were introduced by the early regional programs, very little in the way of actual professional service efficiency was accomplished.

### HOSPITAL COORDINATION AND PREPAID GROUPS

Prepaid groups have always been in a much better position to do this. Permanente, for example, built its own hospitals; because their salaried doctors had privileges in the hospital in which the program operated, for all practical purposes these hospitals served specific communities. Member patients *had* to be hospitalized there, and served by those doctors. It was similar to the European system of full time hospital doctors. The only difference was that in Europe there are separate groups of physicians who work in hospitals and who work outside, whereas in the Permanente system this was blurred, with doctors serving both ambulatory and inhospital patients.

The Health Insurance Plan of Greater New York did not have the same advantages in getting started that Permanente had. In the first place, it was not begun until after World War II and the patriotic enthusiasm had cooled somewhat. Prior to that, it had been hard to push for radical system change in a "win-the-war" platform. The doctors of New York City had reacted very strongly against the suggestion of the development of a prepaid group practice plan, which they called "captive patient" or "closed panel" practice. The implication of their criticism was that with free choice removed, the system would be foreign to American medical tradition. The hospitals, perhaps because of their staff doctors' pressure, were no more enthusiastic. Therefore, a compromise had to be made to win the doctors' cooperation, however grudging. The arrangement was that the doctors who practiced in the groups need not be full-time. The fact that they were allowed to have other commitments made it impossible to put them together into one hospital; the group physicians suffered under the necessity of having their patients admitted to their individual hospitals. If their colleagues in the group did not have privileges in the same hospital, they would not be able to provide care there. The HIP program in New York City limped along at quite a slower pace than the Permanente prepaid group practice, probably because Permanente had all the needed elements of practice in their hands at one time.

It is true that HIP did succeed in a few instances to develop a combined hospital and out-patient group practice that would serve a cluster of patients by a group of doctors working in one place. These successful systems were at Montefiore Hospital in the Bronx and at the New York University in Manhattan. Neither of these survived as unified hospital based groups. Both were eventually closed out; the New York University group separated from the University because of pressure from the medical school faculty, and the Montefiore group failed because HIP was unable to meet financial obligations imposed by this method of practice.

The HIP groups in existence are composed largely of part-time physicians, who share responsibilities for group patients along with their private patients, and are therefore more or less in competition with themselves. The program has never been as successful as Permanente either in attracting patients or in satisfying those who join.

The lesson would seem to be that regionalization, combining the hospital services and out-patient medical care to create an efficient unit for satisfying all patient medical care, is very difficult to accomplish in a basically competitive, independent medical practice system. It could be done, with difficulty, by putting financial and practice restraints on doctors; it could be satisfactory to patients (as the Permanente system apparently is), and financially sound as well.

## ASSOCIATED PRACTICE

In the meantime, the various organizational needs — better management, supervision, fiscal accountabilities — are being attacked from many other angles. New, tentative efforts at redirecting physicians toward an improved organization of practice are now underway, stimulated by federal laws and financial incentive. Some have emerged from the physicians' organizations themselves; these will probably have a greater growth expectancy than those plans emerging from the government or from medical care reformers. I mentioned before, for example, that group practice was at very slow growth in the United States, that even today less than 15 percent of physicians are in group practice. However, varieties of associated practice have been increasing by leaps and bounds. In an "associated practice," physicians may operate as a partnership of two or three physicians who may or may not share patients, though they share office space and personnel overhead. Others may simply occupy office space within the same building; the added convenience of being able to refer to doctors in nearby offices may be important to patients or doctors themselves, without any of the ties of an official group practice arrangement. The increasing number of physician office buildings is noteworthy. Many of them are in conjunction with hospitals and located nearby. The patient has the geographic convenience of group practice: to be able to see his doctor, plus whatever specialist he may need to call upon; and to be admitted or just use the facilities of the hospital more easily than he would in the ordinary, fragmented form of practice.

Partnerships and common office buildings are steps toward group practice, even though they may not have the contractual character or the organizational qualities of group practice. Of course they do not usually have the prepaid insurance aspect, which is of tremendous importance to patients. The values of improved organization of medical practice may not appear as beneficial to a patient as the concrete benefits of an insurance system, where all services are paid for. The financial security of a comprehensive prepaid system is very attractive!

### FOUNDATION APPROACH

There is also a relatively new form of associate practice that medical societies developed on their own, the so-called "foundation." In the foundation, the medical society acts as a paying agent for the doctors and also supervises the care being given. The first "foundation" began in Windsor, Ontario, in the late 1930's. The medical society sponsored a prepaid system for guaranteeing services to people in the community, very largely auto workers, in which the physicians were reimbursed on a fee-for-service basis. Most prepaid group practices in the United States at that time and even earlier had reimbursed the physicians on a salary or capitation basis. Sometimes, as in the prepaid practices of the trade unions (which were generally only specialized consultation services), doctors were paid on a session basis. It was rare in the United States for physicians in a prepaid system to be paid fee-for-service, because the cost of paying a physician his usual and customary fee would theoretically bankrupt the system. However, the Windsor system seemed to thrive; it was argued that the reason it thrived, while American plans failed, was that the patients were Canadians, and therefore sufficiently different from Americans to make the plan work! This, of course, is nonsense. The Canadians involved lived in close proximity to Detroit, and worked in the same industry and had the same pay scales, living standards and aspirations as American citizens. One finds it difficult to distinguish Canadian and American citizens living across the Detroit River from each other. However, the Windsor Medical Care Plan was successful; in the United States little effort was made to duplicate this prepaid plan based on solo practice and fee-for-service, until the 1950's, when the San Joaquin County Medical Society established the first foundation in the U. S.

It proceeded to do substantially what the Windsor Plan had done in Canada. It did not, however, set up a prepaid plan; instead, it agreed to receive funds from the insurance companies and federal agencies supplying patient coverage and to see that the physicians were paid according to a contracted fee scale, established for that community. In addition, the San Joaquin Plan agreed to supervise the quality of service delivered and to see that the system was not abused. This was a real contribution, quite different from anything done previously in the United States. The director of the San Joaquin Plan proceeded to look at the services from the standpoint of "average" services. If a doctor brought a patient to the office more times than the average, or if operations seemed to be performed with greater frequency than the average, the director of the plan discussed this with the physician involved. If it was found that there was insufficient justification for the operative procedure or for the excess visits, he was asked to have a consultation on his next cases before he could undertake the surgery or continue the visits. If he refused he was cut out of the system. Inasmuch as the medical society was controlling the funds coming into the program, being cut off from the system would cut the doctor out of the medical care system in that community. It was a powerful control measure, even with medical society control. The physicians were found to cooperate with the system. Apparently it has worked very well, so that the foundation system is growing in many other medical societies throughout the country, at the county level. The foundation offers an additional step toward eventual group practice. Involved doctors are currently working out of their own offices, but at some future time it may mean that they work in common space as well, and eventually as a true group.

## OPTIMAL SIZE FOR AN ORGANIZED HEALTH UNIT

Putting it all together is difficult, and not only from the management standpoint of trying to organize temperamental professionals or offering to restrict the independence of doctors. Another major problem is the reluctance of people to put *themselves* into a bureaucratic maze. The experiences they have had with bureaucracy, whether it is the government, industry or insurance companies, leads them to be generally wary of the related perils of impersonality, delay and irrelevant response. Too many people are already balking at computer errors in department store bills and credit card accounts. If group practice is to be a success, it has to contain and control its size so as to allow the member patients to remain in fairly constant and personal contact with a small number of known professional people.

Size is an area of great vulnerability in bureaucracy. Maintaining small size relationships in big and impersonal organizations is critical in every area of society, not just in medical care. It has been suggested, for example, that prepaid group practice should be structured as a bunch of grapes, with each grape representing a few thousand people with two or three physicians to look after them. Along the stem would be the ordinary types of specialists to look after these clusters of people — a surgeon and obstetrician, for example — having periodic office hours in each unit. The specialists who see patients more rarely, or who need large and expensive equipment to carry on their job, would give their services in a specialty center to which the patient would be *taken* instead of *sent.* Such specialists would perhaps include othopedists, urologists or neurosurgeons. In the original "grape" office unit, some specialized paraprofessional people would carry on in behalf of the specialists who served only periodically. The overall administration might be responsible for 100,000 or more people, but the patient at the "grape" level would be part of a medical care delivery structure of only 2,000 or 3,000 people, a neighborhood cluster of easily manageable size.

The analogy may not be entirely appropriate, but the idea of having a small cluster of people and a small cluster of physicians, united with similar clusters under an overall administrative process, is very attractive.

# Chapter 12
# The Federal Investment in Medical Care

---

Within the medical care system, the largest part of government payments for patient services derives from the *federal* government. However, the states are also involved, since practically all of the public mental hospital facilities in the United States are state operated and state supported. In addition, at the local community level some of the health services that would not otherwise be available, such as immunizations, emergency services and medical care for some of the poor, will be provided by some local governments.

## THE BEGINNING OF FEDERAL INVOLVEMENT

Because of the nature of the development of the American political system, the federal government was not involved through funding or direct delivery of medical care services to any large extent up until 10 or 15 years ago. In the 18th and 19th centuries the federal Marine Hospital Service, by collecting a few pennies a month from sailors, agreed to pay for medical care for American merchant seamen when they were hospitalized anywhere and at any port. In addition, the government built and operated Marine Hospitals, later called "Public Health Service Hospitals", to provide such care. The federal government also provided medical care and health services for the armed services, for federal prisoners and, in the 20th century, for drug addicts in two specially staffed narcotics hospitals.

Eventually military hospitals in Washington — the Army's Walter Reed, the Naval Medical Center and the Clinical Center of the Public Health Service — began to take care of federal officials: presidents, vice-presidents, congressmen and senators, at a minimal fee to cover hospital operating expenses.

Because of the nature and interpretation of the constitutional mandate, Congress was not inclined to legislate *provision* of health services for the

199

American people.  To many people, so long as physicians, hospitals and other health care resources were publicly accessible, it was not wise or necessary to duplicate the system.  Further, the medical profession insisted, right up until quite recently, that *they* (the doctors) took care of everyone without regard to ability to pay.  Hospitals, too, ran drives and solicited contributions based on the assertion that they took care of everyone, without regard to ability to pay.  Some people doubted the accuracy of those assertions, but the principle was a familiar American one and left Congress disinclined to intervene when it came to medical care delivery.  From Congress' standpoint it was difficult, too; those responsibilities not specifically assigned to the federal government in the Constitution were reserved to the states.  It would have been hard for the federal government to assume responsibilities for the delivery of medical care to citizens who theoretically were wards and responsibilities of the states.    Indians, however, under treaty, were wards of the United States government, so the federal government did have the exclusive responsibility to provide medical care for the Indians.

### THE NEW DEAL AND SOCIAL SECURITY: THE BEGINNING OF WELFARE

American welfare history underlines this shunting of responsibility from the federal level.  The United States did not see its way clear to taking over responsibility for the poor until the 20th century.  The poor were a *local* responsibility: charity hospitals, city hospitals associated with city work-houses, free standing clinics and charitable work of community hospitals were the way in which medical care was delivered to those who could not purchase it themselves.  With the Great Depression of the 1930's, the coming of the New Deal and the implementation of the Social Security Act, this feeling began to change.  The federal government began to provide grants-in-aid to the states to pay for certain categorical aspects of helpless citizens' needs.  Unemployment insurance and pensions for the elderly were part of the Social Security Act.  Categorical payments for the elderly who did not qualify for Social Security and aid to dependent children became part of the New Deal social welfare package.  However, charity medical care continued to be delivered in clinics either associated with hospitals or free standing, or where available for free in doctors' offices.  The states also began to buy medical services ("vendor medical care") in order to insure that poor people would get medical care if they needed it and to put a ceiling on their welfare costs.  Those people who were categorically poor because of unemployment, however, continued to be considered an entirely different kind of responsibility, and neither the federal government nor the states specifically accepted responsiblity for supporting them or paying for their medical care. That continued to be local charge and charity medicine in most instances. The New Deal brought in new concepts of "entitlement" as opposed to charity. But the new ideas were not universally accepted or implemented. If you were a helpless victim — a fatherless child, or old, disabled or blind — you were entitled to some official support. But many people still saw helplessness as partly the victim's fault and there was only grudging assent to welfare payments. Many people resented paying taxes for welfare purposes and their legislative representatives aimed to keep welfare costs down; therefore, the poor generally did not get enough help to keep healthy and well, particularly if they were needy by virtue of physical or mental handicaps. While the social conditions changed, the idea of charity still prevailed.

Physicians generally approved the mode of providing charitable care for the poor. For centuries patients who came to the doctor's office and were unable to pay received care anyway. In depression times, physicians were able to show that from 30 to 40 percent of the bills on their books were uncollectible, that the services that they provided were for patients who were not able to pay.

This has resulted in what is called the "Robin Hood Method" of charges. The doctors, presumably serving an economic spectrum of patients — some able to pay, some without any funds at all and some with limited funds — would make charges proportionate to what the patient's income or ability to pay was. Those people who were well-to-do would presumably pay more, so as to offset the losses of the physician created by those people who could pay only a little or nothing at all.

When the states began to offer reimbursement, it was so small or the appropriations so inadequate that many physicians preferred to take care of the patients without charging the state. These vendor payments turned out to be quite unsatisfactory all around. In these instances welfare departments would augment a client's income by some fixed amount for medical care, just as they would give a fixed amount for rent, clothing or food. This amount was supposed to put him on the same footing with other people in the community who bought their medical care.

The difficulty was that since the welfare grants for food, shelter and clothing were so inadequate, the client was soon using whatever additional money he was granted, such as that theoretically reserved for medical care, to buy necessities. And if the welfare department set up a "vendor payment" medical reimbursement system, instead of giving the money to the client, physicians resented the long forms they had to fill out. In some instances patients could not get care unless it had been previously authorized by the local welfare worker; this created bureaucratic complications in which neither the patients not the physicians were happy.

NATIONAL HEALTH SERVICE AND FEDERAL MEDICAL PAYMENT PROGRAMS

As a result of these difficulties there were pressures on Congress to create a national medical care service; throughout this century, a National Health Service has been constantly promoted by a minority of the people. Agitation and dissent on the part of physicians, the insurance industry, legislators and even some patients, along with the inertia or apathy of a large section of the populace, made it unlikely that such legislation would pass and, ultimately, it did not. After all, it was the poor who needed it the most. The monied majority may have been a little dissatisfied with the status quo, but not enough to agitate for major changes.

At the same time the unsatisfactory system of trying to buy medical care for the poor had to be corrected. A number of efforts were made in this direction between 1950 and 1965, and eventually resulted in the development of the medical payment programs associated with the Social Security Act under Title XVIII (Medicare) and Title XIX (Medicaid). Medicare pays for medical services for the elderly under specified conditions and scope; Medicaid does this for the poor.

Many times the things that people fear come to pass through the very compromises they develop as opposing measures. All of the defects and deficiencies of government medical care services that doctors wanted to prevent and patients feared, and which caused the public at large to be very resistant in implementing, became a reality when the government initiated Medicare and Medicaid. The two laws provide the following, in capsulized form:

*Medicare*

Medicare is the result of a long struggle to obtain a national health insurance program. It is a medical care payment plan for senior citizens (over 65) and for the totally and permanently disabled. It is largely federally funded, paid out of a federal trust fund. Patients have to pay some part of the cost: a monthly premium, a part of the actual hospital cost and a part of the actual physician cost. The hospital care insurance is automatic for all who qualify. The coverage for physician costs, which comes from the monthly premium, is voluntary. A federal agency in the Social Security Administration is responsible for monitoring quality, eligibility, costs and payments.

*Medicaid*

Medicaid is the result of the long-standing concern of welfare agencies to pay for medical care for the poor; not only those receiving welfare (cost assistance), but for the medically needy — the working poor who cannot pay their medical bills. This is a *state* program basically, or joint federal/state. The federal government provides grants, matched by states, for the states to set up programs in accordance with a federally approved plan for paying providers of medical services to eligible poor people. It is a state operated and supervised program, so the nature and content, eligibility, cost control, payments, etc., are under *state* control, varying according to state, and with only moderate federal supervision.

## EFFECTS OF GOVERNMENT FUNDING

### THE BYPRODUCT OF INFLATION

Before the government paid for the poor or the aged, most doctors charged little or nothing for their services to them. Once the government intervened with payment plans, doctors began to charge for all services they performed. Even if they would do no more than they had done before reimbursement was set, even if patients would not seek medical care more frequently than they would have ordinarily since the service was now free, there would still be more money *spent* than before. Two associated phenomena were overlooked, however. Not *all* the poor were being covered by the government, and not *all* the elderly were eligible. And once doctors expected to be paid, all the poor and the aged were expected to pay. This created a new and monumental hardship for people in the twilight zone of being, for example, too poor to afford care, but not poor enough to be eligible for government coverage. Then, because doctors were being paid adequately, there was no excuse for doctors to charge higher fees to their wealthier patients. Or if they did, they at least ought to charge the government less! But they did continue the Robin Hood method of charging some people more than others, and consequently the cost of physicians' office services shot up. In the first year of Medicare, despite the fact that very few additional services were performed, physicians earned a billion dollars more than the year before.

This was the beginning of medical inflation; it has not yet stopped. What had been the ceiling on charges became the floor. Medical costs naturally rose just as the opponents of "socialized medicine" had claimed they would. The officials, medical reformers and health system planners who had based their cost estimates on existing programs found themselves ridiculously out of phase in the light of the skyrocketing costs.

Those who had opposed a government system had said there would be abuses, that patients would make more demands and doctors would tend to take advantage of the system. This latter point was soft-pedaled by the critics, but it was taken for granted that in a human society there would be ways of "getting around the system." In order to augment income, most people would take advantage; and this turned out to be the case. It seemed that many of the people who had not been able to get all they would have liked from the medical care system before, now did so. Whereas prior to

1965, poor people used fewer office services than the middle income or well-to-do and a larger proportion of them were hospitalized and received fewer outpatient services, after 1970 poor people caught up in services. They were getting as many outpatient services as the well-to-do, but hospitalization did not decrease proportionately. Hospitalization continued to increase for *all* segments of the community involving particularly services covered by insurance when performed in the hospital, but not covered outside the hospital.

It is clear that increasing the money available to buy medical services, without putting any constraints on the services delivered or on the charges made, is bound to be inflationary.

### DOUBLE STANDARD OF MEDICAL CARE

Another lesson that was learned, from the addition of federal funds to purchase medical services, was that the care of the poor is not what the private practice of medicine concerns itself with. Although billions more dollars were available to pay for the medical services of the poor, the private American medical system continued to devote the bulk of its energy to the care of middle income and upper income patients. Poor people continued to be served in clinics. Clinic services doubled and emergency room services quadrupled, while physician office service did not increase similarly.

The quality of clinics and public institutions declined. Some of the aspects of public medical care contemptuously referred to as "bureaucracy" and "Army medical care" derive from this classic pattern of starving the public sector while feeding the private sector much more bountifully. While the private sector was paid "cost-plus" or "customary and prevailing charges," the public sector, the bulk of the poor, was on a restricted budget! Public hospitals, for example, began to deteriorate in the 1950's as a result of a complex of circumstances: declining public funding; increasing pressures from the poor; and a gradual shift in medical school graduates' interests — from participation in public medical services of these hospitals to private patient care in voluntary hospitals.

There is a cycle of despair associated with this. As the public hospitals become more impoverished, and the cities provide less money, the maintenance of the institutions deteriorates. The people working in the institutions begin to lose faith and the calibre of performance deteriorates. Physicians who had been devoted to the institution also begin to lose heart and give less and less of their time. It is too unpleasant, no longer satisfying. While the clinics are increasingly more heavily attended by patients they are decreasingly attended by physicians. Patients begin to be seen for only a few minutes at a time. Those doctors who do continue to come become increasingly disgusted with what they are doing and what is being asked of them. A downward spiral of care, sensibility and understanding ensues, with the end result of a very poor hospital and very poor care for poor people.

Physicians continue to resist any encroachment by public officials, or by the federal, state or local government upon the areas of medical practice. Public institutions continue to decline in professional importance, professional quality and professional, as well as patient, satisfaction. More public money is spent with fewer satisfying public medical care activities.

The United States has only rarely engaged itself in direct patient care services. The federal government's role was consistently defined as *paying* for services, and not *delivering* services. This responsibility was left to the private sector; it could be purchased by the government. Except for the armed services, the prisons and Indians, the United States tended to pay for existing medical services instead of providing direct care. This is a defensible social concept and philosophy. But purchased services can only be equitable if the government (the provider) chooses to act in an equitable way. If the provider chooses to give his services only under special conditions and to special classes of people, and the availability of money is insufficient to purchase equity, the poor can never get "equal" medical care from the public system.

If the price the government was prepared to pay really threatened the middle and upper income groups in that the high government prices might attract physicians away, the middle and upper income groups could afford to add a few dollars and outbid the public sector for relatively scarce professional services. As long as the Constitution was construed to forbid the federal government from engaging in the provision of medical services and from entering into a state to give medical services, inequity would prevail. For services to the poor, states would not pay more than their majority citizens paid. Levying taxes to that end was political suicide and any national system had to stay within the same payment structure. So the payment structure would necessarily have gross inequities built into it. Public money could never be adequate to buy for the poor services of the same kind that middle and upper income people could buy for themselves.

American medical care really comprised a double standard: two systems; one for the poor, largely paid out of public funds; and one for the middle and upper income groups, paid out of their own pockets with some public subsidy. This was bound to result in the public medical care system being inferior to the private one.

However, the private system would inevitably become tainted by the same defects and deficiencies that attacked the public system. As the public system deteriorated, the private sector would suffer. The middle and upper income people would also have to use emergency rooms on Wednesdays and weekends when their own doctors were not available. The declining quality of these institutions' provision of care would mean that the middle income and well-to-do, when they required the most urgent, specialized, intensive care, would find themselves at the mercy of inadequate people in inadequate institutions. These were the institutions with the deteriorating facilities, largely staffed with non-American trained physicians or no physicians at all, and an ancillary staff composed of crusty, unhappy, frustrated health workers.

Lincoln pointed out that the world cannot exist half slave and half free. It has become quite clear that if there are to be two medical care systems, they will affect one another in some way. The effect is bound to be to the detriment of the less well financed institution with resulting inadequacies in the fiscally poorer one, so that with less staff and equipment, less enthusiastic or motivated personnel, the institution is bound to become qualitatively poorer as well. It would be wise then for the effort to be made to see to it that the public sector services are as well equipped, staffed and supplied as the private system.

## FINDING THE WAY TO PROVIDE
## GOVERNMENTAL AID

Having reviewed the various problems relating to the reasonably equal access to quality medical care at reasonable cost for all Americans, it is important to discuss how to go about developing the federal resources in a suitable, mutually agreeable way — a very complex problem in itself. It is not only where the money should come from, or how the different parts of the problem should be prioritized in regards to funding. There are more difficult questions with regard to the priorities of development of these resources altogether.

For example, how much money should society spend as a *total* for medical care? It is very easy to protest that since we are the richest country in the world and we spend so many billions for military systems for ourselves and for our allies, that simply by shifting priorities from the military and spending the money in the welfare area we ought to be able to meet our obligations. But it is questionable that we could. In the end all resources are limited. Even if we do not build battleships, there will certainly be increasing demands for education and its improvement, or for a guaranteed minimum annual wage, added welfare and employment demands and housing. Every one of these should have at least as great a piece of the tax dollar as medical services.

BUDGETING/RESTRICTING PHYSICIAN INCOME

Even if we are not too cynical we can recognize the fact that a part of the consideration of cost in either creating or deploying medical resources rests on an assumption that the people working in the field will continue to be paid at a very high rate. For example, physicians are among the best paid professionals in the United States and in the world. It is true that industrial executives make $400,000 or $500,000 a year (plus extras of stock options, pension plans, etc.), but this affects a rather small number of people, and the same may be said for the few thousand athletes and entertainers with very high incomes. When it comes to physicians, the highest paid personnel element of the medical care world, there are approximately 300,000 taking in over $20 billion annually, or about $70,000 per doctor. Even with about 30 percent of a physician's income going for overhead, he still makes between $45 and $50 thousand a year before taxes. The median income in the United States is about $13,000 for a family; the average black family makes just $7800. That means that the average physician in the United States makes approximately four times the family income of 50 percent of the population! Furthermore, since 90 percent of the population makes less than $25,000 a year, physicians, who are just about .1 percent of the population, earn on average more than 90 percent of the population! Some would argue that since society sets its own values and chooses to pay physicians at the high rate they have come to expect, what is wrong with these numbers? Perhaps nothing.

Even the physician in training, who is devoting only a fraction of his time to patient care and the rest to learning about patient care, earns more than the median income. It would appear that with this excessively high value being placed upon a physician's services, perhaps we should think twice about budgeting for enlargement of medical care expenditures. Do we really need to double the supply of physicians in order to assure appropriate access to good quality medical care for every American? Do we need to increase the expenditures (provided that they will be made at current rates) by $20 billion? Should we add another 20 percent to the national expenditures for medical care, thereby raising the proportion of the gross national product being spent on medical services from 8 percent to 10 percent?

In addition, when we realize, as was discussed in previous chapters, that overspecialization of medical practice, lack of proper organization, poor hospital management and fee-for-service all contribute to excessive expenditures for physicians' services, then certainly in our allocation of funds for training of physicians and for the overall medical service resources development budget, we will want to improve economy and performance.

Maybe we should also adapt our ideas about how much physicians should be earning. These are fairly heretical thoughts, I realize, and may not be conducive to the best working relations between the doctors and the public. But on the other hand, it is the sort of realistic appraisal that we must undertake when we look at *other* elements in society in which we are investing. The price of physicians' services and the price of resource development should not be any more sacred from the standpoint of budgeting and appropriations than any other element of public expenditures.

### CUTTING INSTITUTIONAL COSTS

Given facts like these, it is easy to see that we cannot make any firm decisions about how much should be spent on resource development of individual items in the medical care network, without paying attention to all the other elements. If we want to reduce institutional costs, which are the heaviest costs of all, we have to arrange that the medical services now provided in institutions be provided elsewhere. This will, of course, necessitate that different and perhaps additional people work in the community aspects of care. If this could be done through the retraining of people who are now otherwise engaged in institutional care, we would have very little problem with the cost of resource development. If, however, it means that new types of people and training programs have to be created, there will be much educational expense. If we come to the conclusion that the services provided by the most expensive health professional, the physician, can be performed by people with a lesser degree of training, who would then receive a lesser degree of reimbursement, we may save much of our resource allocation. We could then put more money into the training of these paraprofessionals in order to catch up with the current lag in the production of these less expensive people, making it possible to use more in situations handled by physicians.

We cannot make firm decisions about how much should be allocated within the health system for resource development without a prior policy decision as to what resources we want. If we want more community care, we need more community trained people. If we need less expensive people taking care of us than physicians, we want to put more of our money into the training of those people.

### DECIDING WHICH CITIZENS SHOULD PAY

A further factor in assigning costs in federal budgeting for medical care resource development derives from some characteristic American ideas about who should pay for what and when. For example, a large part of the cost of medical care is borne by patients, even in the insurance system. It is not spread evenly over the entire population of insured people; those people who get care pay something additional at the time of service. Under the experience rating system of insurance, those people who have more "experiences" (use more services) pay higher premiums. Should the people who use more services be taxed in some fashion so that they pay a fairer share of the bill for health care and resource development?

There is a typical issue of this kind in the matter of construction of hospitals. If the major part of the cost of constructing hospitals were paid by federal funds, costs would be distributed fairly equally among taxpayers based on their income. However, most hospital construction is not fully federally funded. Even under the terms of the Hill-Burton Act, only a third of the money came from the federal government. Some of it came from the state; in this case it may have been drawn from sales or property taxes, which are not always equitably distributed. Some of the money came from the charges that hospitals made per patient day. Costs per patient day are again unequally distributed, since it comes from out of pocket or the experience-rated insurance premium. But many people argue that this is essentially a fair way of dealing with the problem of medical care institutions; that the user should pay more than the nonuser.

## CUTTING AID TO MEDICAL STUDENTS

In deciding how to pay for the education and training of people who will serve in the medical care field, some of this same attitude is also applied to federal resource allocations. Since physicians are going to be making such exorbitantly great salaries, many of those responsible for developing federal budgeting and appropriations for medical schools believe that the doctors should support themselves in their education and training; society pays them heavily enough afterwards. As a consequence, only a small portion of the medical students' education is supported from federal funds now. Until 1963, there was no federal money available for medical education as such. It is true that a part of medical school support came from the "overhead" charges provided from research grants, but this was in a sense only indirect support to the education. As we shall discuss a little later, it was more of a burden than a privilege and distorted medical education considerably, contributing to our current bitter situation.

At any rate, federal support in terms of direct grants to students to offset the costs of education is very modest. Only about 10 percent of students get total scholarship support and not all of this comes out of the federal pocket. The total amount of money required by the 114 American medical schools to support the medical education process is estimated by the Institute of Medicine of the National Academy of Sciences to be in the neighborhood of $10,000 to $20,000 per student, or nearly a billion dollars a year. Only about 25 percent of that amount comes directly from the federal government. Should the federal government pay all costs of medical education, so that students could go to medical school free, without any additional charges? Some people argue vehemently that it should; that doctors are a national resource and their services are required by all the people. But that argument could perhaps be applied to practically every other professional activity for which there are public needs and for which public resources have to be supplied for training. If medical education is to be publicly financed, it is gradually being realized that many more demands ought to be made on the graduates to demonstrate social responsibility and to fulfill social needs. A doctor who is simply an entrepreneur, earning four times the median American annual income; who displays no regard for social needs; or who refuses to adjust his practice to allow the people's needs to be met sufficiently can hardly justify a national commitment of support for medical education.

If withholding financial support is to be an overall federal policy with regard to tuition support, it ought to affect not only medicine, but physics or chemistry and the humanities. This raises a rather complex question of higher education support that needs to be answered by society: whether a small percentage of the population should enjoy such benefits. But the very large income of physicians colors the argument as it relates to them.

Many of the influential people at the head of government in the Nixon administration seemed to have rather strong prejudices against traditional medical practice and physicians. Strong efforts were made to reduce the amount of money the federal government put into medical education, using the argument that since the physician made so much money in practice, he should be asked to pay his own way in education. The medical schools do not care for this argument because it makes for very difficult budgeting, and they may not be able to attract the most qualified students if those students cannot afford to pay for their own education. Further, it may discourage qualified people from going into that field if they *can* get financial support in other interesting career schools. Withholding financial support definitely discriminates strongly against minorities and women, who still have major difficulties in borrowing sufficient sums to carry them through the long years of education.

The fact is that we would like to have representation from many segments of the population in medical practice, for all kinds of reasons, many of which have been discussed earlier. It is therefore extremely difficult to have a uniform policy on paying for medical education. If scholarships or institutional support are not provided to reduce tuition, we may lose the potential doctors from poor and minority communities. The policy of compelling each student to support himself through medical school might be more easily upheld if society were able to guarantee every family an adequate annual income; then there would not be this kind of burden on the youngster who wanted to go into medicine.

To summarize, the cost of medical education to the student must be kept low to encourage all kinds and classes of students to enter. At the same time the earning level of physicians should be controlled to the same extent. If they have been educated at public expense, they ought to return something to the public for that privilege. In such case resource allocation required for the future might be reduced. Full-scale public payments for medical education would have important implications for the eventual cost of general medical care, and for the possibility of legislating changes in the organizational pattern of health care and the distribution of physicians. For that reason, the decision to finance medical education may be the single most important decision that can be made in the public sector for the realization of equity in medical care.

We have devoted much of the discussion of possible reallocation of government funds to the area of physician training and modes of practice. This has been deliberately emphasized, because physicians are such powerful determinants of what is done in medical care. If the overall system is to be changed, it will not be done without the physicians' participation. Perhaps if we concentrate on changing medical education, it will give us a different kind of doctor, more amenable to social action; more flexible in use of facilities and in sharing responsibility with other medical personnel; and less interested in an exorbitant salary. We cannot focus on other resource needs without taking the physician and his education into account. If we do more outside the hospital, and so need fewer hospital beds, it is because we can persuade the doctors to work that way.

## FUNDING THE ULTIMATE RESOURCE: RESEARCH AND DEVELOPMENT

There is another area of resource development that we are less capable of analyzing so easily. This is the accumulation of new knowledge: biomedical and health care delivery research.

Biomedical research in the United States was a very small-scale operation, funded primarily by private philanthropy, until after the Second World War. In 1937, the National Cancer Institute's budget was only $350,000; even in constant dollars, compared with 1975 expenditures of $2 billion at the National Institutes of Health, that was extremely modest.

A number of things contributed to the phenomenal public funding of research between 1940 and 1970.

SOCIAL ATTITUDES AND TECHNOLOGICAL ADVANCEMENT

One was the realization that we were rich in money, resources and technology. During World War II we made huge financial and technological investments to achieve a successful military objective. We built hundreds of Liberty ships and thousands of tanks and assault boats; we equipped millions of men in our own Army and millions of men in the armies of our allies and sent them all over the world. There was not anything we needed in the way of technology and equipment to win the war that we were not able to produce provided we put up the money. The illusion grew that money itself could solve problems. We even built the first atomic bomb — for $2 billion.

At the same time we were beginning to have experiences with new and exciting developments in chemistry, biology and physics. We were given new, wonderful and terrifying insights into the opportunity for change and improvement in man's condition. When we managed to get inside the atom, we realized the awesome potential and the energy and power of nature itself. Einstein's $E = MC^2$ brought us to the realization that man could master nature; it should be possible to do anything!

New and exciting discoveries in medicine had historic impact on the diagnosis and treatment of disease. Sulfonamides and serum therapy, for example, opened a new world of possibilities in treatment. But penicillin brought the greatest change in attitudes toward medicine and research. The discovery antedated World War II, but laboratory development required for production of it in constant and repeatable form was not completed until the beginning of the War, and full commercial production did not come until almost the end of the War. With it, patients who had lingered for weeks with pneumonia in the open wards of hospitals were now capable of being treated in a few days at home, and pneumonia, "the old man's friend," ceased to be such a killer.

Antibiotics were now here; the great age of miracle drugs had begun. People were clamoring for "the" cure — to everything: heart disease, cancer, anything that interfered with man's ability to live free of illness. Streptomycin and isoniazid wiped out tuberculosis, which had actually been on the wane since the middle of the 19th century, hardly influenced by any of the medical means applied for over 100 years. But the introduction of new drugs caused a sharper decline in its incidence. By the 1950's states and local communities were beginning to close the tuberculosis hospitals or to convert them to other areas of medical need.

The effect of the new drugs is apparent statistically. In New York City in August 1903, 400 out of every 1,000 babies born had died before they were a year old; in August of 1950 in New York City, of every 1,000 babies born only thirty (30) died; in 1975 only seventeen (17) babies per thousand died.

People began to have a vision of life without disease or premature death, and they wanted the vision to become reality. New operations began to be performed. Efforts to change old patterns of sickness, handicaps and pain flourished. Transplants began to make it possible for people who would otherwise die to live out a normal life span. New materials for deteriorated blood vessels were manufactured.

The media contributed to the demand and expectation of cure in no small degree through the widespread reports of discoveries and cures, sometimes exaggerated. Announcement of discoveries created a constant pressure for more discovery.

By 1940, with employee hospitalization coverage fairly standard and widespread, millions of people were suddenly able to afford hospital care; the insurance programs drove them into hospitals for services because outpatient care was not covered. Along with the employee group plans, there were military plans. For example, a program called EMIC (Emergency Maternity and Infancy Care) paid for inhospital maternity care for dependents of the men in uniform. So there were enormous pressures on hospitals for admissions. More hospital beds could not be built because of the wartime freeze on cement and steel.

Something had to give, and what gave was old physiological theory. As an example of the old physiological theory, when I was a housestaff intern in 1939, my surgical patients had to be kept in bed 14 days and were restricted from moving about. The physiological theory at the time was that the healing site had to be kept at absolute rest, or little pieces of clots would break up, go off to the lung or brain and kill or at least incapacitate the patient further. Hernia patients, therefore, were not permitted to cough, and if they did cough or move about too much, we had to keep them in bed an extra two days.

With the pressures of hospital admissions and limited beds, physiologists returned to the laboratory and, regarding the movement of patients, discovered that it was keeping the wound site at absolute rest that was causing fragments to break off and travel through the body, causing further disease or death. They announced that moving the patient about more quickly after surgery was a better method of controlling such thromboses and emboli. The patients began to be walked about within 24 hours after operations. Patients formerly kept ten days were sent home in a day and a half or two days. Hernia patients were operated on and returned home in three days.  Maternity cases were kept overnight.  In England in the 1950's, partly as a result of this kind of experience, a surgeon in the London Hospital published a report on 750 herniorrhaphies that were done in the outpatient department, with the patients sent home by taxi the same day!

One of the results of this, of course, was the reduction of length of stay in hospitals, from 14 to eventually 7 days on average.  But another important and more subtle result was the beginning of an understanding that by bringing certain kinds of pressures from society on medical institutions, imagination and energy could solve any problem.  There was no ineluctable, unchangeable fact of medical practice and medical knowledge. Everything was subject to reinvestigation, reexamination and potential transformation.

### INFLUENCE ON CONGRESS

Putting these things together, we can recognize the social dynamics of attitudinal change that had such a powerful influence in encouraging much more public investment in biomedical research.  There were new drugs that promised cures.  There were new procedures that promised longer and happier, less painful lives.  We could actualize the vision with money, intelligence and energy.  The common philosophy became: if social pressures can engineer these changes, let us press; if more money solves problems, let us put more money into research.

And the philosophy was channeled through an extraordinary group of people in Congress and the federal government, who utilized the sentiments to facilitate the great growth and development of the National Institutes of Health and the investment of the United States in biomedical research. Congressman John Fogarty from Rhode Island, a bricklayer by profession who had never finished high school, had tremendous political zest and understanding.  He became chairman of the Subcommittee on Appropriations for HEW in 1955, a uniquely powerful location for determining health budgets, and made health matters both his career and his hobby.  He was a Democrat with a strong base in the trade union movement, had a standing friendship with most of the Democratic Party movers and shakers and, as one of the elite group of Congressional chairmen with real power and privilege, was in an excellent position to do things.

His counterpart in the Senate was Lister Hill, a Democrat from Alabama. He was chairman of the Senate Committee on Labor and Public Welfare, as well as chairman of its Subcommittee on Health, and of the Subcommittee on Appropriation for Health.  These positions gave him an even better influence on health legislation from the Senate side than Fogarty had on the House side.  In addition Hill belonged to that small group of southern Democrats who share a liberal tradition (except in racial matters), and he had access to the "club," the leaders in Congress. The relationship of these two Washington officials with the party forces gave them an extraordinary opportunity to carry out health policies as they saw fit. Fogarty and Hill, with the appropriate education and orientation, had it in them to transform American medical practice, whether it would be in service, organization, financing or research. For a decade they dominated federal funding in the medical field. The fact that they chose research as the medium for exercising their influence on the ultimate transformation was no accident.

James Shannon, Director of NIH, and Mary Lasker, a wealthy health lobbyist, deserve credit for helping to provide the education that guided this influence, but there is a historic basis for the fact that they were able to have this kind of influence on Hill and Fogarty.

James Shannon became the director of the National Institutes of Health in 1955. He was a physician who learned how to deal with the bureaucracy; if he had attempted to make politics his career, he might have been in the House or the Senate. As a physiologist and physician with a respectable research background, he became the head of the National Institutes of Health when it was still a relatively modest enterprise with a budget of $81 million per year (compared with today's $2 billion), and when it had just survived a rather nasty and somewhat scandalous episode of a badly handled polio vaccine issue.

He immediately set about organizing lines of communication so as to inform and influence the various committees of Congress about NIH activities to insure support. He was particularly anxious that the NIH not suffer as a result of any changed or unpredictable activity by the Surgeon General. When Shannon came to the NIH, the director was a subordinate of the Surgeon General. When Shannon left the NIH 13 years later, this bureaucratic line remained, but Shannon was an equal in prestige and influence. From the beginning he had acted to acquire funds for the NIH. The vaccine scandal made it relatively easier for him to gain such authority, because he was in the eye of the hurricane. His confidence, directness and astute handling of Congress gave him a leadership role that he never surrendered.

The polio scandal had to do with carelessness, lack of supervision, lack of understanding for some of the problems of safety control in vaccine manufacture and a rather cavalier attitude with regard to government-private industry relations. The whole thing was a tragicomedy of ineptitude and unfortunate mischance. What followed was a genteel housecleaning, and even as Shannon succeeded the retiring NIH director, a new Surgeon General was appointed and a new Secretary of HEW came into office. This was all discreetly unmentioned in the scientific or popular literature. The media in those days apparently did not have the same type of investigative, aggressive journalism evidenced 20 years later! The matter was widely known in government circles and in Congress and there was fear that the carelessness, selfishness or inefficiency demonstrated might inhibit continued growth of the NIH. Fogarty and Hill were anxious that the unfortunate incident should not jeopardize the NIH's growth and development, and they were eager to assist the new director of the NIH to achieve the mutual objective.

The other chief influence to Fogarty and Hill was not in the government at all. Mrs. Mary Lasker, widow of the enormously wealthy inventor of modern advertising, used the money she inherited to influence the field of medical research. In a sense, she was the spokeswoman for America's ideas on what medicine and medical research ought to be and do. She wanted to prevent or cure mental illness, heart disease and cancer. With the aid of a newsman, Mike Gorman, an artful purveyor of public relations techniques, she proceeded to inform and educate Congress and the American people in order to continue and augment medical research expenditures. She did this in part by supplying money for political support of selected candidates. Wisely she did not put all the money into the Democratic Party treasury; instead she carefully selected candidates and put up modest sums for each, which made a lot of key people grateful and attentive when occasion arose. In addition, Mike Gorman arranged for conferences and publications that brought before the American people information of what research had done and the possibilities of what research could do. Some of this was done through voluntary health agencies to which Mrs. Lasker contributed and helped to control, such as the Mental Health Association, Cancer Society and Heart Association; and she saw one in particular as a vehicle for public education and pressure on Congress, the Committee for the Nation's Health, headed by Michael Davis. The team of Shannon and Lasker fostered to a large extent the phenomenal growth of the National Institutes of Health, and established the congressional and public support that helped to put American biomedical research into the forefront of world research, both in terms of investment and productivity.

### DISTORTED BYPRODUCTS

In order to do research, people had to be trained, institutions had to be funded and a rain of research gold was needed to revive and develop departments of medical schools and other teaching institutions. Such funding was unequal, of course, since the largesse went into those medical school departments that were able to pick up the kinds of research considered important by the powerful facilitators. Then, because of the support, those institutions were better able to find or develop more and better researchers sharing common goals with the facilitators, and thus draw increasingly larger sums from the treasury.

Older private institutions like Harvard, Yale and Hopkins grew and flourished. State schools that shared the dream, and those in which the states helped to augment the federal support, like New York, California and North Carolina, further distorted the geographic loci for concentration of medical talent and departmental facilities. Large parts of the country were veritable Saharas of research because the water from the federal pump never reached them. Others became research institutes of such magnitude that their research functions overcame all teaching functions. They were medical "schools" in name only; basically they were research laboratories.

And since the schools that had the money and were able to grow and prosper with this golden research shower were the ones that were most in the public eye, their graduates became the professors and deans of the medical schools. Their researchers were the ones who were in the newspapers by virtue of actual accomplishment, or by artful public relations efforts in the Lasker-Gorman axis. Luncheons and dinners for the award of research prizes and medals became front page news. It is no accident that there was a Lasker award for medical news reporting. That encouraged the reporters to remain interested and prolific.

The other schools, even if they did not share in the heavy research funding, chose or were compelled to share in the common aspiration. They may not have been able to do as much research, but they could certainly foster in their students the desire for it, with the wistful view of a potential Nobel Prize.

The distortion of medical education toward research resulted in most of the students learning that research was the most important aspect of the medical function. Direct patient care, the original purpose of medical education, was considered secondary. Emphasis on clinical research skills, to foster or increase new diagnostic and therapeutic opportunities, was magnified. This distortion has had serious consequences in the conflict of expectations between patients and doctors as to just what the function of the physician is. Physicians came to believe that they were to fulfill the social role of "medicine" through laboratory research, rather than through patient care.

A second and perhaps more serious aspect of this distortion, which has contributed to our continuingly inflating cost of medical care, has to do with the increase in the number of specialists. The research aspect of medical education, by forcing emphasis on specialized knowledge, fostered the development of increasing numbers of specialties and subspecialties. The "family doctor" seemed to have no place in medical education. First of all there were no direct medical education funds for him. And secondly the only role models he saw were all researchers or, at the very least, clinical assistants to researchers.

Processes of this kind have a momentum all their own. Let us start with a department of medicine. For the purpose of doing research and investigation, people have to specialize in some aspect of medicine to narrow the field of study. The cardiologist, for example, then has to have clusters of assistants who will help with the research, but he also needs medical assistants to look after the accumulation of patients referred to him as a specialist. These patients will in time be the clinical cases on which the research discoveries will be based. He has to train all of these assistants. Pretty soon instead of interns and residents who are generalized in the department of medicine, there are cardiology fellows and cardiology residents, cancer fellows and cancer residents. While the department may have previously needed ten general residents to serve patients, it may now need seven or eight more in cardiology, seven or eight more in cancer, seven or eight more in lung. Soon what was a 50-bed setup with five people working as house officers becomes a facility of 55 or 60 beds with as many as 50 people working. After training as specialists, they then all go into practice as specialists. The patients learn that they need the specialists for a specific condition, but that the specialists cannot see too many patients. And specialists' fees are kept much higher than generalists' to maintain the prestige and quality of the extra knowledge. Since different kinds of specialists have to be seen, and it takes more than one specialist for certain kinds of conditions, the cost of medical care mounts geometrically and astronomically.

The dilemma was recognized early. Research money was distorting medical education and medical practice, creating an unusual burden of cost and reducing general or family practice to a disappearing commodity.

However, it was a good life for those living it. If changes were to be made to correct the distortion, it was hoped that it could be done by adding on other pieces; that it would not require any change in the investment in research, but an *added* investment in medical care. The argument ran, "it isn't what's being done that is bad, it's that not enough is being done of the other things." There was no recognition of the "system" and interdependence of medical care, medical education and medical research. The proponents of big research, already established in control of the medical schools and supported in many other ways directly and indirectly, made it almost impossible to deal with the problem in any other frame of reference.

### FUNDS FOR CANCER RESEARCH

But when people have a dedication or commitment as these fiercely devoted partisans of biomedical research had, the effect of their activities is both sometimes sterile and other times productive. This was the case of the political fight for the billion dollar campaign for cancer research.

Because cancer is so feared and so often lethal, research toward a cure is bound to have a high priority in most people's minds when there is discussion as to which research efforts should be funded. Therefore, the first unit of the National Institutes of Health was the National Cancer Institute.

Over the years Congress has been quite generous with funds. Research, however, is a fickle mistress. One does not always find what one is looking for, and sometimes it is found only by chance. The scientific name for this is "serendipity," coined after an English politician and writer, Sir Horace Walpole, drew a parable of three princes from Serendip who never found what they were looking for, but who always found interesting things by accident. Hundreds of bacteriologists and laboratory workers must have been discouraged when they saw the clear areas in their agar solution when they were trying to grow colonies of infectious organisms. They not only failed to grow the organisms, but found some colonies mysteriously wiped out when they did. Fifty years may have gone by until Alexander Fleming became curious over this manifestation and eventually discovered penicillin. He was not looking for penicillin; he was looking for an infectious agent, but found a cure. There are other examples. In any case, one of the laws of scientific research might be stated as follows: observe carefully and note carefully; a particular item of information may be of interest even if it is not expected.

This is not to say that "targeted" research is useless. What it does mean is that if one has a fairly good idea about the nature of the target and how to proceed, targeted research can work. An example of this is the "moon shot." We had all the necessary knowledge about escape from the earth's atmosphere, astronomical guidance, rocketry, physics and computer mathematics. The knowledge needed to be refined, of course, and the engineering application had to be developed. This was beautifully organized targeted research.

But the application of this concept as a model for cancer research is false. We do not know the cause of cancer and we don't even know in what direction to look. As a consequence we know very little about what can be done in treatment or cure. If research is to be carried out, it needs to be through basic studies of all the areas of physiology, biochemistry, pathology and epidemiology that might lead to avenues of solution. And empirical tests of a variety of substances may lead us to avenues of treatment. For the "moon shot" it was a question of money. If enough funds were devoted to the engineering application, it was inevitable that a solution would result. No one knows how much money needs to be devoted to finding the cure for cancer, or in how many different directions to look.

These thoughts did not deter the research-minded lobbyists in their pursuit for even larger funds for cancer research. Joining forces were President Nixon who wished to distract attention from his ax-wielding destruction of health program budgets by making gestures in the direction of cancer research and cure; and Senator Kennedy who saw any effort to improve budget and financing in the health field as a positive value. The crusade was launched to obtain one billion dollars — eventually cut to a half billion — for cancer research.

It is not a bad idea to spend a half billion dollars on cancer research. However, it was a mockery to have fastened on cancer research as a solution to the national health problem, given the facts that health budgets were being cut in every direction; that there were terrifying disparities between what people needed in the way of health services; and that the country was being torn apart by the inequitable distribution of all kinds of goods and services. There were not even enough researchers to pick up the money that was already available, let alone the added money that was to be provided by the bill.

The lobbyists won; the half billion dollars was authorized and eventually almost as much was appropriated. The irony is, of course, that we are no closer to a solution three years later than we were at the time the money was provided; nor are we likely to be, unless there is some miraculous breakthrough that may or may not be the result of the heavy investment. More likely, a breakthrough will come from the imaginative insight of some investigator with only a small fraction of the money available, perhaps not even from the appropriated cancer funds! The National Cancer Institute has some difficulty in disposing of its funds and spends some of its money developing plans for getting rid of it.

In essence, research has to be set down in the same perspective as the other aspects of health program development. One may not be able to say how much money should be spent, but one ought to be able to say what proportion of the overall health service and health planning investment ought to be devoted to biomedical research. Research money may actually hamper research activities if improperly appropriated or focused. To put all the research money or any enormous part of it into cancer research may deprive other useful fields of investigators who flock to where the money is. It will distort the overall research effort. Other researchers may be doing work totally unrelated to cancer that might throw great light on the cancer problem and expedite its solution. One cannot haggle with nature on this perspective.

FUNDS FOR MEDICAL SCHOOL RESEARCH: THE ONLY ACCEPTABLE AID

Fear of bureaucracy and socialized medicine kept Congress and the American people hesitant to support medical education directly until almost ten years ago. For example, the American Medical Association, powerful for so many years, was able to use its influence to persuade Congress that the end result of direct support of medical education would be public and bureaucratic control of medical education. Inasmuch as universities have a sacred place in American life and university officials feel the same way about wanting to avoid governmental control, this argument gained a sympathetic ear. Very little effort was made on the part of either university officials, medical school deans or those responsible for medical education to try to promote congressional interest in the direct support of medical education. The first efforts were allowed to be only in the direction of providing funds for medical schools to construct research facilities.

It is important to recognize that Fogarty and Hill had very little else to do, to promote health service in the United States, than to provide funds for biomedical research. They could not go into medical education as there was too much opposition from the AMA and educators. They could not go into medical service because there was opposition from the AMA and from a nation at large afraid of socialized concepts. So they searched for the only area in which they could have an impact. And with the lack of knowledge at the time of what the impact might have of distorting the system by putting all that money into one part of it, they cannot be faulted. It is perfectly obvious that these were well-intentioned people who wanted to do a good job and who had the ultimate goal of curing and helping the American people. The same thing must be said for Shannon and his efforts to promote and develop the National Institutes of Health, and for Mrs. Lasker and her efforts to educate the American people and turn them in the direction of improving research potential and expenditures. All of these efforts were aimed at the improvement of the health of the American people. The evil effect was unintentional.

## FUNDING NATIONAL HEALTH INSURANCE: A LOSING BATTLE

### ANTISOCIALIST THEORY

The great bugaboo of socialized medicine has afflicted the United States since the Bolshevist revolution of 1917. And a national program of health insurance has always been defeated as a consequence.

The idea of a national health insurance program or a national health service has a long history in the United States, going back to at least 1907 or 1909. Theodore Roosevelt's Bull Moose Party in 1912 had a national health insurance plank. A committee of medical economics of the American Medical Association in 1916 recommended national compulsory health insurance as the solution to America's health needs. Edgar Sydenstricker, on behalf of the United States Public Health Service, published a pamphlet in 1916 as an official government bulletin describing possible operation of a national health insurance system in the United States.

However, after World War I, there was a revulsion against this position in the United States. The newspapers had been reasonably sympathetic earlier to Marxism; Karl Marx wrote a frequent column for the New York Herald Tribune in the late 19th century, and John Reed and Boardmann Robinson wrote sympathetic accounts of the Russian Revolution for the newspapers. But the Republican administrations in the 1920's, perhaps in the bitter fight against the League of Nations, became fiercely opposed to any involvement in European ideas and ideals and gave rise to a frantic know-nothing attack on any kind of socialist ideology in the United States. We may recall faintly the Palmer "Red Raids" in which the Attorney General carried out unconstitutional attacks on citizens and groups thought to be even mildly liberal. At one time several members of the New York State Assembly were arrested on the floor of the legislature because they were socialists. Legislation in New York State, which had seemed almost certain to establish a health center program and a health insurance system for the poor, disappeared from the agenda. Socialism was bad; anything tainted with socialism was bad. The Russians had socialized medicine and for that reason alone, we had to avoid it.

At the end of the 1920's the Committee on the Costs of Medical Care was funded by eight respectable foundations, presided over by a respectable physician and university president, Ray Lyman Wilbur. He had been president of the American Medical Association before he became president of Stanford University. His staff included some of the more distinguished members of the professional community, and they reported in a series of 20-odd volumes on manifold aspects of American medical care. Their report suggested, rather mildly, that what the United States needed was voluntary health insurance. The attack on the Committee and the Report was violent; the editorial columns of the American Medical Association carried all kinds of vituperative articles, calling even Blue Cross communistic, and rejecting all recommendations of the Committee.

Over the years the American Medical Association has kept alive inaccurate negative reports on the operations of European socialized medical care systems. Obviously, any system is bound to be defective in one way or another; nothing will ever be ideal or perfect in a human world. But certain kinds of social criteria can be used to judge whether a system or institution meets specified social requirements. "Socialized" systems attempt to spread medical care equally among the population. If the medical care it spreads is bad, at least it will be equally bad; conversely, if the medical care it spreads is good, it will be equally good. The major force of "socialized" national control of health services is to provide equity. The other aspects: the quality of the physicians, the quality of the care in general, its location, etc., are other matters that have to be decided within the framework of that initial decision of equity. Unfortunately, the discussions in the United States about health insurance or socialized medicine never reached the level of trying to judge on the basis of such criteria.

In addition to the American Medical Association, the insurance companies, who were beginning to benefit from the private programs of health insurance, began to add their opposition to a national program, using the same sorts of argument about Bolshevism, socialism, regimentation, etc. The drug suppliers and manufacturers, who had the most to lose in terms of corporate profits, were most vociferous, providing heavy financial support to the efforts of the others. As a result, the United States citizen has been systematically brainwashed about socialized medicine over a period of 40 or 50 years; he is afraid of it.

### ANTIBUREAUCRACY THEORY

And for many reasons, totally unrelated to the possible beneficial or injurious operations of a national health system, most people had had some bad experience with an organized publicly operated system of medical care, whether it was a welfare system, a military system or a Workmen's Compensation or unemployment system, which would mean to them that bureaucracy was the enemy of good medical service.

It is hard to argue with this point because bureaucracy *can* be the enemy of good medical care. On the other hand, any type of institutionalized care is bureaucratic; even the best hospitals are "good" bureaucracies. "Bureaucracy" is a word like "propaganda": it can be good or bad, yet it carries a negative connotation. It does not necessarily follow that a bureaucracy provides bad service; but a bad bureaucracy will provide bad service.

Most ironically, the United States, despite what it believes, has developed in Medicaid a very large-scale and expensive socialized, bureaucratic medical system to care for the poor and the elderly. It is a *bad* socialized medicine system: badly organized, badly supervised, badly operated and inadequately funded.

## THE RESEARCH INVESTMENT: HOW MUCH?

Now having reached this point, what are we to say about what should be an appropriate resource allocation for biomedical research? What is an appropriate congressional appropriation and how should it be divided and used equitably?

Here, I am afraid, I must defer to the economists. How can we know what kind of return we should expect from our research investment — 5 percent, 50 percent, 100 percent? Research is a good in itself and needs to be supported; but I do believe that a limit has to be set on how much will be spent, and I suppose that in some way this should be related to the overall expenditures. If the United States spends $120 billion for medical services, then at least $5 billion should be spent on research and development in the delivery system in order to find new ways of improving the efficiency and economy of delivery. Another $5 billion could be spent profitably in biomedical research so as to reduce the impact and prevent the occurrence of disease and make it possible for things that can't be treated now to be treated in the future. That sort of investment is not being made today at all. We are spending less than $2 billion for all these things; we ought to be spending $10 billion. On the other hand, maybe we should not be spending $120 billion for medical care!

# Chapter 13
# Additional Issues of Financing
# and Organization

## BLOOD TRANSFUSIONS

There are two aspects of the problem concerning blood transfusion that are rather tenuously connected with one another, but ought to be considered separately. One problem is the availability of blood; the other is its misuse. In the United States the collection and distribution of blood has been treated and handled as a profit-making enterprise. As a consequence, in some instances blood is not used or available where it should be; and in other instances it is just too expensive.

Many of the lifesaving measures invented or developed in this century make use of blood in one way or another. Blood is given to relieve anemia or hemorrhage; to reinforce the body's postoperative struggle; to restore and strengthen the tissues in the treatment of leukemia and other blood destroying illnesses; to reinforce circulation during delicate operations such as open heart surgery and transplants. Substances made from blood are used to aid healing, offset the effects of hemophilia, replace losses in genetic diseases, etc.

### SUPPLY OF BLOOD

While blood is "a very wonderful stuff" in Goethe's words, it cannot be stored indefinitely, even if frozen. It is hard to know exactly how much blood is used in the United States, but a 1968 report stated that something on the order of five million pints were collected in a year, of which a little more than half were used for direct transfusions and the rest for the creation of blood products. In our country a large volume of blood is collected by the American Red Cross, and equal or greater amounts are collected by private profit or nonprofit blood banks in various parts of the country. Some regional relationships have been established, whereby blood can be transferred from one place to another as needed, or where central registries are kept so that when particular types of blood are required they can be found. But for the most part, blood banks operate independently.

We customarily recognize four blood types; within limits, people have to be typed in order to assure the safety of the transfusion, since mismatching may result in grave disorders and even death. In addition to the four major blood types, there are subtypes and factors, such as the Rh factor; there are other factors that we still know too little about. Sometimes even carefully typed blood will produce a reaction in the recipient.

In the United States blood is collected from people who are paid (professional donors), from those who give blood as a replacement for what they have received in the past or expect to receive in the future; from those who donate in return for transfusions to relatives or friends; and from volunteers who give their blood simply as a public service. There are a number of subgroups of these major donor groups, but for all practical purposes these constitute the major sources of blood. In the United States, less than 10 percent of the blood collected is from volunteers, and more than half is from paid donors. Because this blood is donated for the purpose of getting money, and since there is in many instances a desperate need for the blood, the care required in examining the donor for the protection of the recipient may be less than optimal.

Probably as a result, hepatitis following transfusions has soared and has become a virtual epidemic in the United States. We are still not sure what the relation is between transfusion hepatitis and the hepatitis commonly associated with the injection of infected material. Malaria, syphilis and other infectious diseases have been known to be transmitted in transfusions. The desperate search for blood has led to certain kinds of corrupt practices, whereby United States agencies seek out paid donors in developing countries, among impoverished and undernourished people, who can scarcely afford to lose the blood that they sell. In a sense they become "wells," tapped from time to time by the United States agencies to supply some of the blood we require for processing or direct transfusions. The possibility of bringing in added disease to the recipient is, of course, not unlikely.

OVERUSE OF TRANSFUSIONS

The evils of the blood transfusion system in the United States are not limited to the entrepreneurial collecting and distributing mechanism; related to this is the fact that physicians are either overzealous in recommending transfusions or somewhat careless in deciding on its necessity. During the War, signs saying "Is this trip necessary?" were posted in many places to discourage careless overuse of the transportation facilities. Such a sign might be helpful to physicians and surgeons when it comes to transfusions. Under the best of circumstances an occasional mismatching must occur; but the devastating effect of an improperly given or matched, possibly diseased blood transfusion, when it was not truly necessary in the first place, cannot be overestimated.

Richard Titmuss, in a profoundly thoughtful book, *The Gift Relationship,* measures the effect in the United States, Britain and the Soviet Union of the differing policies with regard to transfusions. There are far fewer transfusions proportionally in Great Britain, and far fewer evil consequences. Titmuss feels that this is because the British system is entirely a voluntary one, whereas the United States and the Soviet Union depend on paid donors. While the Soviets are more careful than we are, the end results show that paying blood donors is a bad policy, with almost catastrophic social consequences. Blood, like medical care, needs to be taken out of the market place.

## PREVENTIVE MEDICINE

Preventive medicine is one of the things toward which medical education is supposed to condition a doctor. Unfortunately, the type of education we emphasize today unconsciously neglects that important element of practice and does not train the doctor to serve important clusters of people. For example, doctors generally do not like to take care of patients who have mild, nonspecific complaints. Of course, they also do not like to take care of patients with cancer or other fatal diseases when there is no possible optimistic outcome. They do not like to take care of old people. They do not like to deal with sex education and they do not like to take care of well people at all, which is probably part of the reason they do not like to do preventive medicine.

### THE ARGUMENT AGAINST PREVENTIVE MEDICINE

As a result, some of the important preventive services that could contribute to the reduction of disease treatment go almost entirely without consideration in modern American medical practice. It should be understood that there is some justification for the physician's cynical view of the lack of effectiveness of preventive medicine and the consequent lack of attention he pays to it. Many investigators — among them Thomas McKeown, Professor of Social Medicine at Birmingham, who edited a book entitled *Screening in Medicine,* and Archie Cochrane, another English Professor of Medicine, who wrote *Effectiveness and Efficiency* — take up this matter of what can or ought to be done in the way of preventing disease, and of what use these things are from a scientific standpoint.

The really serious diseases, cancer and heart disease, are generally not preventable. It is true that the evidence seems to be overwhelming that cigarette smoking is a cause of cancer of the lung, and that the elimination of cigarette smoking *might* reduce significantly the incidence of cancer of the lung. Cancer of the breast and uterus in women, cancer of the rectum and colon in men, the solid tumors (the largest contributors to cancer deaths), and cancer of the blood are all of unknown etiology; prevention is clearly not yet within the realm of possibility.

However, early diagnosis is theoretically possible as a second level of prevention, provided that patients are examined carefully at suitable intervals so as to detect these diseases early enough. The first symptoms may be so subtle as to be missed at a preventive examination and, when found at the next examination, be in full blossom. We simply do not know at what intervals people need to be examined in order to catch these diseases early enough to offset lethal effects. That does not mean that the preventive examination is useless; it means that it would be a mistake to persuade people that, if they did have early or frequent examinations, they would be absolutely saved from death from cancer. Further, there is a suspicion among students of disease that there are at least two different kinds of cancer: one that grows rapidly and metastasizes early, spreading throughout the body before any overt sign can be detected; and another kind that grows relatively slowly and does not metastasize until quite late. It would be logical to expect that there is a kind of "normal curve" of distribution of the benignity or malignancy of tumors. In that case, the idea of prevention of cancer through early diagnosis is worthless. The statistics seem to show that survival rates from most cancers have not changed enough in recent years to justify the emphasis on frequent examination as a sound preventive measure. Furthermore, to be cold-blooded about it, the added number of examinations that would have to be done, the repeated use of technical instruments and the cost of the laboratory tests, etc., might make the prevention of one case of the disease so fantastically expensive that society would be unwilling to pay the price.

While the same is not entirely true of preventing deaths from heart disease, it is very largely true. We do not know what the fate will be in the long run of those people who are treated for early hypertension, since long-term drug treatment is still in its early stages. It remains to be seen whether the early use of drugs to keep blood pressure down will result in fewer cases of stroke and early death from the heart disease that traditionally follows prolonged hypertension. If so, examination in early life, which would indicate the beginnings of high blood pressure and dictate continuing drug treatment thereafter, as in the case of diabetics, may be a lifesaving procedure; we should know about that soon. There are arguments from some investigators that the drugs used are not safe themselves; that those that lower blood pressure produce effects sometimes as dangerous as the disease. But this, too, remains to be seen.

To summarize, the arguments against preventive medicine are as follows:
(a) There is very little that can be prevented
(b) Early diagnosis is difficult or impossible in most instances
(c) The intervals during which the preventive examinations have to be made are not clearly known
(d) The cost of prevention might be so expensive as to be prohibitive
(e) The treatment may result in effects as dangerous as the disease

### THE DOCTOR'S NEGATIVE ATTITUDE

In other areas, the care of patients with mild or nonspecific complaints arouses irritation in the doctor. It is too "trivial." The unwillingness of the doctor to concern himself with these matters derives in part from the emphasis in medical schools on strange, exotic, complex diseases that stretch the physician's imagination and skill to make a diagnosis and give him great satisfaction in solution. He sees medicine as a sort of contest of wits, an intellectual competition that he wins by making an obscure diagnosis. There is considerable ego satisfaction in being able to meet and conquer a strange, difficult disease, a worthy opponent. The challenge of well people and nonspecific complaints is not such as to encourage a doctor to be content handling them.

However, it is perfectly clear that people do not go to physicians unless something is urging them to ask for help, a situation they cannot handle or define for themselves. The appearance of "wellness" or the vagueness of the complaints do not necessarily represent the true nature of the unease or *dis*ease that actually motivates the patient. I am not speaking here of subconscious "sick" motivation, but the normal emotional or mental discomfort; the feeling that induces a kind of fear in people, a distress they do not want to think about, try to relegate to the subconscious, and yet feel sufficient pressure so that they seek professional help. The *good* doctor, the idealized healer, is expected to have the wisdom, understanding and sympathy to recognize that a patient comes distressed, and to seek delicately to establish what might be the true motivation. Elderly patients are sometimes demanding and thoroughly dislikable in their self-concern and idiosyncrasies. Medical education needs to emphasize the fact that nothing is to be overlooked when the patient enters the office, that an effective relationship between doctor and patient must begin with the doctor's willingness and desire to extend help, no matter what the patient's complaint is or how serious it appears to be at first inspection. This will require an entirely different kind of orientation in medical education, and it is unlikely that it will be accomplished as long as the model of the physician as seen in the medical school is the researcher and conqueror of obscure disease.

In short, since prevention is largely a social act — abolishing the cigarette industry, for example, or air, water and food pollutants that contain carcinogens — emphasis on prevention as an *individual* action is largely misplaced. However, the possibility of utilizing a visit to the physician to discuss some annoying or unusual symptom *is* a valuable preventive measure. If we had a universal comprehensive medical care system, providing for a periodic visit to and discussion with a physician, some symptoms might be elicited at such a "well-adult conference" (maybe as a family conference on a regular basis, and including other health workers in addition to or instead of the doctor). This could be a sound basis for a preventive program.

## SEX EDUCATION

I find it hard to explain why physicians are so reluctant to deal with sex education and can think only that this may be a relic, a residual character-istic of the Calvinist American response to anything that has to do with sex. Physicians recognize from their medical training that there are emotional problems that might even cause or intensify disease, deriving from the sexual life of the individual. They know that sexual satisfaction and the ability to realize one's sexual identity plays a large part in overall health. Providing information and education to patients is extremely important. "Know the truth and the truth will make you free" seems to be the motto derived from the psychoanalytic process and modern psychiatry. It may be so, but most physicians do not feel responsible for this area of patient services. Consequently, a host of specialized therapists and counselors have become established. Some are physicians, but by and large it has become the province of psychologists, social workers, sociologists, anthropologists, self-educated groups, etc.

Perhaps sex education and therapy are not necessarily medical specialties or responsibilities. For a long time practically everything that related to the human body or brain was considered to be the responsibility of the physician. However, it may be that there are areas of responsibility that need not be related to the medical model at all. There are some people who believe, for example, that psychiatry, especially those aspects dealing with emotional difficulties that influence an individual's performance in society and in the family, may be totally unrelated to illness and outside the medical model altogether. If that is so, the people who should be making the diagnosis or providing treatment should not be physicians, and physicians perhaps should not meddle in this area. There are even those who believe that the adoption of the medical model in psychiatry has been a crucial error; that diagnosis and therapy, even in mental illness, do not apply in this area. They believe that the subjective therapy of understanding, confrontation and adjustment are much more relevant in the treatment of mental and emotional difficulties than medical prescriptions or therapy. The responses of an individual do not have to be considered in either the category of "sick" or "well."

I find it difficult to sort out exactly where I stand on these issues, but I must confess that when I see to what lengths those who are not physicians go in attempting to "help" people who have emotional difficulties, either with the job, with the family, or with living in society altogether, I am not at all sure that there is a model other than the medical model which can be more successful!

# Chapter 14
# What Happens in Other Countries

---

## THE AMERICAN MOTIVATION FOR
## SEEKING SOLUTIONS ABROAD

As there is increasing expression of dissatisfaction with the defects of the American medical care system, many experts are turning to analysis of foreign systems for possible solutions. As we discussed earlier, these medical care system defects are most apparent in uncontrollably mounting costs, poor access and an overall growing lack of confidence in the physicians or hospitals. So we are beginning to take seriously the fact that we are the last "developed" nation in the world without an organized and structured health service. Practically every member of a congressional committee that deals with health has made a trip to one or more European countries, and recently the medical care systems in Canada and Australia have been carefully analyzed.

There is something wryly amusing about this situation, since for so many years most legislators were terribly disdainful of the European systems. Following the lead of the American Medical Association, everybody spoke with great contempt of "socialized medicine." You only had to mention a European country and its medical care system at a discussion of these matters, to be overwhelmed by a tidal wave of pejorative comments, regardless of the fact that most of the commentators had had no personal experience with any of the systems. Everyone had read the horror stories: the English patients waiting in line for hours or even days to be seen by a doctor; the many months of waiting for elective surgery; the jokes about queues for the National Health Service. For the thrifty-minded there were stories of the luxuries of wigs, multiple sets of false teeth, or having the same leg amputated twice or three times, etc. Socialized medicine was a staple subject for lots of stand-up comics and humorous feature writers, for columnists in conservative newspapers and magazines and, of course, for

233

legislators who wanted to protect the entrepreneurial interests and traditions of the American system.

One will not forget very soon the endearing editorial that Dr. Fishbein published in the *Journal of the American Medical Association* in December 1932 denouncing the Report of the Committee on the Costs of Medical Care, mild as it was, as "Socialism and Communism — inciting to revolution." Of course, today we are afraid he may turn out to be right for entirely different reasons: the failures of the private insurance schemes and Blue Cross and Blue Shield to provide us with suitable protection against the cost of medical care may well lead to some sort of stringent governmental action.

In any case, just as we did in clinical medicine a hundred years ago, we now turn to Europe for a look at the medical care systems there, to see what we can learn, from their successes and failures, what we should do — or not do! — in developing a system of our own. We look to their methods of combating inflation of costs; improving access to care; stabilizing sporadic or uncertain availability of physicians; assuring quality; and relieving what for many people seems to be total unresponsiveness to their health needs.

## AMERICA VS. EUROPE:
## COST CONTROL IN PERSPECTIVE

It is only since the 1920's that Americans have been really satisfied with the American medical educational system as the best in the world, which means trusting physicians who were trained wholly in this country. Before that, most Americans preferred doctors who had some or all of their training abroad; foreign-trained physicians were considered to be superior to American-trained ones. It is only since the growth of laboratory and clinical research orientation in medical education in the United States and the building of hundred million dollar hospitals and medical care complex research centers, with consequent medical miracle stories in the media, that we have come to put the European model behind us and consider it a less worthy reflection of modern medicine.

The fact is, of course, that European medical education did not keep pace with the advances and developments in American medical practice and education; as a consequence, many of the virtues of American medical developments, in terms of quality and competence of practitioners, did not affect Europe. The doctors graduating from European schools could not all hope to become specialists as they could in the United States, by spending three or four years in intensive training after medical school; they could not hope to be other than family doctors, general practitioners and primary care physicians. Europe, therefore, has been better supplied with physicians at that first contact level, despite the fact that there were fewer physicians altogether in proportion to the population. This was entirely fewer *specialists.* Yet the numbers of specialists that they did produce seemed more than adequate to take care of the specialized needs of their population. And although European medicine has tended to lag behind America in research orientation and specialist production, this is not entirely true, since medicine in Scandinavia has kept up admirably with American advances. Swedish technology is not only equal to, but perhaps in some ways, *superior* to that of the United States.

European and American practice and education began to grow apart at the beginning of the 19th century. In the middle twentieth, the gulf was very wide. Perhaps before we enter into specific discussions about the situations of particular countries, it might be well to have a look at the general differences between European and American medicine, emphasizing the fact that American medicine developed in response to different kinds of stimuli and pressures in the 19th century, and later to a different magnitude of financial investment and technological development. The following figures illustrate health care expenditure differences between the United States and foreign countries.

FIGURE 14-1:   Proportion of GNP Spent on Health Services (%)

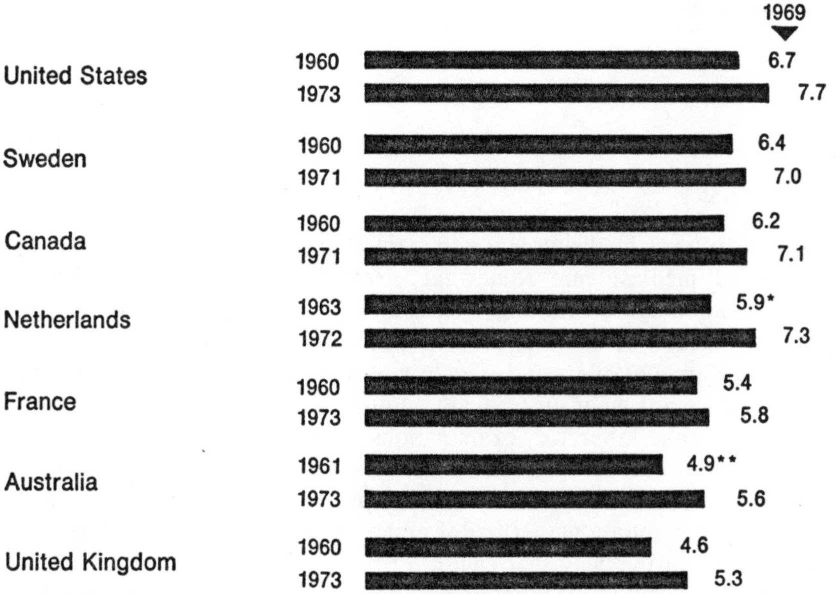

| | | 1969 ▼ |
|---|---|---|
| **United States** | 1960 | 6.7 |
| | 1973 | 7.7 |
| **Sweden** | 1960 | 6.4 |
| | 1971 | 7.0 |
| **Canada** | 1960 | 6.2 |
| | 1971 | 7.1 |
| **Netherlands** | 1963 | 5.9* |
| | 1972 | 7.3 |
| **France** | 1960 | 5.4 |
| | 1973 | 5.8 |
| **Australia** | 1961 | 4.9** |
| | 1973 | 5.6 |
| **United Kingdom** | 1960 | 4.6 |
| | 1973 | 5.3 |

\* 1968
\*\* 1970

*Source:* Adapted from R. Maxwell, *Health Care: The Growing Dilemma,* McKinsey & Company, 1974, p. 18.

FIGURE 14-2:   Annual Health Expenditure per Person (U. S. $)

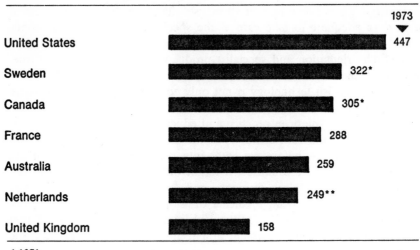

1973

| | |
|---|---|
| United States | 447 |
| Sweden | 322* |
| Canada | 305* |
| France | 288 |
| Australia | 259 |
| Netherlands | 249** |
| United Kingdom | 158 |

\* 1971
\*\* 1972

*Source:* McKinsey Research Department (calculations from total expenditure and population statistics)

*Source:* Adapted from R. Maxwell, *Health Care: The Growing Dilemma,* McKinsey & Company, 1974, p. 18.

LACK OF SPECIALISTS MEANS LOWER COSTS

That European medicine tends to train fewer specialists serves to keep the cost of medical care somewhat below that of the United States; specialists not only demand higher fees than general practitioners, but they have to be served by an army of technicians and paraprofessionals, as well as by a vast amount of expensive instruments and equipment. Consulting a specialist does not mean just having another doctor look at you; it means more x rays, more laboratory examinations, more tests of various kinds that may include advanced diagnostic procedures (even surgery). These steps would not be taken if it were not that the specialist was trying to refine that diagnosis. It is not altogether bad, I agree. In many instances a diagnosis will be made in this way that could not be made otherwise. However, a very significant part of the inflation of medical costs in the United States has to be attributed to the large numbers of specialists that we have encouraged through exceptional opportunities for training and then freely allowed to be paid at their own valuation in our entrepreneurial medical care system.

### SALARIES VS. FEE-FOR-SERVICE

Another significant distinction between European and American medical practice stems from the fact that to a very large extent hospital physicians in Europe are more limited in number (this, of course, is also a reflection of the fewer specialists) and tend to be salaried rather than fee-for-service. General practitioners as a rule do not practice in hospitals. While there may be private hospitals to which some specialists take their patients for necessary care, to a considerable degree in practically all European countries, patients are referred to hospitals where salaried specialists work. The American system allows access to the hospital to all physicians who qualify and become members of the staff; we do not have salaried physicians responsible for patients admitted. As explained earlier in the book, the open nature of American medical education and the resultant physician/hospital relationships created the trend of entrepreneurial physicians working in hospitals quite early in the 19th century; it has never changed.

### PUBLIC VS. PRIVATE PAYMENT

A third distinction has to do with the way in which medical services are paid. In practically every country in Europe, hospital services for the bulk of the population are free, or at nominal cost. For over a hundred years, it was the habit of the well-to-do to receive care in private hospitals and, since it is only after World War II that a prosperous middle class of any significant size has developed in Europe, the number of people who took advantage of the private hospital system was always very small. Therefore, Europeans generally share a tradition and expectation of *public* hospital care, paid for out of government funds, either from special hospital taxes or general revenues. Additionally, most physicians in Europe have been accustomed to receiving a part or most of their income from the government. Health insurance of one kind or another, subsidized or even wholly supported by the government, was a characteristic of European medicine from the middle of the 19th century.

### DIFFERENT PATIENT PERSPECTIVE

Taking the above differences into consideration, it must be obvious that the European patient sees his medical care in a somewhat different perspective from that of the American patient. Very little has changed for the European patient in over 100 years; the same sort of first contact physician looks after him, and he sees a specialist only when his family doctor wants him to see a specialist. If he is hospitalized he expects to go to a public hospital and be treated as a general hospital patient without private care or care by physicians whom he chooses. This is the type of care his father received, and this is the type of care his children will probably receive. It is true that the physicians' offices are now more modern, with more equipment. It is true that they now provide much more in the way of laboratory examination, x rays, diagnostic tests, immunization, etc. Perhaps the European doctor has begun to take on some of the technocratic qualities that we object to in American physicians — a bit impersonal, a bit too busy to pay sympathetic attention — but the nature of the structure has changed very little.

### DIFFERENT PHYSICIAN PERSPECTIVE

For the European doctor, the situation is substantially the same for him as it would have been for his father or grandfather as they came into practice. There are limited opportunities for becoming a specialist; the general expectation for a doctor is that he will be a family physician. If he does become a specialist, he will expect to do at least some of his work, at part or full salary, in a public or government-controlled hospital. And, of course, he expects to obtain part of his income from government payment for care of government-insured patients. He may take a full-time job in this capacity, with no loss of prestige.

## EUROPEAN AND AMERICAN MEDICAL EDUCATION

### BASIC DIFFERENCES

The relatively unchanging quality of the European medical care system and practice derives in part from their relatively unchanging medical education. The European starts medical school at 18 or 19 years of age, the equivalent of an American high school graduate, although the gymnasium, upper school or lycee education that the European undergoes is of somewhat greater depth than American high school education. However, when he goes to college, he goes directly into a medical school that is part of the university, and spends the next five or six years learning to be a doctor. The first two years he takes courses that are basically similar to American premedical training, but he gets some experience with patient care. In the last three or four years, he has full patient contact, learning and practicing all aspects of their care.

There are notable differences between the American and European medical school experience: teachers in European universities tend to be more formal in their relationship; there is less research going on and more attention to the clinical aspect of patient care; there is less experience for the students in touching patients directly. The student watches more than he participates in most instances, and he tends to be reminded more of the need for using his eyes and hands than elaborate and expensive equipment and machines.

The American physician is not taken into medicine at such a young age. His expectations are different because he has been given to understand that everything is changing and changing very rapidly. Perhaps even in his own lifetime he has seen how medical education and practice have changed, and the kinds of arguments and discussions that have gone on have given him a feeling that the ground on which he stands is a little shaky. What he is learning now may not be what he will practice; what doctors are doing now is not what they may be doing in the near future. There is an uncomfortable feeling of mobility or insecurity in the American doctor's life, rather than the stable and traditional life the European doctor has been educated to expect.

I think that taking the student into medicine at 18 perhaps offers greater possibility for assuring that he will carry on in a traditional way; a student at 21 may be less likely to be putty in the hands of the teacher and the institution.

Be that as it may, American doctors are clearly educated differently than the Europeans. After a four-year college experience of rather broader and more general education than the European medical student, he gets a much deeper and broader clinical experience. The American medical school tends to give the student much more opportunity for personal contact and exchange with the patient. He is expected to take care of patients, to report on his methods and to learn by doing.

Very early in his training, the American student learns to distinguish between what is education and what is practice, and a little of the paradoxical inequity of this democratic country creeps in at this point. Inasmuch as the European student learns on *all* patients who are admitted to the public hospital, almost all the people admitted to hospitals are exposed to medical students. In the United States, generally the student is taught on the bodies of the poor; that is, on ward patients or patients of teaching services. These represent only a fraction of the people admitted to hospitals and this gross inequality in approach tends to give the student a different view of his responsibilities. During his training period he sees the difference in the way in which doctors treat "teaching" patients and their private patients; what he is permitted to do and the expectation of the amount of diagnostic and therapeutic activity that is carried on for private patients, as against what he sees is being done to the poor people who are the "teaching material." A great deal more may be done, extravagantly so, for the sake of learning, rather than for the sake of actually helping the patient. This distinction between what is education and what is practice conditions him in a way for private practice and for the care of middle-class paying patients. A great deal of bitterness is, of course, also engendered in the poor people, particularly in the minorities, who, as "teaching material," are the subject of "learning" by the students and house staff.

There is considerable irony in the American argument that socialized medicine is "undemocratic," in view of the truly undemocratic nature of American medical education as opposed to the rather more democratic nature of European medical education.

It stands to reason, then, with a different type of medical education, a different focus on the physician's responsibility in medical care and a different organization of medical practice for over a hundred years, that physician and patient attitudes in the medical care systems would differ in Europe and the United States.

## EFFORTS TO IMPORT OR COPY FOREIGN SYSTEMS

It has been said that "revolution can be neither exported nor imported;" nor can social institutions be exported or imported. No matter how much we admire or respect what is being done in another country, if we would try to bring the institution (whether it is education, medical care, welfare services, religion, government, or whatever) into our own country, we would have to modify it in accordance with our own traditions, history, social attitudes, cultural makeup, and so forth, so that it would end up being more "ours" than "theirs."

### EASTERN EUROPE AND THE SOVIET SYSTEM

An interesting observation in this regard relates to the history of medical care organization in eastern Europe. After World War II the Soviet Union became the leader and model for the Eastern European People's Democracies. Enthusiastically they began to develop a Soviet-style medical care system, modeled after the Russian Socialist medical care system that had been in operation since 1917. In Czechoslovakia, particularly, the government in exile translated Henry Sigerist's *Socialized Medicine in the Soviet Union* into Czech so that their partisan medical care planners in England would be prepared to put that medical care system into operation in Czechoslovakia the minute they were reinstated after the defeat of the Germans.

In the 1960's, some 20 years after the adoption of a Soviet model by the Eastern European Socialist People's Democratic Republic, I visited a number of these eastern European countries. It was a most illuminating experience. Despite their efforts to copy the Russian system, each of the European socialist democracies had developed a somewhat different approach to socialized medicine.

For example, the Soviet Union's medical care system forbids private practice by a physician, yet in a number of the People's Republics, private practice is permitted and sometimes encouraged. In Poland, it was necessary to encourage private practice in order to provide for rural medical care. The Polish government had not been able to impose a governmentally controlled agricultural system on the peasants in the same way that Stalin had imposed it upon the Russian peasants. As a consequence, 85 percent of Polish farms are not controlled by the government, and the Polish farmer is essentially a free agent. Therefore, a medical care system supported by taxes was simply not applicable to the Polish farmer. Some change had to be made in the system to provide the independent Polish farmer with medical care; private practice was the answer. In addition, because the Germans had been so savagely destructive of the Polish intellectual and professional class (just as they had destroyed the Jewish professional class all over Europe), there were very few Polish physicians available for the development of a socialized system. The doctors had to be encouraged to work part-time in the socialized system on salary, and part-time as private practitioners on a fee-for-service basis. To enable all the Polish people to have access to physicians would not have been possible if the doctors had worked only the seven-hour day of other workers.

Despite the fact that in the Soviet Union there are never any charges for medical services, in East Germany the medical care system does permit some charges.

In Yugoslavia free choice of physician is permitted and there are no polyclinics on the Soviet model.

Even some of the better aspects of the Soviet system have not been uniformly adopted or exactly replicated, despite the fact that they represent significant advances in medical system quality. For example, the continuing educational program of the Soviet Union, which involves bringing doctors back to post-graduate courses at regular intervals, and provides for comprehensive supervision of the doctors by their superiors through the polyclinics, has not been followed in Yugoslavia. This is probably because the resources for the creation or development of such programs simply were not available. The Czechs have developed an excellent continuing education program on this model.

### AMERICA AND THE EASTERN EUROPE SYSTEM

While we may have a great deal to learn from the European experience, particularly the relationships of physicians to government, education to medical practice and methods of payment to methods of practice, there is much that is simply not applicable. The benefits of various methods of practice in the European countries should be observed carefully and the lessons absorbed in order to develop the best possible medical care system for the United States. However, at the same time, we should be aware that the systems in operation today in Europe grew out of events not duplicated in our own country; therefore they are not systems that can be simply transplanted onto the American soil and expected to prosper and serve our needs as they serve theirs. We are different in many ways — in our expectations, historical development and world view; in our attitudes toward doctors, hospitals and medical care; in the way in which we view methods of payment, money and success; in our social and cultural attitudes and values. It is therefore necessary for us to develop our own system.

But specific elements of the various European systems may have excellent effect in stimulating our thinking toward potential change and improvement. For example, decentralization and unit management on the Yugoslav model are very appealing; can we replicate it? Is revenue sharing a potential vehicle for local control and local support? Continuing education on the Czech model, with house staff supplying the *locum teneus* ("substitute doctor") when a family doctor is away relearning his craft, seems a thoroughly useful American possibility.

On the other hand, let's face the fact that government control of a medical care system in a monolithic way frightens a lot of Americans, and I do not believe they will ever accept it. Furthermore, there is a faction that argues the United States *has* socialized medicine now in Medicaid, and is doing a very poor job of it.

### MEDICAL SYSTEMS IN ENGLAND
### AND WESTERN EUROPE

European experience may give us patterns against which we can measure our expectations and aspirations, although not necessarily our exact plans.

So let us now, for the sake of trying to explore some of these things, have a look at a few of the different methods of medical practice and education and at the attitudes with which patients accept, adopt or complain about the medical care system in their countries.

### PAYMENT FOR SERVICES: AN OVERVIEW      *Fee for Service*

Let us begin by looking at the European experience first from the standpoint of payment for services. European nations began with a social security system for payment for medical services early in the 19th century. The Danes were first in the 1830's, developing a system of employers setting up employee sick funds to be used by the employees to buy medical services when they needed them. It had no governmental indulgence or contribution at first, but it was encouraged by the government, and a similar system was used for buying medical care for the poor. In England, the "Friendly Societies," associations of working people, did approximately the same thing: collected money from employed people to create a fund that would be used to buy medical services when needed.

By the 1880's, in the wake of the industrial revolution, the working people of Europe had organized into unions and became essentially political, even forming political parties based on union affiliation. The Social Democratic Party in many parts of Europe and the Labor Party in England agitated for widespread social welfare programs based on government-sponsored, employer-employee contributions for medical care and other welfare services.

Such a movement was paradoxically supported by the German Chancellor, Prince Otto von Bismarck, while advising and guiding William II, the young monarch who had just succeeded in the unification of Germany. Conservative in outlook and hostile to the radical activities of the burgeoning Social Democratic movement, Bismarck suggested to his king that a two-pronged attack be mounted to disarm the Social Democrats. He pointed out that it would be ironically shrewd to adopt their social welfare platform, throwing them and their allies into disarray, while at the same time pursuing a pugnacious and belligerent foreign policy to establish Germany as the key power in Central Europe. The strategy worked. Bismarck introduced social security, including pensions and unemployment and health benefits. The Social Democrats railed against it in vain, recognizing the subterfuge for what it was; that his program on the domestic scene was to win the confidence and support of the majority of the German people so that they would also support his foreign adventures. But Bismarck's introduction of social security was a radical step, even though it was used to further reactionary ends.

This social security program became a powerful lever for the introduction of social security programs, particularly health insurance, all over Europe. When a struggle took place between Germany and Denmark resulting in the German occupation and possession of Danish territory, the social security program was introduced into that province. Soon programs trickled over into the rest of Denmark. The Germans held Alsace and Lorraine following the French defeat in 1870; after World War I when Alsace and Lorraine were returned to France, the Alsacians and Lotharingians refused to give up the social security that they had under the Germans. As a consequence, all of France eventually adopted social security in the 1920's. As of 1911 Britain also had a national health insurance program. This was a goal for which the other countries of Europe aimed, and finally achieved in one fashion or another by World War II.

The changes that have taken place since World War II represent modifications of the original Bismarckian program. Under that system, workers and employers paid a certain amount into an insurance fund. In the beginning, these insurance funds were related to particular industries or even to particular places of employment; consequently there were thousands of different funds, duplicating but not displacing the small Friendly Societies that had grown up all over Europe with the beginning of unionism. When a man changed employment, or lost his job, he lost his health insurance benefits. Not all the funds offered the same benefits or were equally scrupulous in payments or supervision. It was not too  different from what many employed Americans find today!

The difference in approach was that the government undertook to guarantee basic standards or floors as to what constituted appropriate benefits under the programs. There would continue to be different insurance companies, but all of them had to offer the same basic insurance benefits. Furthermore, since the unions were negotiating these insurance programs, generally they all had to accept the same kind of premiums. Even before World War II many of the health insurance programs in Europe had identical premium structures and identical benefits within a particular country. Furthermore, between World War I and World War II, because inflation caused disastrous bankruptcy in some of the insurance programs, the government stepped in to pay some part of the cost in order to protect the various insurance companies and the workers who were covered by them. As a consequence, by the middle of the 1920's most of the health insurance systems were basically supported by the government; while the insured may have paid into their own particular industry, they were actually part of a larger national system. If they moved from one industry to another, they continued with the same coverage; they did not lose their investment in their health insurance. For all practical purposes, therefore, health insurance under social security for most of the European countries, even before World War II, represented a kind of national health insurance progam in which the workers were covered for clearly determined basic health needs, to a fixed level of payment guaranteed by the government.

You can see from this that most people growing up in Europe since 1920 were covered by an insurance program for some or all of their medical services. They were free to go to any of the doctors and hospitals that were part of the insurance system. Doctors were generally paid by *capitation,* out of the sick chest fund. It made hardly any difference that the funds were contributions from several sources, partly supported by the employee, the employer and the government. The sick chest itself negotiated arrangements with the doctors to pay them. For the family doctor, the physician with whom the patient would have to have first contact, the capitation payment was so much per month per patient. He had responsibility for all patients for whom he received monthly payments. This varied, of course, in that in some countries the doctor might continue to be paid a small amount by each patient at time of service; in other countries this was not so. It was felt that some fee for the service creates a special bond between doctor and patient — each knows they share a responsibility.

Unfortunately, however, in some countries the doctors never received a sum they considered satisfactory for the services performed to the insured patients. Doctors felt they had to do something more than simply participate in that medical care system in order to achieve a financial standard consistent with their expectations. In some countries, some of the doctors refused to participate in the system at all and limited their practice to taking care of only the wealthier patients who paid full fees. In some instances, they continued to practice privately in addition to working in the insurance system. In some places the doctors insisted on being allowed to take money from the patients who were covered by the insurance. With the exception of Denmark, most doctors in most European countries have expressed dissatisfaction with their country's system of paying them. While *they* are dissatisfied, in most places the patients are satisfied.

### ENGLAND

It is important to touch a few historic points in order to understand the National Health Service of England. The beginning of unionism in the early 19th century brought the development of the Friendly Societies and small health insurance funds, as well as efforts to persuade health departments to take responsibility for medical care. Then at the time of the Boer War it was discovered that more than half of the young people who were brought up for military service failed to pass the physical examination. A Parliamentary inquiry found that very few of the working people in the country had the money to buy medical service for their children. As a result of the study and after much parliamentary discussion, England decided to institute a National Health Insurance program supervised by the government, in which the employer and employee would contribute funds to allow a sick worker to be cared for without any expense to him. This in turn would leave him free to be able to use his own money to buy services for his family.

The National Health Insurance System began in 1911 after considerable opposition, but it never worked properly; between 1911 and World War II there was much criticism of the system. During World War II, Parliament appointed the "Beveridge Commission" to study what should be done after the War to improve health services. They came up with a proposal for a comprehensive national health service, paid for very largely out of tax receipts, to cover all the people in the country. This plan was finally put into effect in 1948 and, with modifications in 1974, has continued to this day.

It is a *service* instead of an *insurance program;* the difference is that the benefits are not limited. The amount of service that a person needs is to be provided without regard to cost. The individual does not pay in accordance with the risk that is involved, but only a token amount; the bulk of the costs is paid for out of general treasury appropriations.

Every person in the British Isles, whether he is a resident or a visitor, is entitled to all the medical care he needs without charge, except for some modest payments for prescription medication. He is entitled to consult a primary care physician or a specialist; to be hospitalized, including surgery or other types of examination and treatment; to be kept in the hospital as long as is necessary; and to have all his medications attended to, including mental health and ophthalmological services. All this is paid for out of a government fund, about 90 percent of which is from general taxes and 10 percent a contribution out of wages.

In this system, family doctors (primary care physicians) are reimbursed on a capitation payment. They have a "list" of patients who are their responsibility, who are registered with them and for whom they receive a fixed sum every month. The specialists are on a salary based on the number of sessions they provide by working in hospitals, either in the outpatient department as consultants, or in the hospital as physicians to bed patients. A full-time consultant is paid on the basis of "eleven elevenths." That is, the week is considered to have 11 sessions (six morning and five afternoon); a full-time physician serves all 11 and receives a commensurate salary. Most British specialists prefer to practice on a part-time basis of nine-elevenths, serving a mix of nine mornings and afternoons a week. They then work as much additional time as they like in their private offices, where they can charge fees to those patients who come to them outside the National Health Service system.

I will not go into the amount of money that the doctors receive in Britain because it would not be relevant to the American context. Their tax structure, standard of living and relation of reimbursement to other professionals is quite different. The average doctor, if he is fully salaried, will make about a third of what his American counterpart makes, and pay much heavier taxes. However, a physician's income in Britain compares favorably with the rest of society proportionately, even as an American doctor's does.

Specialists tend to make considerably more than general practitioners. This gives rise to dissatisfaction, particularly since general practitioners generally do work harder than specialists, given the circumstances under which they work. The general practitioners' grievances have been expressed forcibly and frequently to the Minister of Health. Negotiations have taken place on a number of occasions, and parliamentary inquiries have been made to try to satisfy them, but they are still not satisfied. They feel that too many demands are made on them and that they are not paid sufficiently. The specialists, on the other hand, have been reasonably satisfied with their reimbursement. The fact that most of them are nine-elevenths means they can also maintain a lucrative private practice.

However, because it is a closed system, a fixed number of specialists are appointed to the hospitals in accordance with a table of organization developed by the Ministry. A great many of the graduates of British medical schools have to spend many years working as residents in British hospitals at relatively low salaries before they can be granted official status as assigned consultants within the system, entitled to the salaries of specialists. Consequently, the hospital staffs have been very restive; on a number of occasions they have threatened to strike, and in 1975 there were strikes by junior house staff against the system to try to get more consultant places and better income. Perhaps as a side effect to the lack of specialist openings, a considerable number of young British medical graduates with specialist aspirations emigrate, and come to the United States and Canada.

British specialists can also receive "merit awards." This is a method of rewarding excellence by adding a percentage of income in three categories, the highest of which doubles one's salary. The awards are decided by an anonymous committee and the names of the recipients are never made public. Mostly university professors are said to benefit from this award system.

The patients, in general, seem to be quite happy with the system. We are told that 98 percent of the patients and approximately the same percentage of physicians are registered with the system.  There are therefore about 50 million resident citizen patients in England, and about 50 thousand physicians.   Patient satisfaction, despite the grievances of the general practitioners and the hospital residents, tends to support the idea that the British system is working reasonably well.

Parliamentary appropriations to the Ministry of Health pay for a variety of other services that the patients may need: pharmaceuticals (over the counter and prescription drugs), according to listed prices plus a small profit for the dispenser; nursing services in the home; ambulance services; and all the public health services, such as epidemiological, sanitary and environmental control.   Although to a great extent these public health services are paid for out of local taxes, the national government does participate to some degree.

A small number of doctors, perhaps 500, practice completely outside the system.  They see only a few hundred patients, those of considerable wealth or prestige who do not choose to participate in the national medical care system.  They charge very high fees; do a reasonably good job of care even by American standards, using the same technology, equipment, etc.; and represent a kind of elite medical force.  There is a much larger number of specialists who participate to some degree in the system, but who also look after private patients who may or may not be part of the system.  These patients choose to see a specialist on their own; they "jump the queue" as the British say, so as to avoid waiting for quite a long time or having to see a physician not of their choosing.  There are about two million of these patients.  They are usually part of a kind of combined Blue Cross-Blue Shield system of insurance for which they pay a modest annual premium that covers physician and hospital bills.  Approximately ten percent of the beds in British hospitals are called "amenity beds" and are open to private patients.  There is considerable argument about this at the present time; the Labor Party government is attempting to wipe out these "amenity beds," but they continue to exist.

What we learn from the British system is that *quality* can be maintained, *access* can be increased and health service *equity* can be provided in a nationalized medical care system.  In essence, government control yields a *democratic,* rather than totalitarian, system.

The English system works.  It provides equal access for all citizens, and an opportunity for all physicians to participate.  It keeps a relatively tight hold on expenses by severe budgeting in parliamentary appropriations, which have sometimes produced awkward constraints and dissatisfactions in the system, but not enough to threaten its existence.

SCANDINAVIA

There are certain differences in the way in which the separate Scandinavian countries carry out the directives of their individual health insurance programs. These are not health "services" in the British sense, but health "insurance" programs. However, the modes of operation differ to a degree that renders them only slightly different from the British system. There is a difference in the way in which the money is collected and a slight difference in the way in which the money is divided or distributed among the doctors, but the patient care system remains very similar.

### Denmark

In Denmark the "sick chests" are almost entirely united into one central fund, to which employers, employees and the federal government contribute. All the people who work are covered; this means that about 85 percent of the Danish population benefits by the health insurance system. The general practitioners are paid on a capitation basis, as in England, by the number of patients on their lists. In some of the isolated rural parts of the country the doctors may charge the patients a small additional amount at time of service. The Danes feel that the physician who has a limited number of people on his list in a sparsely settled area should also be able to make an income equivalent to that of colleagues in more densely populated areas.

All hospital physicians are salaried and full-time. Patients are referred by the general practitioners to the hospital outpatient department for consultation; they are admitted to the hospital for service. The general practitioner never works in the hospital; he gets reports from his colleagues at the hospital, but basically the two systems are quite separate.

The Danish system seems to work almost perfectly. Practically everyone is covered and takes advantage of the system by using it; complaints are rare. General practitioners seem to be well-trained. There is particularly good use of preventive services, and high quality care in both doctors' offices and institutions.

### Sweden

In Sweden, the system works a little differently, perhaps because the national health service is relatively newer than Denmark's; it did not go into full operation until the 1950's. The doctors and specialists in Sweden do not tend to practice as individual general practitioners as they do in Denmark; they are more likely to be practicing in "polyclinics." These are large office buildings where doctors are concentrated. Although hospital physicians are full-time and the patients are referred to the hospital for service, patients may also be referred to specialists in polyclinics, rather than to the hospital as they are in Denmark or England. Doctors are reimbursed more on the basis of fee-for-service than they are on the basis of capitation per patient. And this makes a significant difference in the way in which the physician earns his living. However, the earnings of Swedish specialists and general practitioners seem to be fairly equal.

In Sweden, funds for the national health insurance scheme also derive from employer, employee and government contributions.

*Norway*

In Norway, the health insurance scheme is part of a trade union program rather than a national governmental program. Otherwise the system is similar to the Danish system. The general practitioners are reimbursed on a capitation basis, and some general practitioners are permitted to charge a small additional fee at time of service. All hospital services are free and provided by full-time house staff physicians.

In Norway, as in Sweden, there are large, sparsely settled areas in the north, occupied largely by Laplanders. In order to provide equitable medical services there, they have developed a special health service system. The government pays a base salary to a health officer for living in these areas. He is expected to provide the necessary services, and is assisted by public health nurses associated with his health center. In addition to his base salary, he is permitted to charge a fixed rate established by the government for the medical care services he provides. A similar service, with similar payment features, applies to the islanders off the shores of northern Norway.

In the Scandinavian countries, as in England, the medical care system has tended to spread the medical services broadly and evenly over all elements of the population. In these countries, the patients are remarkably satisfied with the system. To a very considerable degree, the physicians are also reasonably satisfied. There are elements of dissatisfaction, stemming from conditions of work, system of reimbursement or inequities between general practitioner and specialist salaries, but these dissatisfactions are minimal when compared with the overall doctor and patient satisfaction.

In all these countries, the hospitals are well-equipped, the physicians are well-trained, the medical care and medical education systems are up-to-date and the amount of money that is being spent is considerably less than that being spent proportionately in the United States.

## FRANCE AND GERMANY

While a very large proportion of the population in France and Germany may be covered by health insurance, there are significant operational differences between their systems and those in the Scandinavian countries and England.

There is a form of compulsory health insurance, with employee contributions (based on salary) and employer contributions. However, in these systems the fee at time of service that the patient is expected to pay is not simply a token payment, as it is in the Scandinavian system. For example, in France, when a patient is admitted to a hospital, he is expected to pay the hospital charges. He will then be reimbursed from Social Security for about 80 percent of the cost if he has been treated in a public hospital (where most patients go), or less than that if he attended a private hospital where the charges are higher.

Doctors' fees are negotiated by the medical society and the government; this is also true in the Scandinavian countries. The patient pays the bill and is reimbursed by Social Security for up to 80 percent of the bill, except when the doctor has not agreed to accept the Social Security scale. In this case, the patient receives only 80 percent of the accepted scale and has to pay a much larger part of the actual cost.

Aside from this difference in the payment mechanism, the systems are very similar to those of England and the Scandinavian countries. The Scandinavian system tends to be more inclusive and certainly works more in the patient's interest, since the health insurance system pays the doctor directly, rather than forcing the patient to put up the money and then wait to be reimbursed some part of the cost.

### HOLLAND

As I pointed out earlier, tradition and history in the development of a health service will have a great effect on its ultimate form. The designers of the system may aim to replicate the system of another country, but the best they will actually manage to accomplish is to bring their own existing system somewhat into line with the foreign ideal. They can rarely create an exact duplicate.

This is clearly in evidence in Holland, where religious tradition has had a very strong influence. The religious orders have contributed a large share of voluntary health services and have built and developed charitable institutions over the centuries, thus maintaining a very powerful effect on the shape of the present Dutch medical care system. Much of the health service is out of the hands of the government altogether; almost all of the general hospitals are run by voluntary, nonprofit organizations, particularly the organizations of the Roman Catholic and Protestant churches. The government does run some general and psychiatric hospitals, but the majority are by religious orders.

Even so, most of the hospitals select a full-time staff of house specialists. In some instances, the hospitals permit a qualified specialist who has been approved by the particular hospital managing board to work there independently; the patient then pays just for the room services, and the specialist is paid through the insurance. The Dutch insurance system pays for chronic illness and surgery, or what might be noted as "heavy" medical needs. This national social insurance is financed the way the United States finances social security. However, for routine medical care, the patients are insured under the sick funds to which, as in Scandinavia, the employer, employee and government contributes. In addition, those people who are self-employed take out private insurance with the same kind of coverage. In any case, the sickness funds in Holland are not controlled by the government, although the standard criteria, or even charges, are set in collaboration with government agencies.

### A REVIEW OF WESTERN EUROPEAN MEDICAL CARE

Taking western Europe as a whole, one can say that health insurance against the cost of routine medical services and hospital care is covered for almost all the people to such an extent that the possibility of bankruptcy by illness has been altogether obviated. Because of differing arrangements for paying physicians (capitation, per session, salary, fee-for-service, co-payment by patient, etc.), there is some loss of control over inflationary rise of medical care costs. This is naturally greater in those countries where the fee systems tend to be more open-ended; there the rate of inflation will approximate that of the United States.

Because government controls the hospitals to a very considerable degree in most of these countries, the inflation of hospital costs has been controlled to a far better extent than it has been in the United States. However, in some instances the control has taken the shape of reducing expenses without sufficient regard for the danger of obsolescence and decay in physical facilities. This is particularly true in England. In addition, insufficient attention has been paid to alternatives to hospital care in most of these countries; therefore, the opportunity for cost control by trying to maintain outpatient facilities is lost. This is not uniformly true, of course; in the Scandinavian countries and Holland we do see striking evidences of excellent community medical services, such as the use of paraprofessionals in nursing homes, that make it possible to reduce the volume of hospitalization.

There are 50 percent fewer hospital workers proportionately in Europe than in the United States, which of course reduces the cost of hospitalization there considerably, since personnel costs represent more than two-thirds of the cost of hospital operation.

One more thing has to be kept in mind. Many families in Europe contain more than one breadwinner, a matter that is also becoming increasingly prevalent in the United States. It is therefore very difficult to arrange for home care of sick people; consequently, length of stay in European hospitals will tend to be longer than length of stay in American hospitals.

## MEDICAL SYSTEMS IN SOCIALIST COUNTRIES

We have already discussed the American antagonism to socialized medicine as an aspect of Soviet socialism, but it would not be fair to leave the discussion of the European programs for insuring medical care without devoting some attention to what goes on in socialist countries.

### STRUCTURE AND ORGANIZATION

The situation, of course, is quite different from ours because of the kind of control that socialist governments can maintain over budget, priorities, manpower, organizational decisions, etc. In the Soviet Union, the system is very highly structured; operational decisions are made through planning groups existing at all levels of government and, since the government is hierarchic, the decision tends to be made from the top down. There is a Ministry of Health of the USSR, a Ministry of Health of each federal Republic, a Minister of Health of every district, and equivalent officials in the counties and local communities. All of these have something to say about policies and needs. The information goes up the hierarchic ladder, and while there may be some negotiations, basically the budgeting is done from the top down. This pattern tends to be followed in Poland, Czechoslovakia and Bulgaria. There is considerably more leeway in the organization and structure of medical service in Yugoslavia. Here, the Titoist variant of Marxism had made a strong effort to decentralize through "polycentric" planning, which means decision-making at the lowest levels.

In the Soviet Union, patient care is mediated at the primary point of contact, usually through general practitioners and specialists at polyclinics. The Soviet citizen belongs to a polyclinic by virtue of his neighborhood or his place of employment. He must go there for his initial service. If he is to be hospitalized, he will be sent to a hospital responsible for his area. One does not choose one's physician, specialist or hospital in the Soviet Union. However, practically all the people have access to an institutional arrangement of the kind described, although unfortunately the Soviets also have some problems about staffing the rural and isolated areas, despite lavish encouragement, political stimulation, etc. The Soviet Union is well-supplied with general hospitals, mental hospitals, rehabilitation centers, various types of care institutions for children and pregnant women, as well as recreational and convalescent facilities. They are also well-supplied with medical manpower; there is considerable question about the proportionate supply as compared to the United States, because of differences in language, definitions and hours worked.

In Yugoslavia, the local social security board covering the "commune" (perhaps a quarter of a million people) arranges to pay general practitioners who work in groups of two or three in communal clinics with a paid nurse. This is treated as a separate "institution," and the local social security board negotiates a capitation rate with them based on so much for each patient. The board also negotiates with outpatient departments to pay fee-for-service for patient consultation there. The general practitioners refer patients to the outpatient service, but do not work there themselves. Hospitals are paid on a per diem basis (so much per bed per day). However, there has been some experimenting with methods of budgeting payment per case, in an effort to keep costs down. How successful these efforts will be remains to be seen.

### PAYMENT SYSTEMS

Soviet doctors are all paid on a salary basis, corresponding to the level of specialty training and experience, and the location of the physician. Yugoslav doctors are paid differently. The family doctor gets paid on a capitation basis; the specialist in an outpatient department is paid out of the fee-for-service pool; and the hospital doctors are paid by salary. However, the major difference in the Yugoslav system is that each of these separate "institutions" has to negotiate its arrangements with the social security board and then negotiate with committees within its own staff for payment procedure and working conditions. This kind of self-government makes for variations in salaries and is supposed to be an important stimulus to good service. In addition, in the Yugoslav system, each of these self-supporting institutions has to make a decision as to personnel matters: whether they want to hire someone else, or whether they want somebody with a different sort of training; if so, they pay for his training with the understanding that he will come back to work for them.

You can readily see that the incentive system in Yugoslavia — based on the small unit, self-determination, institutional self-sufficiency and local planning — is totally different from incentive in the Soviet Union, where the physician drive is for greater advancement through improvement in skills or experience, but without an opportunity of advancement in practicing level. It is much harder to be a participant in a large-scale, hierarchic scheme than it is in the decentralized scheme. Of course, in a polycentric plan it is also more difficult to set uniform standards and see that they are maintained.

The chief lesson learned from observation of the Soviet and Yugoslav medical systems is the difference between two types of socialist medical practice; we cannot merely pigeonhole systems in socialist countries as "socialized medicine." We can also see the differences between the socialist countries and the western European countries, with their large-scale insurance schemes or national health service. All systems — East and West — operate in totally different ways, yet all seem to have the elements of equity in distribution of services.

### EMERGENCY CARE

One superb characteristic of the socialist countries' medical care system that should be carefully studied and emulated is their emergency medical system. In most of the Democratic People's Republics this is a separate medical care system, distinct from the routine office and hospital system. Physicians may be the same ones who work in the offices, making extra pay by undertaking to serve so many hours on emergency call. The service has small emergency cars to transport doctors and nurses; ambulances; and sometimes even their own hospitals. The system tends to be efficient and very dependable.

## MEDICAL SYSTEMS IN CANADA AND AUSTRALIA

In many ways it can be seen how much the Canadians have been influenced by England in their social and welfare policies. They have a much stronger social welfare system than we do. They now have a comprehensive national medical insurance scheme, in which the Dominion pays half the cost and the provinces pick up the rest of the cost; every Canadian is covered for care received in the doctor's office, in the home and in the hospital.

The provinces independently make whatever arrangements they choose in order to assure that every person is covered. They may collect taxes from individuals, enforce employer-employee contributions or pay the bulk from general revenues. They also elect the method of physician reimbursement. They may pay fee-for-service, capitation or salary. Some of the provincial systems seem to be working extremely well, after some initial hesitancy and even brief strikes in Saskatchewan and later in Quebec.

The system in Ontario is different from the system in Saskatchewan, but at the same time the similarities are such that the difference reflects only different historical tradition in the two provinces. Saskatchewan has a long socialist history, but Ontario has traditionally been a stronghold of the Dominion government.

In any case, the Canadian system seems to work reasonably well, with contentment among Canadians that they are getting what they are entitled to: good medical care without the threat of bankruptcy. Both the Dominion and the provincial governments seem to feel the system is working. A number of American admirers have attempted to introduce legislation in the Congress proposing programs similar to those of the provinces. Recently a bill drawn from the experiences of British Columbia has been introduced as a model for national health insurance for the United States.

The Canadian experience is important to examine for two reasons. One is that having established national health insurance, Canadian public health people, including the Minister of National Health and Welfare, are taking a long look at ways in which *health* — not just medical care — can be improved. Perhaps, if we ever get to the point of dealing with matters of payment, we will also be able to come to terms with the reality of health system needs instead of medical care needs. The other thing we can learn from Canada is the effective focus upon child health. We do so little for children in the public arena. The Canadian child health service tends to be separate, with its own specially trained doctors, nurses and dentists. There are special feeding programs and special medical services for the handicapped. It may be that we could adopt this emphasis without any change; that this is one instance of a health system that can be readily transplanted.

Americans are also beginning to look to Australia for clues as to what we might want to do in improving our medical care system. The Australians have been legislating a complex of payment schemes for almost 40 years, constantly amending and revising the laws. This patchwork of layers of "solutions" does many of the things that need to be done: gives the poor access, pays for expensive medications, reduces hospital expenses and takes the fear of bankruptcy away for most working people. They have created a mixture of public and private payment: out-of-pocket, insurance, government subsidies, etc. It may be that this type of mixture is our ultimate fate. But if so, it will be with something less than what the Australians have. They have fewer specialists to start with, and a different tradition of equitable care; therefore, the vast difference between private practice and Medicaid does not exist there, nor would it be tolerated. If we eventually work out a complex patchwork similar to the Australian model, we had better do something more to equalize the delivery system as well. The Australians are less satisfied with their system than either the Canadians or the British; that should be warning enough.

## AMERICA'S HEALTH PROBLEMS IN THE
## PERSPECTIVE OF FOREIGN NATIONS

In general, some of the problems such as manpower shortages and inflation that plague us also plague the citizens of foreign nations. It is not easy to get people to work in isolated, sparsely settled places like Swedish Lapland or Eastern Siberia. Sweden, Norway and Russia all have to use a variety of techniques and incentives to try to get their manpower evenly, or adequately and optimally, distributed. No one seems to have solved the problem completely. There are also problems concerning prescription drugs. Too many prescriptions are written; the doctor-patient encounter is rarely terminated without one or two prescriptions. The use of generic prescribing is not widespread, and inflation of medical costs is difficult to control. In many countries leeway is left to physicians to order or prescribe things that they think would be useful and necessary, to avoid the taint of narrow control over doctors. Consequently, cost of drugs remains a problem.

Some of the other American problems are not shared in other parts of the world. An overuse of diagnostic tests, x rays, laboratory work and specialist care is hardly a problem in Europe at all. And our drive for consumer participation or control of the medical care system seems to leave Europeans puzzled. They don't understand why our elected officials cannot be permitted to cope with this. The idea of public participation in health service organizations and the planning and implementation of reform is not very high on the European agenda. Also, the feminist rebellion against male domination is not as strongly visible in European medicine, perhaps because women are much better represented in the medical fields than they are here. Nor is the campaign to "humanize" medicine and motivate physicians to achieve a more effective doctor-patient relationship as prominent there. Either the doctors are more concerned, or appear to be, or the doctor-patient relationship expected here is not expected by Europeans.

All in all, the excellence for which the United States seems to have striven in medical care is defined by enormously well-trained physicians and technologically perfect institutions. The emphasis on research and equipment, and on the development of new and more useful drugs, reflects the aggressiveness of the entrepreneurial system. The Europeans seem to have concentrated on equity, giving quality a lower priority. This is not to say that European medicine is of a generally low quality. As a matter of fact, in most of the hospitals in western Europe, the level of medical care is as modern as that of most places in the United States. Perhaps there are one or two great teaching institutions here that are superior, but it is quite likely that there are one or two European medical schools that are equal to our best. The difference is that a *quality* emphasis is based on limited economic access to that high quality, so that large numbers of people may be barred from access. An *equity* emphasis means that everyone has access to approximately equal services; these may not be of the highest technical achievement of the top level in the *quality* emphasis systems, but everyone is afforded equal access. Perhaps if we thought that the difference between the very highest quality of modern medical care and the average quality of modern care really didn't matter so far as survival, disability or satisfaction were concerned, it might not seem worthwhile to make the enormous investment that we have made in the development of our high quality system at the expense of equity.

# Chapter 15

# The Process of Creating Health Legislation
# and Policy

For those who are preparing to draft national health legislation and for those who are watching as one bill after another is reported in the press, it may be worthwhile to review the elaborate process by which ideas become bills and bills become laws.

### INTRODUCING A CONGRESSIONAL BILL

There is an orderly procedure by which congressional bills are written, introduced, considered, voted on and, if passed, become laws. Bills can be written by anyone, of course, but the language has to be clear and precise enough so as to ensure that unintended effects will not be obtained. Every once in a while that happens, even though the bills are drafted by cunning and experienced legal draftsmen! Bills can be introduced only by legislators. Furthermore, most bills have to be considered by committees of appropriate reference before they come under consideration by the entire legislative body. And bills applying to either raising or spending money have to go to appropriation committees for consideration. Even if a law is passed authorizing "X" million dollars to be spent for project "Y," no money will be spent until it is officially appropriated by an appropriations committee for that agency of government and passed by both houses of Congress.

Under ordinary circumstances, bills are therefore prepared by Representatives or Senators because of their specific personal interest in a subject or their membership in a congressional committee interested in that subject. Sometimes they are asked to submit such a bill because it represents part of their party's policy.

If the President and his Cabinet are not of the same party as the congressional majority, legislating becomes complicated; different bills, with different force although apparently similar aims, will appear and have

259

to be considered.   Both parties try to make the situation as difficult as possible for the other.   The Executive Branch has to carry out the law, if and when it is passed, so arguments against the congressional version have to be considered carefully.   The result is sometimes a stalemate.   In the recent combative period between the Nixon Administration and a Democratic Congress, for example, appropriation legislation didn't pass for HEW for three years!  HEW continued to operate on a "continuing resolution," allowing it to spend no more than it had spent in a previous year and to spend no money on anything that was authorized under a lapsed law.   It made the job of the agency officials very difficult; there was continuous debate as to whether they should start new programs, continue old ones or promise anything for the future.   Yet hospitals, doctors, neighborhood health centers and schools needed to know!

If the parties are the same in both the White House and Congress, the ritual of legislating has become fairly well fixed since Franklin D. Roosevelt's time.

## THE PROGRESSION OF A HEALTH BILL

There is a major rhythm in the routine of preparing a legislative program.   The following is a simplified example of the pattern of development of Administration health authorizations and appropriations in connection with HEW.

### STEP 1:  PROGRAM GOALS VS. BUDGET ESTIMATES

At the beginning of the fiscal year, from just before July 1 through September, the agencies of the Department of HEW would be busy preparing a program describing what they thought ought to be recommended to the next session of Congress.   This was based on rough estimates of their next year's budget provided by the Bureau of the Budget (currently called the Office of Management and Budget).   The Department fiscal staff, conferring with the Secretary and his policy staff, would then assign equally rough budgetary estimates to the agencies in the Department.   These would be arranged to conform with the Bureau of the Budget's overall HEW expenditure proposal; "next year's" budget will look not too dissimilar from "this year's" expenditures, at least in the kinds of programs being considered.   In recent years, the Secretary's evaluation and planning staff also occupied itself, in cooperation with agency officials, in working out five year program plans, into which this next year's budget would be fitted.   Some old programs might be dropped, new ones adopted, or continuing ones adapted.   But the budgetary allocation would relate to the figures given.

From September through December, these plans would be hammered out, in consultations among HEW agency heads with the policy staff from the Secretary's office, the fiscal people and the Bureau of the Budget. During that time, memoranda would begin to go back to the White House staff, usually as a result of peremptory orders by the presidential assistant in charge of preparation of the budget, reading: "you will provide, by (a certain date), a program (along these lines), and (according to this outline)." This would occasion numerous meetings at HEW, the White House, or the Executive Office Building. People rush back and forth — to "BOB" (Bureau of the Budget), "OMB" (Office of Management and Budget) or "EOB" (Executive Office Building).*

STEP 2: ADAPTING PROGRAM GOALS TO FIT THE BUDGET

By December, the exact limits of the budget for the next year would be reasonably well-known, and expendable portions of programs began to be cut away. If programs were not reduced piecemeal, whole areas would be extirpated. A program upon which one had spent the best part of six months to outline and develop might be completely gone, or so reduced that it would be nothing more than a faint gesture or hope. For example, in 1966, when we got word that President Johnson was interested in reducing infant mortality, that he was shocked and distressed that we were 13th (or 15th or 18th) on the list of rankings in infant mortality in the civilized world, I was delighted to be able to proceed with the development of a mother and child care program. I had many times requested top priority consideration for this type of program. The reason for the uncertainty as to our infant mortality international ranking is the variation in the process of computation by different national and international statistical agencies. However, after our own staff analysis, we were convinced that the United States was seriously worse off than most Western or European countries, and that we ought to have an all-out mother and child care effort. So we developed a bolder and more sharply focused attack on infant mortality than any in current use — with a relatively modest budget request — but the program mysteriously went down the drain before it was firmed up into final form. When tentative budgets are trimmed like this, new programs are usually the first to go.

---

* In my experience, if I were talking to someone I wanted to impress, I would say that I was going to the "White House." To be admitted, one had to have a pass or at least be expected, with one's name on the list at the gate. Our secretaries always told the people who called while we were out that we were "at the White House."

## STEP 3: DRAFTING THE PROPOSAL

By Christmas, the critical issues and program outline, along with approximate budget, would be ready. This was done so that they could be incorporated into drafts of the President's State of the Union message and Health message. For the State of the Union message, the health material had to be compressed into a few paragraphs. In the later Health message, the specifics of the intended new authorizations or appropriations would be expanded.

These draft messages then also shuttled through the message centers of the Department and the White House with erratic speed. This time of year was the most agonizing, because it meant being constantly on the alert (far into the night!) for at least a month. Requests for changes — whole new sections, language and program ideas — would be frequent. We were saddled with only a minute piece (the health segment) of the action, but the presidential assistants and their associates were massively preoccupied with *every* agency program from *every* Department, with the mammoth budgetary considerations from every Department, fitting them together with all the financial and political consequences of what was to be done or not done! It was no wonder that calls came at nine or ten o'clock at night for presentation of a brand new draft the next morning at nine, or that a leisurely Sunday afternoon with the New York *Times* was turned into a nightmare of feverish activity. Various agency heads would be called into the office to rewrite, redefine and provide accurate statistics, costs, estimates and numbers of all kinds off the top of their heads; or to find the book, report or person with the information! Great fun! As a matter of fact, it was. One felt at the very heart of the political process in the course of legislating benefits for all humanity — or at least for the American part of it.

And so while we cursed, groaned and made unflattering comments about the intelligence or humanity of the White House aides, as we moved wearily to the recurrent task, occasionally (but not too frequently, I admit) there would flash across my mind a wave of sympathy for the White House staff. Whatever we were suffering in the preparation of our "black book" (the top secret notebook with the program, financial plan and background information), they had a truly ghastly chore involving 30 or 40 such books! The wave of sympathy didn't last long, it is true. In retrospect, I marvel at the diligence and dedication — and the results.

In addition, my immediate superior was a perfectionist concerning anything he presented to the White House. The special correspondence paper used exclusively for messages bearing the Secretary's signature, or for messages to the White House, did not react well to erasure; even one correction left a slightly ragged look to a document. So one mistake meant that the whole page was to be redone. This put a high premium on extremely accurate secretarial work, and the secretaries were accustomed to the demand and reacted to it automatically. They also had to be willing to work the same unreasonable hours we did. However, the job offered added status and money, so that we never lacked for first class help.

### STEP 4: PREPARING THE FINAL LEGISLATIVE FORM

Once the messages were locked in, from late December to February would be occupied with preparing legislation in appropriate form to submit to Congress to follow immediately upon the Health message. (Draft bills will appear in the Congress either on the initiation of a member or upon request from the President.\*) This, too, would be a hectic time, because the language had to be carefully composed; the wording of legislation can make a great deal of difference in its effectiveness. The lawyers who read the law, or those who draft it, decide on the practical interpretation of each line of a law. And there will be bureaucrats at all levels who will stubbornly stick by the letter of the law, and judges who will interpret what was "intended" in the wording. Whatever we may think about the spirit that gives life, it is the word that kills, and we spent anguished hours over the words.

### STEP 5: DEFENDING THE LEGISLATION

The last phase would be defense of the legislation, involving preparing briefs for the Secretary and staff in preparation for congressional hearings, along with testimony and supporting documents that would be used to convince the Committees and Congress of the value and necessity of proposed laws and appropriations.

Between February and May, theoretically, Committees hear witnesses, search out their own data and eventually "mark up" a law. This is voted upon by the Committee, and since we are talking about a bill prepared *by* the party in power *for* the party in power, it generally will pass the Committee and be reported to the House or Senate. In the House, bills so passed by Committees must be ushered onto the floor through the Rules

---

\* Sometimes by "Executive Communication," a letter from a Cabinet officer or the President to the Speaker of the House and President of the Senate and so to Committee; otherwise an Administration stalwart is given the honor of introducing the draft and the bill will be known by his name.

Committee. This Committee establishes the priorities of which of the thousands of bills get to the floor at all, and in what order. The Senate is less ceremonious; by voice vote, a bill that passes a Committee can be brought to the floor of the Senate.

### STEP 6: VOTING A BILL INTO LAW: AUTHORIZATION

Bills may be initiated in either the House or the Senate, of course, but there is a degree of protocol involved. Anything that will involve taxes (including Social Security funds) must originate with the Ways and Means Committee of the House. In any case, after a bill is passed by one, the identical bill must be passed by the other before it can be authorized into law. If the bills passed by the two houses are different, a Joint Conference Committee is appointed with representatives from the Committees of both houses that originated the bills. This Joint Conference Committee attempts to reach an acceptable compromise, and if it does, both houses then vote the compromise. There is a kind of "gentleman's agreement" in this, so that a compromise bill will be voted positively by both houses, as a show of faith in the appointed negotiators. Of course, if they can't reach an acceptable compromise, there's no law.

### STEP 7: APPROPRIATION OF FUNDS

After the passage of the authorization of the new laws or amendments of old laws, the Appropriations Committees meet to decide on how much money should be allocated to these programs. They may appropriate *nothing;* in this case, even though there may be a law allowing something to be done, nothing *can* be done. They cannot appropriate *more* money than the law allows, but any amount up to that.

In previous years, the Committees and Congress were rather careless about paying attention to what the total appropriated expenditure added up to as they passed authorization after authorization and appropriation after appropriation. (Many authorizations for health laws came from different Committees. Most public health and research laws came from the House Committee on Interstate and Foreign Commerce, because the federal government cannot interfere in state affairs unless *other* states are also affected. Child health laws came from the Ways and Means Committee, because originally child health legislation was part of the Social Security Act (Title V) and, therefore, the tax committee's prerogative.) The President had to take responsibility for the eventual bill in the budget as passed by congressional appropriation. If the appropriation exceeded the budget, added taxation would have to cover the balance. That created much friction between President Nixon and Congress, for example, in that he simply went ahead and forbade the executive agencies to spend all the money Congress appropriated. This made Congress furious. President Ford vetoes all the legislation that appropriates more money than he thinks we should be spending.

Congress has recently passed a law to police itself on expenditures, through a Congressional Budget Office. The leaders of Congress, with the help of this Office, establish a ceiling on expenditures (just as the President does, but it may not be the same ceiling), and try to set limits and priorities on Committee expenditures. It will be a tough, thankless job, considering how jealous Committees and their chairmen are of their prerogatives.

There are years when hearings, debates and conferences for compromise and change go on long after the legislative cycle is supposed to be over for that year. That complicates life, too.

## NATIONAL HEALTH POLICY FORMULATION: SPHERES OF INFLUENCE

### INFLUENCE IN THE EXECUTIVE BRANCH

Health policy formulation has a rhythm of progression too, but not as cyclical as the pattern of health legislation. At different points, the policy that influences legislative and administrative decisions cuts across the legislative cycle, with an irregular rhythm. Policy decisions are influenced by spheres of influence. Even as the Secretary has a policy staff, the Secretaries of the various Cabinet Departments are a policy staff for the President. But the President has the advice and counsel of his own staff, and often one was led to wonder whether the White House staff, with its greater and more constant access to the President, didn't have greater influence than the office of a Cabinet Secretary. In addition, there were the other influences on Cabinet Departments, on the White House staff and on the President himself — of the friends, acquaintances, paid lobbyists and influential members of the community. While these sources may have had more influence on Congress than they did on the White House, there was a definite stream of information, ideas and attitudes that also flowed that way. The Office of Management and Budget is set up like the Cabinet Departments, with examiners and chiefs who parallel the Departments. And they are not simply reactive; they are usually staffed by knowledgeable and experienced people who know perhaps as much, if not more, about Department workings, popular needs and program possibilities as the staff people in the Departments. Their input into policy decisions may often be crucial, and perhaps even decisive.

INFLUENCE IN CONGRESS

Congress is in another parallel circle of action and influence. There are committees of the House and Senate who concern themselves with elements of the programs and Department policy. The chairmen of these committees have had long experience, and they have their prejudices and pet hobbies. They tend to know Department programs well. If they do not, they have staff assistants who do. Their ideas and attitudes have to be considered and the Chairman consulted or the Administration will rue the day the bill comes up for consideration! Generally, therefore, before a bill is put into final form, or even in the late Fall days when a program is just being crystallized, Administration stalwarts in Congress are briefed on what may be coming. Their advice never goes unheeded. They may need to be persuaded, and this may take a word from the White House; they cannot be ignored. Powerful anti-Administration stalwarts are also consulted, perhaps not until after the legislation is completely decided upon, but surely before it is set in the concrete form of an enrolled bill.

So policy is a mightily worked and reworked thing with multiple sources, colored by both the variety of Executive Branch influences and Congressional influences. Nothing better illustrates the excellence of the pluralistic democratic process, nor its faults. You can imagine the difficulty with which a new idea passes through all these channels and people to become a program. And perhaps it will be easier for you to understand, as it came to be understood by me, why radical change is so tortuously slow in coming, even though the recognition of the need may be years old. We do not have an effective, properly organized medical care system in this country. The labyrinth of policy formation and legislation is one reason.

# Chapter 16
# Regulation

## PHYSICIAN ACCOUNTABILITY

After all the matters of structure, philosophy, money and tradition in the medical care system have been disposed of, there remains the matter of discipline. If a patient is not dealt with justly, what recourse does he have? And how can one know what course of medical treatment should be taken, and if it was?

In a word, doctors must provide patient *accountability*. The patient should know what his condition is, what options in treatment are possible, what course of action his physician is taking, and why. He should understand and agree, or disagree and find another doctor. And when treatment is received, the patient should know that what was supposed to be done *was* done, and done correctly.

If the patient does not recover, or do as well as he might, but the above considerations have been well attended to, the physician cannot be held at fault; no man is perfect.

The physician's ethical and moral behavior mandate includes, then, informed consent, skilled attention, and proper therapeutic management.

It may be that a good many people have turned away from traditional medical practice because of dissatisfaction or bad experiences as well as generalized distrust of physicians, as in George Bernard Shaw's indictment in *The Doctor's Dilemma* — physicians caring more for their fees than for their patients. Evidence does appear in thousands of law suits that doctors, on occasion, do things that are not in the best interests of the patient, due to ignorance, greed, carelessness or incompetence. Tightening up the system of supervision may provide for greater accountability. Physicians who know that others will be looking over their shoulders will tend to be a lot more careful.

The trouble is that "supervision" as visualized by the doctor is one thing — he does not believe in people looking on and telling him what to do.

267

"Supervision" as visualized by the great payer of bills — the federal government — is quite another thing. Government is less interested in whether the physician did a good job than whether it got its money's worth! Professional supervision and financial supervision do not provide the same protection to the patient, nor the same kind of accountability.

We cannot expect physicians to do everything correctly; but the question remains as to how much leeway can be tolerated. We would like to believe that physicians can be omniscient, and that by paying more attention they will diagnose and treat everything correctly and bring about a favorable result in every instance; this is sadly not the case. There remains too much that we do not know, and with which physicians cannot yet deal; for many diseases we must be prepared to say that a good result is as yet impossible.

### BEST TREATMENT AS LEAST TREATMENT

In an interesting article in the October 1974 issue of *The Yale Scientific Journal,* entitled "Iatrogenic Disease: The Physician as Pathogen," a medical student named Alan Colner pulled together many references to show that advances in medicine can bring about problems also. Although increasing the number of transfusions may result in saving the lives of those who might otherwise die of anemia or hemorrhage, the risks of viral hepatitis following blood transfusions raise grave doubts as to whether there isn't such a thing as overuse of transfusions. The following anecdote illustrates that professionals tend to take the easiest or most routine course and that sometimes the lay ignorance of the consumer may have an unexpectedly wise effect.

A young boy with congenital heart disease was failing rapidly and required open heart surgery. The surgeons were accustomed to using eight pints of blood in such operations to compensate for blood loss and also to maintain "extracorporeal" (outside) circulation while the patient was undergoing surgery. In this case, however, because the family belonged to a religion that banned the use of blood transfusions, the surgeons could not get consent. There were increasingly heated arguments between the surgeons and the family. Eventually the surgeons began to back off; they offered to withdraw the child's blood prior to surgery, circulating it outside the body in plastic containers while they circulated a complex salt solution through the child's blood vessels during surgery. Afterwards they would restore his own blood into his body. The parents agreed, provided that the blood was never wholly removed from the child's body, in that a needle would remain in the vein so that there would be continuing contact. To the parents, this meant that the blood he received back would be his own blood and not a foreign substance. The surgeons agreed, and the operation was performed in this way. The child survived and the surgeons learned from this experience that they could dispense with the eight pints of blood; transfusions would now be needed only rarely during this type of open heart surgery.

### SIDE EFFECTS OF DRUGS

The same kinds of stories might be told about a variety of other miracle substances without which one would think that modern surgery or medicine could not be practiced. Antibiotics, for example, are probably used too much. Sometimes even the wrong ones are used when another (or none) might be required. Chloromycetin, which is essential for the treatment of typhoid fever, should not be used in the treatment of any other disease that is not life-threatening, because in a significant number of cases this drug may paralyze the bone marrow, producing a lethal anemia. Even some necessary drugs carry with them perceptible dangers of morbidity or fatality. If the patient is told of the possible consequences and still elects to have the drug, then the physician has certainly done his duty. The patient has been warned and freely chooses to take the risk. Anesthesia, for example, carries with it dangerous side effects. However, during surgery anesthesia is generally required. The least dangerous and most carefully controlled use of anesthetics is recommended, of course.

There are also instances where treatments intended to help patients are later found to be dangerous or destructive. In the early days radiotherapy was used rather widely, before the long-term effects were known. Radiation of pregnant women to determine the position of the fetus was considered extraordinarily useful and even necessary in obstetrics. But it turned out that a significant number of children who had suffered this radiation *in uteri* later developed leukemia. In the early days enlargement of the thymus gland in the chest, whose function was unknown, was considered to be the cause of a variety of illnesses in children if it did not regress normally. Consequently, many physicians recommended radiating the thymus in order to reduce its size. Many of those children later developed cancer of the thyroid. Parenthetically, we still have no idea as to the use of the tonsils, although we have been removing them for generations in carload lots — to the great advantage of the tonsillectomist and to the questionable benefit of the tonsillectomized.

The story of synthetic estrogen (stilbestrol) is very similar. It was used in pregnant women who suffered from threatened abortion. This is a clinical description of a situation in which a woman starts to bleed early in pregnancy, with a strong possibility that she will lose the child. The use of stilbestrol stopped the bleeding and seemed to allow the woman to continue to carry the child to term. It was used almost routinely and somewhat carelessly whenever women in early pregnancy complained of cramps with the threat of abortion, even if they did not bleed.  Recently it has been shown that the use of stilbestrol in early pregnancy resulted in a significant number of the children born developing genital cancers in early adult life.

Many other drugs have harmful side effects to the patient.  Where their use is absolutely necessary and the patient has been warned of the possibilities, certainly the drug could be used.  The problem is whether we know enough about the effects and values of drugs to be able to weigh risk versus benefit and proceed to recommend them.  It may be that in the long run the best treatment is the least treatment.  It may be that the wisdom of some of the older practitioners who relied upon *vis medicatrix naturae* ("The Healing Power of Nature"), should be applied more frequently today, especially since 25 or 30 percent of patients in hospitals are there because of something the doctor did; it must be added quickly that it is not necessarily because of something he did wrong.

## MALPRACTICE

To complete the discussion of regulation it is important to discuss malpractice.  It is a crucial matter, having increasing publicity in the media.  "Malpractice" is a generic term used to describe action by a physician that is contrary to accepted medical practice; an action that does damage to the patient and for which the patient can seek redress under the law.  A massive study on malpractice, ordered by Secretary Elliot Richardson of HEW and completed in 1973, contains enough basic information to help portray the problem and offer possible solutions.  The report reads in part:

> Medicine, too, for all its widely heralded accomplishments is still more art than science.  And because no two human beings are alike, the art of medicine in everyday practice involves countless individual judgments by doctors.  There are many variables in every treatment situation which must be considered in making a proper diagnosis and instituting appropriate therapy.  Inevitably, the degree of delicacy required for so many medical decisions and procedures, combined with the inherent dangers of uncertainty of modern medicine, must produce occasional errors or failures in treatment.  When these occur, when the patient suffers an adverse result in the course of therapy, with or without negligence on the part of the person rendering that care, then the stage is set for a malpractice attitude.*

---

* Medical Malpractice, report of the Secretary's Commission of Medical Malpractice, Department of Health, Education and Welfare, Washington, D. C., DHEW Publication OS73-88, January 16, 1973, Introduction, I, 1.

The report further notes that out of 12,000 claims reaching settlement in 1970, only about 10,000 were truly claims; the other 2,000 never completed filing. Forty percent of these resulted in payment to the claimant, either through a settlement or by jury action. The total amount of money paid out was more than $80,000,000 with over $10,000,000 in costs.

### PATIENT VS. DOCTOR VS. LAWYER VS. INSURANCE COMPANY

The cost of malpractice insurance has become so high in many specialties that one orthopedist said, "I have to earn $900 a week before I can start making money for myself." Doctors blame the frequency of suits and the consequent high price of insurance on the trial lawyers who take cases on a contingency basis; that is, they get paid only if their client wins the case. According to the physician, this encourages the lawyers to "sue on anything," even when a case is clearly not one of doctor negligence, in order to obtain a settlement. Lawyers, on the other hand, claim that the problem is ineptitude, carelessness and greed on the part of the physicians, causing them to stumble into situations for which patients require legal redress. Both blame the insurance companies, who in turn protest that the reason they have to keep the premiums so high is because cases can be brought long after the incident has occurred, giving rise to unexpected damages or costs years later. An insurance company is never sure from one year to the next how much money it is going to have to pay out.

The situation requires a number of different approaches. Clearly, the injured patient deserves redress. If what was done was the best that medicine could offer, perhaps the patient's redress might be paid out of tax funds, even as victims of crime or accident may be reimbursed by the state. If there is negligence or other fault on the part of the doctor, then clearly he should be liable to suit; and it is this situation that necessitates insurance. In order to judge where and if fault is present, however, it seems reasonable to have a preliminary panel of disinterested doctors and lawyers meet with representation for the client or the public to sort the facts and send only justified cases to court. Reasonable solutions like this will undoubtedly come eventually, but at the moment doctors are trying to get the community to bear the bulk of the burden; the lawyers are unwilling to give up the lucrative aspects of the negligence cases; and arbitration is a long way off. However, there are models in the United States of similar successful approaches to the problem, and one or two states have already legislated in that direction. Perhaps with a national program of this kind, malpractice will sink back into the quiet backwaters from which it so recently emerged.

### OTHER FORMS OF CONTROL AND REDRESS

But this should not dissuade us from considering what needs to be done in the way of protecting patients against incompetence. For a long time the

272 A Spy in the House of Medicine

only recourse that patients had if they felt injured or mistreated by a physician was to go to court. There was no recourse elsewhere. Theoretically, the medical profession was policed by the profession itself. This is one of the earliest definitions of a profession, that (a) it has a recognizable discipline that can be taught to others; (b) that the profession itself decides what is wrong and what needs to be done to correct it; and (c) that the profession polices itself. But the profession's self-discipline was never a very solid activity. From earliest times different schools, espousing different methods of diagnosis, prognosis or treatment, lined themselves up against one another so that physicians could always find other physicians to justify what they had done — short of deliberate and unprovoked murder! As a consequence, nothing much could be done.

When licensing was introduced in the 16th century by Henry VIII, it was with some idea of assuring accountability; the bestowal or withdrawal of the license would guarantee the competence of the individual practitioner. However, in a short space of time different licensing bodies established themselves, with different standards and varying conceptions of competence, so that the degree or the license it represented came to mean very little in terms of protection. As a matter of fact, even until the present day, I believe, the Bishop of Lambeth in London may give an honorary M.D., thus permitting a person to practice. While I doubt that many "Lambeth degrees" are floating around England today, I suspect that there are still a good many questionable practitioners here and there who do not get tried by a "jury of their peers," to be found guilty and so lose their license. As licensing grew up in the United States it became established as a state function. The medical society, the profession itself, did not have direct control of licensure, although usually the medical society sufficiently controlled the members of the licensing board, so that action that was taken was as the society wished.

It is not only the extreme license revocation that is the issue. Perhaps some doctors are less qualified or skillful than others; how can the patient know? The medical societies have shied away from setting up a "Guide Michelin" of competent doctors, with one, two or three stars to indicate excellence of quality, and two, three or four dollar signs to indicate expense. Nor is it common for a physician to lose his license unless he is caught committing murder, poisoning a patient, dealing in narcotics or taking advantage of a patient sexually (although I understand that this is now a tolerated psychiatric procedure!).

There has been no carefully structured, graduated program of punitive measures by which a physician could guide himself. If he fails to take proper care, or displays incompetence, there should be degrees of punishment fitting to the degrees of carelessness or incompetency: fines of anywhere from $100 to $100,000; loss of license for one month to two years; or "reduction in rank," whereby he would be compelled to return to a hospital, undertake further training and be approved by his supervisor before he could be licensed as a free practitioner again. None of these punitive measures exist.

In certain minor ways, aspects of such controls have been applied. For almost 50 years, obstetrical units in hospitals have held monthly maternal mortality meetings spurred on by city health departments; the pediatric departments of hospitals have had monthly infant mortality meetings with the same stimulus. Doctors have to explain why mothers died in childbirth or why infants did not survive in that brief neonatal period of hospitalization. If the explanations are not satisfactory and the event occurs more than once, that physician might be edged off the staff and lose the privilege of operating in that institution. As I said, this occurs rarely. And however embarrassing or humiliating it has been, it has not stopped the physician from working in some other hospital, particularly if it were an "open staff hospital" and perhaps proprietary, owned by other physicians, where the single objective was to keep the beds filled and not to worry too much about quality of practice.

More recently, surgical divisions of hospitals have begun to hold mortality conferences dealing with operative procedures or anesthetic mortality, which surgeons naturally preferred to use in their statistics rather than "operative mortality." The same sort of process would take place: rarely has a surgeon lost his privileges; if he were to lose them, he could certainly find another hospital in which to work. Discipline by the profession was really a paper tiger.

## THE GOVERNMENT ATTEMPTS
## QUALITY/COST CONTROL

With the advent of Medicare and Medicaid, as the federal government began to pay a larger and larger share of hospital expenses and physician costs, Congress began to be very uncomfortable with the open-ended nature of the payment mechanism. A quick glance at the monthly or yearly financial reports showed quite clearly that the fiscal intermediaries, the insurance companies, cared little about quality of service; they merely paid the bills. They had been put in the center of this operation as a pass-through between the federal government and the providers so as to protect the doctors and the hospitals from the presumed harsh or "socialized" domination of the federal government. But they made no effort to determine whether they were paying for what was actually done; if done, whether it was necessary; and, if necessary, whether it was done properly. So Congress began to legislate amendments to these laws, providing for more supervision and control.    The organized profession resisted this vigorously, claiming that *they* were the logical supervisors; even some within the profession claimed that doctors, by nature a virtuous breed, required *no* supervision. Consequently, the control measures legislated by Congress had to be very delicately and subtly applied.

### UTILIZATION REVIEW

The first of these measures, called "Utilization Review," did not seem to have anything to do with quality standards whatever. It was purely a cost control measure.    As a matter of fact, it had been introduced by the American Medical Association itself many years before, as a means to rationalize the admission policies of hospitals.  Under Utilization Review, at the end of a fixed period of time of 12 days to 14 days, the reasons for a patient remaining in the hospital were to be examined in order to determine that he was reasonably and legitimately retained in the institution.  Patients who stayed *less* than that were not reviewed; inasmuch as 90 percent or more of the patients in general hospitals stay less than ten days and the average duration of stay is now seven to eight days, the likelihood that a patient would come up for Utilization Review would be fairly small.  But there it was.  Once one started looking at why he continued to be in the hospital, however, one might find that he had not been treated properly; that he was there because of something the doctor did rather than something that fate or nature had done.   Following up on this, the imaginative leadership of the San Joaquin County Medical Society quietly imposed a new rule, so that surgeons who seemed to show up fairly regularly in the Utilization Review were not to operate without a second opinion from a consultant.  The practice spread, and Utilization Review, designed as primarily a cost control device, became a mechanism of some degree of quality control as well.  However, it is perfectly plain that this was a very small contribution to a very large problem.  And one or two medical societies began to oppose the matter more vigorously, hoping to forestall the eventuality of more rigid federal control.

It may be a myth or it may be a quaint and curious fact of history, but some of the more radical or progressive legislation is traditionally introduced by very conservative and even reactionary governments.  There are usually complex reasons for it; we need not review history in broad detail, except to point out that one of the more important pieces of progressive legislation in the 19th century was the Social Security legislation in Germany in the 1880's, instituted by Prince Otto von Bismarck, a leader of the Imperial Conservative forces.  In an effort to spike the guns of the Marxist Social Democratic Party, he deliberately forced Social Security legislation through the Diet.

PROFESSIONAL STANDARDS REVIEW ORGANIZATION

In any case, after the relatively innocuous Utilization Review, the ogre that came down the road most recently has been the Professional Standards Review Organization (PSRO). It was tacked on to the 1972 Social Security Amendment by Senator Wallace F. Bennett of Utah, a conservative Republican who was very concerned about the open-ended public expenditures for health care, and who modeled the national amendment after a similar program in his state. The American Medical Association's vociferous opposing efforts to use their long-term commitment to the Republican Party as leverage to modify or wipe out this legislation were unsuccessful. The bill became law, although it still has not been implemented; reams of bureaucratic forms and endless committee meetings have yet to be undertaken.

Under the Professional Standards Review Organization law, clusters of 300 or more doctors were to arrange themselves in an organization, funded with federal money, to review hospital records in a continuing, integrated way. The amount of money required to maintain this system is fairly heavy, of course, since much data would have to be maintained and collected for applying the concepts of "Peer Review" (judgments made by individual peer physicians). Briefly, the PSRO system would require use of explicit criteria and standards for reviewing length of hospital stay, evaluating the medical care provided and maintaining "profiles" of physicians in each PSRO unit to establish norms from which to judge individual behavior. The law provides for only hospital review at present; but certainly if National Health Insurance is established, the likelihood is that PSRO will extend into the physician's office as well. For example, a pneumonia patient's record would be examined for justification of admission, length of stay, validation of diagnosis, quality of therapeutic services performed and whether any were contraindicated, specifics of the discharge status, complications, etc.

PSRO has elements of a powerful tool for bringing doctors into line and rendering them accountable, but PSRO regulations as issued so far do not offer a perfect or even serviceable mechanism for precise accountability. As presently set up, the boards do not contain any consumers; the physicians are still able to deal with their own, in their own way. However, the results of hearings (with physician's name omitted) are to be public, since the documents are not exempt from disclosure under the Freedom of Information Act. If clear evidence of misconduct can be found and disciplinary hearings by state licensing boards have not yet been called, the PSRO board and the licensing board will undoubtedly be subject to law suits brought by activist community groups.

## ELEMENTS OF ACCOUNTABILITY

In the long run, a whole range of activities will have to be carried out if the accountability of physicians and hospitals is to approach justice to patients:

(1) *Informed consent* of the patient should ensure that he has all the information at his disposal before surgery, treatment of one kind or another, or even diagnostic activities are performed. It has been suggested that the patient be given his record so that he can see what has been found and what has been done and, if he chooses to see another doctor, bring his record with him. While this is being tried in a few places, it is unlikely to be popular with many physicians.

(2) The state should provide an *ombudsman,* a person who is not responsible to state governments or to any private association, but is a protector and a defender of the individual patient's rights. He may call to account the government or individual bureaucrats who fail to carry out their obligations. He is the person whom a patient can consult for advice and help when nothing else avails.

(3) There needs to be a *grievance mechanism* through which consumers are represented to deal with physicians, hospitals and other institutions. The patient who has tried to make a case before a medical society grievance committee, in which only physician members of the society are present, will understand how important it is to have equal representation by consumer members.

(4) The *medical societies* need to develop better methods of policing the ethics and practices of their membership, even without PSRO, and with the appropriate punitive measures as indicated earlier.

(5) *Licensing boards* should have the power to punish equally through fines, suspension of license, sentence to public work, expulsion or loss of license.

(6) The *"Intermediaries"* must be compelled to scrutinize the behavior of the providers whom they pay, and not be merely a middleman mechanism for federal money. They must keep records along with the PSRO, the medical society itself and the licensing board, in order to provide the widest range of public information concerning provider behavior. Failure to follow through should result in heavy fines to them.

(7) *Insurance commissioners* must see part of their role as riding herd on insurance companies and the intermediaries.

(8) *Health Departments* must see part of their role as quality control assurance among providers. They should not merely license hospitals or other institutions that fulfill minimal requirements.

(9) The *Joint Commission on the Accreditation of Hospitals* must provide for consumer membership on its board and not, as they currently do,

represent only the AMA, the American College of Physicians, the American College of Surgeons and the American Hospital Association.

(10) In addition to malpractice suits, there needs to be an *arbitration mechanism* to screen and reduce the malpractice case load on the courts.

(11) Finally, there ought to be some *central grievance point* where an individual can register a complaint and receive some assurance within 24 hours that something can or will be done. Too often bureaucratic mechanisms fail to accommodate client or patient satisfaction; they should provide effective channels to resolve problems.

In Pennsylvania some years back, Dr. Thomas Georges was both Secretary of Health and Secretary of Welfare. He ordered the hundreds of Pennsylvania welfare offices to be the recipients of any grievance about the need for medical care or the failure of the provision of proper medical care. The various offices were ordered to send these complaints in duplicate to Harrisburg immediately, to demand information from the accused individual organization immediately and to report back to the client within 24 hours. It may not have been perfectly successful but I am sure it was much more successful than most other mechanisms.

At times, some individuals have demonstrated how effective attention to the various details of accountability can influence the whole of the structure. I mentioned earlier Dr. Donald Harrington, who established the first Medical Foundation in San Joaquin County, California, and compelled the physicians to accept both fee schedules and the supervision and restraints imposed by peer judgment. Another instance was that of the Insurance Commissioner of Pennsylvania, Herbert Dennenberg, who made himself thoroughly disliked by successfully challenging insurance companies, physicians, Blue Cross and the hospitals.

# Chapter 17
# Glimpses of a Brighter Future

It would be unfair and misleading, in writing a book about the American medical care system and how it works, to leave the impression that everything is wrong; that everyone trying to make change is helpless; that the "good guys" are restrained or asleep while the "bad guys" are riding around supercharged, preventing improvements. It is true that it is easy to criticize clear-cut adversary or inequitable situations. However, the facts in complex social institutions usually reflect so much good in the worst of things and so much bad in the best of things that we can only hope to accomplish reasonable compromises on our way toward a utopian ideal. In the meantime, we might try to see social advance in Yale's political scientist C. E. Lindblom's term "disjointed incrementalism," in which little pieces move into place with some degree of continuity over time, resulting in some minor and major improvements. We are never quite as bad as we were; we are never quite as good as we are going to be. As John Gardner used to say, it may be that those who profess to know the perfect answer probably don't understand the question! They seem to be unaware of the fact that the key element in human society is its dynamism, its constant state of change; that what may have been a suitable response in the past may be totally unsuited to the present or the future. Marx understood this. He talked about *quantity* of individual changes eventually resulting in an overall change in *quality*. But some socialist societies profess an ideology of uncomplicated perfection today; perhaps they should take note that today's perfection may be tomorrow's problem, that we are always in a state of becoming.

This should not hinder us from trying to do different things, of course. We dare not believe that no matter how bad things are today, they will be different and better tomorrow if we just wait. We have to make judgments about today's defects; examine different ways in which they might be corrected; weigh potential benefits against further defects; and proceed cautiously and intelligently.

In any case, the point is that, even within our disorganized, unbalanced and defective medical care system, there are things worth preserving. There are little bright spots here and there — new growths — that ought to be retained, improved and extended. It will be useful if we discuss some of these bright spots from the standpoint of their *intended* and *actual* value.

## MONEY: COSTS AND FINANCE INNOVATIONS

Everyone is concerned about cost: the apparently uncontrollable inflation; the expense of health insurance premiums; and the fact that most insurance does not cover enough of the costs faced by the average family.

### FOUNDATIONS AND PREPAID GROUP PRACTICES

In a number of places in the United States, types of insurance are available that, if purchased through joint employer-employee funds, are not overwhelming in cost to an individual. Most of the general costs of medical care are covered, with no threat to the physician of change in the organization of his practice, and no threat to the free choice of the patient. Most of such types of health insurance contracts are handled through what are known as "foundations" and represent the effort of the medical profession itself to come to grips with the financial pressures on patients. Such a plan was pioneered in Windsor, Ontario, forty years ago and the Windsor Medical Services is still in operation. Under this foundation system, the physicians agree to some sort of fee schedule and agree to have their bills monitored by the foundation administration. In other words, the doctors have put themselves under supervision and control, by their own medical society, which is the least onerous to them. The oldest and most successful plan of this type in the United States is the San Joaquin County program in California; about a hundred such foundations are now in existence in the United States.

Not all medical societies are willing to undertake such a role. Some of the foundation structures are shaky and doctors grumble about the rule that a second opinion must be sought before surgery, a way of reducing unnecessary surgery. Also, many of the patient service deficiencies of the present system of medical care are not corrected by merely improving the insurance coverage.

A more comprehensive attack on costs and coverage is represented by prepaid group practice, which is much older than the foundation and recently popularized as "HMO" ("Health Maintenance Organization") by the Nixon administration. Prepaid group practice was discussed at length in an earlier chapter; the most successful model is the Kaiser-Permanente plan. A very successful *cooperative* prepaid group practice model is the Group Health Cooperative of Puget Sound in Seattle.

The principal obstacle to growth for both of these prepaid schemes is the high cost of the insurance and the lack of incentive for physicians to undertake such initiative on their own. Physicians have to be particularly social-minded to allow themselves to be placed under even the relatively light discipline of the foundation, or the more comprehensive supervision of a prepaid group practice. Since 1968, there has been agitation from the presidential administrations as well as Congress for a federal program of incentives for the development of prepaid group practice and foundations, and monitored insurance programs for the delivery of comprehensive care. However, sufficient monies have not been made available either because of presidential vetoes or congressional inaction; or, when money has been made available, the directives and regulations as set up within the Department of Health, Education and Welfare have been very difficult to comply with. At present only a handful of these prepaid group practices or modified foundations have received the necessary federal support to get started. The numbers of people now covered either through foundations or prepaid group practice is probably less than 10 million; this is certainly not enough, in view of the needs of the country's 200 million people.

In any case, the foundation and the prepaid group practice represent significant existing attributes that ought to be preserved and perhaps modified, but certainly utilized in future developments for the improvement of medical care for all our citizens.

### COMMUNITY HEALTH NETWORKS

Another development stems from the government's efforts in the 1960's to build in community participation and control, as part of the Office of Economic Opportunity programs. These were not cost control service units and, inasmuch as they were funded by the federal government, are not in the same category as the insurance-type programs aimed at the majority of the employed. However, there are lessons built into this kind of program that could be utilized in the area of cost control in the future.

Prepaid group practice and foundations are both based upon what the middle class has been accustomed to buying and using. These were generally professionally organized and directed. But the OEO neighborhood health center plan was conceived by the federal government to provide suitably directed and supervised medical care for those in lower income groups or isolated geographic locations who could not be made part of the other types of programs; as such they represent an important parallel development. Although the OEO neighborhood health center was intended to involve much community participation and perhaps even control, to a very considerable degree medical schools and teaching hospitals were the initial professional base in their development. But the OEO philosophy of "maximum feasible participation" mandated that the community become involved and, as a consequence, large-scale community involvement was realized in the program organization; how could this be built into all plans in the future?

A step in this direction is underway in Rochester, New York, where there is a network of neighborhood health centers, a community-based prepaid group practice program operating from the university and a physician-controlled foundation-type insurance program. This unified system makes it possible for union welfare funds or clusters of workers or residents to choose the kind of facility in which to receive care, as well as the kind of insurance program they want.

In New Haven, three similar kinds of programs are in operation, although each program is directed at different elements of the population, so that people cannot specifically choose from among them. Poor people are generally restricted to a neighborhood health center; unionized workers to an HMO; and Yale students and faculty to a special Yale HMO. Still, there are the neighborhood health center and two prepaid group practice plans in operation; these may eventually provide general residents with a similar choice. The same type of setup in Boston makes it possible for working people, community residents and the Harvard community of students and all university employees to take advantage of a common HMO.

These network approaches promise a way of coming to terms with America's difficult problem of pluralism, where the expectations and needs of different groups in the population cannot be met by a single-faceted program. You and I, very knowledgeable about medical care needs, dangers of inflation under professional control and the need for supervising the quality of care, may believe that we know *the* perfect way of organizing and underwriting medical care. However, it would be perfect only for the likes of us. There would be at least as many people, and maybe more, who wouldn't like our solution. And the model system of medical care for the future has to take into consideration the varied and pluralistic needs of *all* people: those who want care; those who have to pay for it (that is, the government and us); and those who have to provide it (that is, the doctors, nurses, administrators, etc.). Given that set of circumstances, the systems of Rochester, New Haven and Boston are probably the most promising.

If we put this together with what we have learned from Kaiser-Permanente, the foundation experience in San Joaquin County and the increasing willingness of organizations like Blue Cross to undertake coverage on an HMO basis for more and more elements of the community, it would seem possible that a national health insurance program could exhibit considerable plurality with a great deal of satisfaction to the diverse elements of the population. In other words, national health insurance does not have to be a mechanical monolith.

One of these programs of promise that failed still had redeeming qualities that are noteworthy for our discussion. This was the very ambitious program, organized in Governor Reagan's administration in California, which created multiple sites of comprehensive group practice for patients who were eligible for Medicaid. (Medicaid in California is called Medi-Cal.) The plan itself was quite simple. Every person who was eligible for Medicaid received a card, similar to a credit card. The state government, through the Welfare Department, made contracts with a number of companies which promised to deliver the services covered under the Medicaid program. The patients had restricted choice, of course; they could get their care only from the physicians, hospitals and other institutions that were part of the contracted agencies. The system did not work for a number of reasons. In the first place, the state officials who developed the program were so anxious to save money (Governor Reagan's administration was dedicated to saving money) that they failed to examine the capability of the contracting companies or groups very carefully. Some of these groups were more ambitious than scrupulous, and as a consequence, they promised more than they could, or would, fulfill. They failed to provide a sufficient number of adequately qualified physicians, and, by cutting such corners, made it difficult for the eligible patients to receive the contracted care that they needed. It turned out to be a gigantic financial windfall for some of the contracted groups, but a disastrous situation as far as welfare medical care was concerned. An investigation by the government accounting office disclosed horrible details that forced the state to begin a careful review of what was happening and to take corrective steps.

This failure should not obscure the fact that a state *can* take measures to create programs to provide organized comprehensive care for their eligible constituents. It does prove that such programs require considerable and continuous supervision and control. It was pointed out in Britain in 1947, when their National Health Service went into effect, that if the government takes responsibility, the government has to see that the responsibility is carried out. Setting up single source programs for beneficiaries forces an additional obligation upon a public or official agency to see to it that the single sources provide exactly what they are being paid to provide. If, at some future time, we do have a national health program in which the government (state or local) undertakes to select the groups of institutions that are to give the medical services, the government will be obliged to see to it that the medical care is carried out adequately and scrupulously by those agencies.

## ORGANIZATIONAL INNOVATIONS

### STATE, REGIONAL AND INSTITUTIONAL MODELS

We have mentioned networks of health centers, a sort of regional grouping of prepayment mechanisms, making available clusters of sophisticated specialists. In one area, the first step was to organize and produce that cluster of sophisticated specialists.

Thirty years ago Hunterdon County, New Jersey, had no hospital and practically no specialists. It was largely rural, but it was also a bedroom community for New York City. With the help of a philanthropic foundation, the Commonwealth Fund, New York University Medical School and local interest groups, that county now has a hospital and a full-fledged group practice. They have not gotten around to prepayment yet, but they do have the salaried base of specialists to do it.

Other communities have achieved hospital services in different ways. Tufts University and the New England Medical Center undertook to provide specialist services for the rural hospitals in the state of Maine by rotating faculty and house staff through those hospitals. An on-going program for consultation and recruitment of doctors for Maine is still underway in that collaborative arrangement.

Health departments have undertaken to intervene in areas that are poorly supplied with doctors and other medical resources, and in many cases too impoverished to help themselves. The Tennessee Health Department supports a combined health officer-practitioner in eastern Tennessee, who serves a wide area with the help of public health nurses, bringing modern medical care to a rural area that could not otherwise be served. The combination of salaried health officer and practitioner, some of whose services are paid for by the state Medicaid programs, is similar to the system discussed in Chapter 14 in Sweden and the Soviet Union.

In the northern counties of Florida, for many years the Department of Obstetrics at the University of Florida Medical School (Gainesville) took responsibility for prenatal and delivery services. Obstetrics professor Harry Prystowsky insisted that students, house staff and attending staff all participate in offering not just occasional clinic visits, but the whole range of comprehensive medical care for poor black women in those counties. In addition, they developed a transport service and provided hospitalization as needed in the University Hospital in Gainesville.

So there is a corps of professional people, community people, hospitals, health departments and university teaching institutions all trying to make change in the direction of improved organization — some cost control, some extension of health insurance — all aiming at a more general contribution to equity in medical services. There are also community

efforts, without any federal participation, in which self-reliant people
attempt to develop their own program, such as the La Clinica del Pueblo de
Tierra Amarilla, New Mexico. These are truly isolated instances, but the
innovations in organization and financing are a healthy approach to the
future.

ORGANIZED ALTERNATIVES TO HOSPITALIZATION

As critical as the development of comprehensive services and appropriate
manpower resources may be to fulfill medical needs, suitable attention will
have to be paid to the fact that expensive types of services are being used
perhaps unnecessarily because of our love affair with technology. There
was a time when people hesitated or were even afraid to be admitted to a
general hospital or mental hospital. Every effort was made to keep people
out. Today, the impulse seems to be to drive as many people into
institutions as possible, due to reasons already discussed: because we do not
have sufficient community services; and because out of hospital services are
rarely covered by insurance.

But there are a number of significant developments in this area of
institutional alternatives, some of them in existence for many years. One of
the most noteworthy, of course, is the Montefiore Home Care system,
discussed at length in Chapter 4, providing for the health needs of
chronically ill people in their homes, the social, recreational, physical and
occupational therapy needs, as well as a consideration of the *family's* needs.
This is an extremely effective model program, utilizing the family as
primary care providers, constantly and responsibly backed up by needed
professional care, which would provide, for example, for periodic patient
institutionalization during family vacations, and continuous home visits
during regular times. But the fact is that much of what is done in the
medical care system today frustrates the possibility of home care becoming
an effective mechanism of institutional alternative. Both Medicare and
Medicaid would resist, for example, placing a home care patient into an
expensive institution, even for short periods, unless there were clear medical
need. Obviously, there would be no clear medical indication or the patient
could not be kept in the home at all. What is needed is a national approach
to a "trade-off" of cost of maintaining a patient at home with infrequent
hospitalization, and the cost of maintaining a patient in the hospital the
whole time. With such rational concerns as the norm, home care might
become an important community adjunct to care and a large-scale substitute for institutional care.

Of course this could be accomplished just as easily for mental patients, as
is demonstrated in the Amsterdam First Aid System in Holland, in
operation for many years. In this system, a psychiatrist and social worker

team sees a patient on an emergency basis upon request, and then acts as a "triage" — a sorting out point for decision as to what the future care of this patient should be. In a few instances the patient may be sent to a mental hospital or to the ward of a general hospital for short-term care. But in most instances the patient is kept at home; treatment is suggested to the family physician, and he and the family work together.

There are important values in maintaining a patient in the home, but unless there is a comprehensive service in which all the elements of needed care are integrated — all relevant professionals and the family — such community services cannot work. In the United States today, with the individualized efforts of all necessary components, it is almost impossible to orchestrate an effective home system. The key element that is missing is financial; but the crucial, economic grease for making the system work may become available with the introduction of national health insurance or a national health service. As a consequence, the lesson of the Montefiore Home Care Program and the Amsterdam First Aid System may become integral elements of the comprehensive system of the future.

Other American alternatives to hospital and institutional care also exist. Outpatient and community care for the mentally ill is more commonplace, but sadly enough it is being done without conscientious attention to the needs of the mental patient outside the hospital. But excellent programs run by the English and Dutch governments, involving family doctors, outpatient facilities and half-way house programs, provide constructive models. With a better organized family doctor program in the United States, a better community health program might be brought into being.

Another interesting alternative to institutional care is the "Surgicenter," a very descriptive trade name of the Ambulatory Surgical Facility (ASF). Many surgical procedures could be done just as well, and perhaps better, in an outpatient situation with follow-up treatment at home. In Britain for almost 30 years, ordinary hernia and varicose vein operations were done in the outpatient department. Many pediatricians assert that for psychological reasons, most surgical procedures on young children should be done that way, so that the mother can look after the child in familiar surroundings. And for children the amount of required nursing care, other than mothering, may be small.

In the United States, such an effort was begun in Albuquerque, New Mexico, and has spread all over the country. It can have a very significant impact on hospital occupancy and save much expense without endangering patients' lives one bit. The evidence is overwhelming that most surgical procedures do not require prolonged institutionalization.

It should also be mentioned that in the past ten years an interesting and useful federal program of organized care has been developed in a hundred different locations in the United States for selected pregnant women and

children.  These programs are of two kinds:  one is called the Maternity and
Infancy Care Project, aimed specifically at pregnant women and infants up
to one year of age; the other is called Children and Youth Project, aimed at
children from the ages of 1 to 19.  In both instances, beneficiaries were
expected to be from poor families or at least from families living in
deprived or depressed areas.  The programs are principally associated with
teaching hospitals and large city health departments.  Only a fraction of
those who should be eligible are receiving care because of the limited
numbers and locations of these units.  However, these projects point to the
possibilities of specifically designated comprehensive service centers for
restricted elements of the population.  In most of the discussions in this
book "comprehensive care" meant "across the board" provision of care to
all elements of the population.  However, some of the people who propose
comprehensive programs think in terms of programs aimed at specific
elements of the population, or specifically deprived areas, as in the
successful model of the OEO neighborhood health centers.  Others have
suggested specifically rural models, like the Rip Van Winkle Clinic with its
satellite programs, or the Clinica Cooperative in New Mexico.  A third
possibility is to concentrate on a specific age group; the children's model
demonstrated in these projects is very appealing.  But because it would
mean using specially trained pediatric personnel and would therefore be
somewhat limited in overall service scope, it has not been widely considered
as an effective approach to a national health program.  There are some
people in Congress, however, who think that the approach to a national
health program should be gradual, aking it up a slice at a time, and they
have considered using children as the introductory step.  They would
propose to extend programs to other elements of the population later.
Many European countries have developed separate children's health
services and school health programs, although they have national health
insurance for everyone.  If there will be in this country separate consideration of children because of their special needs and disadvantages, it may
be that the federal Children and Youth Program will serve as a model, and
will be extended to include an effective school health program to make sure
that at least children get a fair shake in the delivery of medical care.

## WOMANPOWER INNOVATIONS

### FAMILY HEALTH WORKERS AND PHYSICIAN EXTENDERS

Another limiting factor in improving medical care availability is lack of
manpower in some areas.  Other resources are less critical.  Federal
programs have improved hospital distribution in rural and deprived areas,
even in ghetto areas, over the past 25 or 30 years.  However, the manpower

situation has become critical, due to increasing specialism and the diminution of primary care physicians. Also, specialists tend to be concentrated in the suburbs or around teaching hospitals in the big cities. This has made it extraordinarily difficult to provide adequate medical care in the ghetto or rural areas, even where organized programs are in existence. Efforts have been evident to increase the number of needed medical personnel of all kinds; to improve their distribution into deprived areas by incentives; or to substitute paraprofessionals to offset the lack of professionals. Some of the new kinds of manpower were developed in response to community involvement, based on assessments of cultural need and demand. The origins of the "family health worker," as an integral part of most OEO neighborhood health centers, is an example of this.

The Family Health Maintenance Demonstration at Montefiore showed that the use of a specially trained public health nurse for prenatal and well-baby care could be an important contribution to both the immediate patient and the concept of team practice. This use of paraprofessionals as an augmenting force has been very slow in taking hold, largely because of physicians' unwillingness to share responsibility for patient care; but the increasing complexities of the delivery of modern health services requires this team approach. The Montefiore team, consisting of a doctor, nurse, social worker, public health nurse and pediatrician or obstetrician, seems a logical and a useful device for sharing responsibility. Some small cost control elements were demonstrated as well, as patients saw doctors less often and nurses more, but the major improvement was in patient satisfaction and in the reduction of the unnecessary use of medical specialists in routine care of pregnancy and infancy.

The growth of the physician extender, or physician assistant, owes its progress largely to professional agitation and intervention. The pediatric associate program at the University of Colorado, the physician assistant program at Duke University and the "medex" program at the University of Washington in Seattle all derived essentially from professional pressures. There is still an unresolved issue as to whether the family health worker (the *community* response), the physician assistant (the *professional* response) or the physician himself should be the point of primary contact. Not enough experience has been collected as to the quality, acceptability and eventual trade-off in terms of capability and funding to be certain as to what needs to be done. What evidence there is seems to show that the physician assistant can do a capable job of primary care, and that he is reasonably satisfactory to the people he serves. The same is true of the family health worker, *within a team setting* with physician and nurse.

It is not clear yet whether the use of these added or substitute paraprofessionals really serves to reduce or even contain costs, or whether they are just added structures that will ultimately add *further* costs. Some observers and experts in the field believe very strongly that the use of physician assistants will merely drive up the cost of physician care; that it will add to the number of services and result in increasing disparities in income because the physician assistants will be exploited at lower levels of income, acting as a screen for what the physician will eventually do anyway. This belief is reinforced by the larger numbers of physicians now being turned out and the strong congressional efforts to redirect new physicians to careers in general practice. If in the next ten years there will be significantly larger numbers of doctors, particularly in the primary care area, what role can physician assistants play?

A similar argument is used against proliferation of family health workers by the people who believe that the future of improved medical practice depends upon increasing education of *patients,* as to personal care in preventing disease, etc. They are joined by those who feel that today's doctor is better educated to cope with the cultural needs of his patients than the laboratory-oriented medical graduate of the past 25 years. Further, there is some feeling that lesser practitioners ought to be used only in a team setting, in order to have available support and consultation.

Socio-cultural issues of this kind cannot be settled by fiat. Doctors certainly ought to be able to relate better to the cultural needs of their patients and be more understanding of the underlying personal and psychological factors that contribute to the reason they seek help. It is unlikely that within the foreseeable future all doctors are going to be converted to this utopian ideal. It may still be that some kind of intermediary will be needed, particularly where the cultural differences between the provider and the consumer are very great. It is equally unlikely, however, that introduction of physician substitutes at that level, for educational or translational purposes, will serve to reduce the cost of medical care. Be that as it may, the likelihood is that future medical services will have to take advantage of less expensive trained personnel to do the portion of medical care that does not necessitate a specialist.

### MIDWIVES

The feminist rebellion has turned many people's minds, and not only women's, toward the values that might be obtained in returning to the use of midwives. People are asking themselves whether childbirth isn't really a normal process that should be withdrawn from the medical and hospital setting altogether; many popular books are being written on the subject. Yale University is teaching midwives, and there is great demand for their services. So many young women are refusing to go to a hospital or a male physician to have their babies, that programs are opening up to provide midwife delivery services *away* from the hospital. New York's Maternity

Center Association has just announced such a program, and other cities also have them.

Cases assessed as "high risk" may still be cared for in-hospital by obstetricians (many more of whom will soon be women!), but it is likely that millions of babies will be born away from hospitals, with far less anesthesia to the mothers and far less instrumentation to the babies.

Consonant with this, the University of Mississippi, with the active participation of the federal government, has created a network of midwives in Delta regions, where hundreds of thousands of poor people have lived with little or no access to medical care, because of poverty, racism and consequent resource limitations. Here midwifery is essential to the provision of proper care; it may also be the answer for many other rural areas.

### NATIONAL HEALTH SERVICE CORPS AND INCENTIVE LEGISLATION

Congress has worked in other directions to increase manpower in deprived areas. A National Health Service Corps has been established, sending volunteer professionals into these areas. This represents a way for people to play some social role in the discharge of their professional obligations. They can join the Corps for two years or longer, and be assigned to underserved areas; in return for this they are granted loan-forgiveness for the loans they have taken to pay for their professional education, and they also receive salaries for the Service Corps work. The Service Corps experiences and satisfactions may encourage the doctor to remain, but even if he does not, these experiences will serve to improve the caliber and quality of the service he performs wherever else he settles. The National Health Service Corps can also become a valuable adjunct to any national health program of the future.

New manpower legislation is offering tempting incentives for young doctors to become family practitioners rather than specialists. The same law will penalize medical schools that don't train family doctors, and hospitals that train too many specialists.

## TECHNOLOGICAL INNOVATIONS

Many people hope and believe that machinery and technology will be the salvation of the medical care system and the people it is intended to serve. I don't really believe that, but obviously technology has much to offer us.

Technical equipment should be used much more than it is in diagnosis, especially for rural and deprived areas: closed circuit TV for diagnosis and consultation; computer read-outs of blood cell analysis; ECG reading by telephone; and x rays. However, there is a note of warning that has to be sounded: if there is a machine, it will be used. Doctors will use it not only when it is clearly necessary, but to forestall law suits, to show off, or just because they're lazy. Patients will demand the latest. An EMI, for example, is a brain scanner combining x ray and computer; it is unbelievably accurate, and it would seem that everyone should have his head examined this way. But it radiates dangerous rays, and we are not sure that it is worth it, that we need it or that the expense is comparable to the benefits or risks involved.

Technology is a good servant but a bad master. There will always be more, and maybe too much! Logan Airport in Boston and experimental programs in New York use closed circuit TV and dozens of hospitals now have the EMI scanner; the future seems full of machinery.

## ADMINISTRATIVE INNOVATIONS

### LEGISLATION

Some of the more important developments in the past few years with implications for future national health insurance or national health services programs have to do principally with the provision of federal funds for the purpose of establishing planning and evaluation capabilities within states or communities. They are intended to examine the process of medical care delivery as a system, to determine what specifically needs to be changed, and what might be the best way of changing it. The Comprehensive Health Planning Act of 1966 was not entirely successful because effective state plans had not been developed. But since then a great deal more has become known about the deficiencies in the medical care system, and we also have a fairly comprehensive view of what the actual resources are. The plans, polemics and proposals of earlier years were sometimes based on very rough approximations that often suited the writers' points of view. Today we are much more aware of what the actual problems are, their magnitude and their location; and what the realities are of costs, access and availability of resources. Therefore, those engaged in large-scale decision-making on public health or medical care programs are better able to make judgments as to what can and what should be done.

The same applies to evaluations of the success or failure of particular programs. We are now aware of the fact that simply depending on the analyses or judgments of participating providers is a poor way of deciding whether a program works or not, whether it is satisfactory to clients and whether it should be continued or extended. Under such circumstances, the existence of laws like PSRO (Professional Standards Review Organization) and UR (Utilization Review) offer opportunities for deciding on the appropriateness and timeliness of diagnosis and treatment and even on the validity of location of care.

At the present time, most of the evaluation mechanisms authorized by government tend to be professionally dominated and controlled, so that much of the more useful data will still be absent from public knowledge. There are serious limitations, therefore, in the value of PSRO or UR as instruments of evaluation; however, they represent a good beginning.

### THE PATIENT'S BILL OF RIGHTS

Another beginning is in the drive for patient orientation in institutions and even in ambulatory medical services. The use of the "Patient's Bill of Rights," for example, is an effort to educate people about what they are entitled to and whether they're actually getting it. Again, many of the efforts for ensuring patients' rights derive from the OEO neighborhood health center activities; the first patients' rights pamphlets were created and distributed there. Some of these pamphlets may have been too complicated or inflammatory, but the motivation represents an important forward step. The American Hospital Association has urged constituent member hospitals to distribute a Patient's Bill of Rights to all incoming patients. Physicians and hospital lawyers have been protesting this because it may serve as a basis for malpractice suit. However, the American Hospital Association is persisting, as are many community agencies equally interested in improving the patient's position in obtaining appropriate medical care. Future national health programs will certainly include a Patient's Bill of Rights or its equivalent.

### THE OMBUDSMAN

Another development is that an "ombudsman," a patient representative, has been authorized and paid for in many institutions. The problem, of course, is that if the institution pays for the ombudsman, the probability is that whoever pays the piper, calls the tune. Much information that ought to be given a patient about negligence, improper handling or inadequate care will be withheld out of deference to the institution. After all, if the patient is given that information, the institution, if sued, would have no ground for defending itself against the charges.

### EMERGENCY CARE INNOVATIONS

In the United States, emergency medical care is one of the most neglected areas of medical service. Although some hospitals have an ambulance service, in many instances they do not. In some instances, the city may maintain an ambulance system, but in most instances it doesn't. Ambulance services are generally the prerogative of fire companies, funeral parlors or volunteer or profit-making ambulance companies. In some instances the persons who man the ambulances are trained to take care of specific patient emergency needs: coronary infarction, stroke, fractures or hemorrhage. But in many instances, the ambulance people are inadequately trained.

A massive national effort funded by the federal government and also supported by the Robert Wood Johnson Foundation is underway to provide training opportunities for emergency technicians in all communities, to make sure that the patients are properly handled in transport, and given appropriate care at the site. Efforts are also being made to train emergency room personnel more fully. A national network of communication is being set up so that injuries on the highway or in isolated places may be picked up quickly and cared for adequately. Some thought is also being given to the use of special kinds of hospitals for special emergencies. For example, pioneering work is being done with burns at a special burn hospital.

In the future development of a national health program, it is quite likely that special emphasis on emergency needs will be made. In European countries, the emergency medical services are kept separate from the routine services. The socialist countries maintain a very elaborate system of emergency care. It is quite possible that we may be able to undertake something similarly effective ourselves.

We have discussed a variety of current medical care attributes, in the way of funding, organization, administration, community participation, manpower development, quality control and cost control, that show the way that might be taken for a national health program. The use of existing knowledge from present pilot programs might go a long way toward the improvement of health services in every dimension for the better care of all the people in this country. We ought to keep in mind, when we come to a new system, that different elements of what constitutes a good system have already been tested and ought to be put to use. We may never attain a perfect system, and some of the pilot programs may not be perfect either, but we certainly have a lot of working programs and experimental areas to develop. We can start with these ideas and expand, keeping within the framework of the familiar and secure. This will keep the boat from rocking too much. If we want to decentralize medical services or develop multiple systems of care, we have those models. There is no reason why an American medical care system, based on American traditional methods, needs, aspirations and expectations, cannot be as successful as the most successful European system. We have ways of financing, organizing and providing our resources; we can put them to work.

# Chapter 18
# Reviewing the Medical Care Situation

---

## THE OVERALL PROBLEMS

In the review of the situation of American medical care that we have undertaken throughout this book, it should be clear that the topics discussed cannot really be separated and catalogued individually. The chapter topics have attempted to subdivide the overall field into individual components; but it actually cannot be done. The issues, the elements, the individuals and the settings are all interdependent.

We have been primarily concerned with access, availability, cost and quality. We recognize as participant problems: numbers of doctors and other workers; distribution by specialty and geography; expensive equipment and technology. We recognize that effective patient utilization of services depends on a complex of knowledge, expectation, access and personal qualities in addition to "medical need." In providers we see patterns imposed by training and education, social expectation, socioeconomic background and professional expertise. There are American social attitudes that condition all these things: who is selected to be a doctor, nurse or technician; the pattern of suburban migration; the obstructions to equity in education and cultural advantages.

To focus on medical care organization and delivery as such, without reference to the topics of general social welfare discussed earlier — nutrition, housing, education, employment, welfare reform, family allowances — may seem either hypocritical or contradictory. It is neither. Just as there is no intention to offer you a recipe manual for medical care organization, this is not intended to be an oversimplified answer column for national grievances either. I prefer to assume that a nation concerned enough to plan and carry out equitable distribution of medical care services will not ignore:

- Nutrition for those particularly vulnerable groups (the children, the pregnant and the aged)
- Decent housing for everyone
- Meaningful jobs for those who can work
- Social assistance for families through day care and after school centers

However, a complex society does not lend itself to easy definition of problems, clear-cut classification, simple diagnosis of illness and simple specification of solutions; therefore, human problems rarely have perfect solutions. But they may have better modes of solution than those currently practiced! Our job is to identify the elements that *can* be improved, and to try to select the components within these elements that will offer the best leverage for change or influence.

## ACCESS: THE GREATEST PROBLEM; POSSIBLE SOLUTIONS

Access, the key to equity, should have the greatest emphasis in our consideration: greater than cost control, greater than quality, greater than physicians' freedom of choice regarding location of practice and type of specialization.

### MEDICAL TEAMS

We may have to envision a system of clusters of doctors and other health workers, selected to carry out clearly defined tasks as a unified team. Lest this appear too utopian a recommendation, let me make the following points:
Today:

- 15 percent of doctors are in group practice
- More than 50 percent of doctors are in some form of associated practice
- 300,000 of the 1 million trained, licensed registered nurses are not working
- There are thousands of college, junior college and university programs that could train medical assistants
- Most doctors have trained and are using medical assistants
- There are 18,000 pediatricians already in the process of reorganizing their practice to become team practices

The difficulty is not the utopian character of the recommendation; it is instead the inertia among doctors, patients, government officials, congressmen and medical reformers that creates a barrier to action. The lessons are there; they are clear and their path is well-illuminated.

### LOCAL CONTROL OF MONEY AND ORGANIZATION

*Money* is what most people think of as the real obstacle: how and by whom such proposed programs will be paid for, and under what conditions. But money isn't the obstacle at all. We are spending as much as is needed — perhaps more than would be needed — to finance a health service equally accessible and qualitatively satisfying to everyone. The difficulty is that those from whom the money comes and those to whom the money goes are all terrified that substantial changes in the system will do harm to the currently existing, albeit unsatisfactory, system. They fear the devil they know not, they prefer the devil they know. So the measure to be taken must reassure all the participants: patients and providers; government and populace; consumer and administrator; professional and non-professional; insurer and insured. They must know that the changed circumstances will not do serious damage to their situation, and may even improve their existing situations, if not their income.

*Control* is the key to this adjustment. It is a poorly kept secret that no one is really in charge of the medical care system and, as a consequence, no one can make any guarantees; or, if promises are made, no one sees that they are kept. The situation is very much like that of a transportation network. There are tracks, trains, stations, equipment of all kinds, trained and skilled people; but if there were no control intelligence to plan routes, scheduling, stops or communications, can you imagine the chaos, the frightening and hilarious consequences?

In the American medical care system, each element is an independent piece of the pattern, able to make its own decisions: the doctor — if and how he sees you and for what price; the hospital — whether or not it admits you, what it does and when it discharges you (although the doctor plays a part in those decisions, too). The nursing home, the pharmacy and the technicians similarly are afforded a large degree of autonomous decision.

The decision to improve access will require a decision on how the system is to be controlled. And this in turn will require negotiations and agreement among all factions involved as to who shall control, and to what extent.

The sensible approach will have to be decentralized, *local control* of medical care delivery units. There is no way that the huge, American bureaucratic machinery can be coordinated into a series of compromise arrangements on such a large scale. But at the local level, the amount of "give" and the resulting compromise will be one that local people can live with. This compromise may be different in every locality; it will be one that each locality judges suitable for itself. Compromises on the local level could involve:

(1) *Money* — to be raised locally to match federal and/or state grants (as in Canada) or the whole amount as a per capita budget assignment made from national trust funds. This would be a national decision, of course. But in the use of the money, local priorities could be set up; health personnel and institutions could decide locally on professional needs and reimbursement; the community as a whole could decide on whether or not they wanted nonphysicians in primary care, better transport or more and smaller health service centers, fee-for-service ambulatory care, nursing homes or community services — and how much of each.

(2) *Manpower* — which will powerfully influence how soon and how fairly the "equitable" solutions can be carried out. While it is true that physicians are a national resource and to a very great extent federal and state funds will be needed to support medical education, local participation in funding may establish a pattern of community selection of candidates for medical education.

Although universities and colleges are now widely dispersed, community college systems are an integral part of the educational patterns in most communities. The nonphysician health workers required to bolster the medical care system can be developed locally, according to national professional standards, and accredited by institutions wherever they work. The Veterans' Administration hospital network could also be decentralized in its operations to become part of the community network of health care, medical education and training.

(3) *Organization of Services* — to promote efficiency and economy. For example, *Emergency Care* should undoubtedly be organized: doctors and assistants on duty 24 hours a day; taxi and ambulance services to and from homes; trained volunteers situated in work places and residential areas. On roads and highways special call stations and trained services should be available. Helicopters and aircraft should be used in addition to land vehicles.

Similarly, *Child Health Services,* particularly in schools, can be organized without too much opposition. A combination midwife-nurse-physician assistant can be trained to look after infants and pregnant women. Pediatric assistants can look after children of school age.

*Mental Health First Aid* can easily be organized into a system similar to the Amsterdam First Aid System. Again the prototypes in the existing Community Mental Health Centers lend themselves to role transformation: a team of a social worker, psychiatric case worker or nurse, together with a psychiatrist, would be on call for specific regions of the city 24 hours a day. On demand, the team would visit, diagnose and give emergency treatment in case of mental illness. Thereafter, the patient would be expected to be looked after by the family physician or community health service, however organized. Of course, if when first seen the patient appears too sick to be kept in the community, he would be sent to a general hospital for short-term care or, most rarely, to a mental hospital for long-term care.

*Regionalization* of hospitals, despite the important vested interests of existing institutions, would probably also take place fairly early on in the development of organized community health services.

*Group and team medical practice* may be the last element to become organized, since many doctors, products of present selection and education, will resist the resultant demands and discipline of supervised intergrated service. However, younger physicians, incentive payments, and tougher political stance on the part of some communities may bring this about in more and more places and eventually become standard. The groups visualized will probably not be the large "firms" of 100 or more doctors. The lesson of public service is that service units must be kept small, close to the people served and as informally organized as possible. Groups may be large administratively, but the service units must be small, with the "grape" analogy structure mentioned previously.

## SUMMARY

In short, equity achieved by way of improved access will require decentralized, local control of funds budgeted to provide specified kinds of medical care on the basis of national standards. The methods of organizing, staffing and administering those standard service requirements must be left to the communities themselves. The federal role is threefold: (1) agreeing upon standards and levels of funding; (2) supervising implementation; (3) providing services to areas and groups that would otherwise be unable to implement the law or meet the national standards.

I'd like to include a paragraph from an article I wrote some years ago proposing consideration of changing the medical care delivery system along these same lines:

It is not only the maldistribution and unavailability that make for the crisis, therefore, but the inequity. It is highly unlikely that the resource distribution can be regularized within our lifetime, or that it is politically feasible in any case. But the inequity can be struck down tomorrow by legislative mandate. At least everyone will be in the same boat. All will have the right to call on a doctor, have access to a hospital; all will have to wait, if anyone waits; all will take "fair shares."

Finally, as evidence that availability of resources is not the dominant factor in deciding on a national health service, the analogy and historic precedent I draw upon is the experience of the British National Health Service.  In 1944 the British government announced:

> "The Government have announced that they intend to establish a comprehensive health service for everybody in this country.  They want to ensure that in the future every man and woman and child can rely on getting all the advice and treatment and care which they may need in matters of personal health; that what they get shall be the best medical and other facilities available; that their getting these shall not depend on whether they can pay for them, or on any other factor irrelevent to the real need. . . ."
>
> "To ensure that everybody in the country — irrespective to means, age, sex, or occupation — shall have equal opportunity to benefit from the best and most up-to-date medical and allied service available." (Ministry of Health, "A National Health Service" London, HMSO, Feb. 1, 1944, pp. 5, 47.)

Curiously, it may not be the obstruction of the medical profession or other related interest groups, such as health insurance companies or drug manufacturers, that will slow up the possibility of accomplishing those objectives.  Too many Americans do not trust local government; they have had too many personal or related experiences with corruption, incompetence or "insolence of office" by state and local officials.  It will take time to overcome the stereotypes.  But in recent years a series of events give promise of the start of a new cycle of responsibility, allowing more confidence to be placed in local government.  Evidence of corruption and insensitivity to local needs by the federal government; growing competence of state governments; and revenue sharing and its success, where public participation has been allowed to mold its priorities, all provide the possibility of more careful, workable local controls.  The bugaboo of decentralization may hold this aspect of the solution up for a while, but increasing evidence of democratic success will facilitate such response.

Franklin Roosevelt said we had nothing to fear but fear itself.  All aspects of the models suggested for providing fair shares for everyone in medical care are known and have been tried somewhere in America: group practice with prepayment; regionalization of hospitals; local control of health center activity; etc. We have nothing to fear but fear itself in designing a medical care system that will give the medical care we need to all of us.

# INDEX

## About the Author

After graduating from Jefferson Medical College, Dr. Silver began his career interning in a small community hospital. For three years, prior to World War II, he had a general practice. During the War, he served as a medical officer with a field hospital in various countries. When he returned from the War, Dr. Silver began working with the Migrant Labor Program as Regional Medical Officer. Dr. Silver then earned a masters degree in Public Health from Johns Hopkins University. He then worked as a local health officer in a rural county in Maryland, later to become a district health officer in Baltimore, during which time he taught at Johns Hopkins University. In 1951, Dr. Silver became the Chief of Social Medicine at Montefiore Hospital in New York, where he built the prepaid group practice, home care program, and Family Health Maintenance Demonstration, which were its component parts. At the same he taught Administrative Medicine at Columbia University School of Public Health. After that he became Professor of Social Medicine at the newly organized Albert Einstein College of Medicine. In 1965, Dr. Silver moved to Washington, D. C. to become the Deputy Assistant Secretary for Health in the Department of Health, Education and Welfare. In 1968, he left to join the former Secretary of HEW, John Gardner, to head up the health program of Urban Coalition. He stayed there until he took his present job in 1971 as Professor of Public Health and International Health at Yale University. Currently, he is also a consultant to WHO for medical care organization.

Dr. Silver has authored two books on the Family Health Maintenance Demonstration, both called *Family Medical Care*. Appearing ten years apart, the most recent was published in 1974. He has also published works on medical care problems both here and abroad in professional journals, and in *The Nation,* and as chapters in books.